The
Psychoanalytic
Study
of the Child

VOLUME THIRTY-FOUR

The
Psychoanalytic
Study
of the Child

VOLUME THIRTY-FOUR

New Haven
Yale University Press
1979

Designed by Sally Harris
and set in Baskerville type.
Printed in the United States of America by
Vail-Ballou Press, Inc., Binghamton, N.Y.
Published in Great Britain, Europe, Africa, and
Asia (except Japan) by Yale University Press,
Ltd., London. Distributed in Australia and
New Zealand by Book & Film Services, Artarmon,
N.S.W., Australia; and in Japan by Harper & Row,
Publishers, Tokyo Office.

Contents

EARLY NORMAL DEVELOPMENT

APPLICATIONS OF PSYCHOANALYSIS

Contents

THE DEVELOPMENT
OF BLIND CHILDREN

Foreword

ANNA FREUD

THE HAMPSTEAD CLINIC'S INVOLVEMENT WITH BLIND INFANTS, BLIND children, and their mothers began approximately 20 years ago for a stated purpose. We were, at that time, very conscious of the quandary of the child analyst who, faced with the whole complex fabric of the developing child's psychic life, is unable to isolate any single determining element sufficiently to study its specific impact on normal growth. We turned, as a proposed remedy, to the clinical example of children who, by the action of fate, are deprived of some single, vital factor, such as constitutionally of the full use of their sensory apparatus or, environmentally, of the presence of one or more caring adults. The very absence of such a significant variable would, we hoped, highlight its specific contribution to development under normal conditions.

In the case of children born blind, or losing part or the whole of vision in the first years of life, this led to pinpointing the role played by sight in certain important developmental respects: the unfolding of the mother-child relationship; turning the infant's libidinal interest increasingly from his own body and self to animate and inanimate objects in the external world; the developing ego functions of grasping and orientation in space; the laying down of the memory traces which build up the child's representational world; and the processes of imitation and identification which lead toward the normal construction of a superego.

As the four papers in this section demonstrate, our interest soon went beyond this original topic of the role of vision in the sighted and turned to the blind child's alternate means of achieving per-

Director, Hampstead Child-Therapy Clinic, London.

sonality growth. The contributions collected here are concerned
with such problems as: how far contact with the mother's voice
and the sound of her footsteps can substitute for eye contact;
whether acoustic stimuli can promote grasping and reaching out
as the visual ones do, or whether delays in these functions are
caused by the change in the type of sensory perception; how far
the absence of vision affects the blind child's ability to play; or
how far the apparent lack of spontaneity in this respect results
from inappropriateness of the toys provided and from the sighted
educator's inability to interpret the cues which betray the blind
child's inner wishes and concerns. Gaps between the mental life
of the blind and the sighted become even more obvious in the
study of speech which is, as under normal conditions, acquired by
imitation, but which only in part corresponds with the mental
processes in the blind, i.e., with their mental thing representations
that are formed on the basis of acoustic and tactile, not on the
basis of visual, memory traces. There is, finally, the whole fasci-
nating question of the blind child's enforced adjustment to a
world which differs from him in essential respects, which mis-
judges and underestimates many of his abilities and achievements,
and which is, at one and the same time, needed, rejected, envied,
admired, and longed for.

The purpose of these essays will be served if they provide even a
single step toward better understanding of the blind child's
arduous path toward achieving personal growth, and toward his
increasing acceptance into and integration with the sighted world.

To Be Blind in a Sighted World

DOROTHY BURLINGHAM

OUR OBSERVATION OF BLIND INFANTS AND CHILDREN OVER A NUMBER of years has served a manifold purpose: to gain some idea how development proceeds without the assistance of sight; how the absence of vision influences the functions of the other senses; how the blind construct an image of the world which diverges from that of sighted people; and how at the same time they manage to adapt to their sighted environment.

The blind child's image of the world may be unique. It is certainly limited compared with that of sighted people. The important point is, however, that it reflects the blind child's specific needs and specific capabilities.

PRECURSORS

Divergencies from the sighted begin early in the infancy of the blind. The blind infant's isolation begins when his mother handles him according to her own, different, sensory equipment. The impossibility of eye-to-eye contact makes her feel a frustrating lack of rapport with the child. As a result, she may either withdraw from her infant, or initiate inappropriate stimulation to which the infant cannot respond. Instead of the close mother-infant interaction which normally governs development at this juncture, there now exists, on the mother's side, a limited ability

Dorothy Burlingham is Coordinator of Research of the Study Group for the Blind at the Hampstead Child-Therapy Course and Clinic, London, which was maintained by the Grant Foundation, Inc., New York, and by the National Institute for Mental Health, Bethesda, Maryland.

to understand her blind child, his developmental needs, his thoughts, and, later, his speech. The child on his side is forced to initiate his own ways and means of satisfying his specific requirements.

Outside the realm of vision, a close relationship between infant and mother may be promoted through touch and hearing. Skin contact between child and mother can do a good deal to substitute for eye contact. The child's listening to the mother's voice and movement imparts information about her bodily tensions, her moods, and movements. Nevertheless, stimulation of this kind does not prevent an impairment of the relationship, nor does it prevent important differences in basic personality development from that of the sighted.

HEARING AND LISTENING

The sense of hearing, once awakened, is of inestimable value to the blind child. As there is scarcely a moment without sound, stimulation is continuous. Thus, hearing does for the blind, at least in part, what vision does for the sighted infant: it deflects attention and cathexis from the body and attaches it to events in the external world. The blind child begins to register what is going on around him to gain information and to satisfy curiosity. The sense of hearing becomes sharpened by continued use.

An unexpected disadvantage of listening is the fact that concentration on sound is helped by immobility. This contrasts with the motor development normally expected at this period. It also creates an appearance of utter passivity to which mothers react in different ways. Some remark that their infants are "ever so good, never cause any trouble at all." Others are worried by their infants' quietude, taking it as a sign that the children not only are blind, but possibly mentally deficient. Attempts to stimulate them into activity as one would a sighted child remain without response. The difficulty here is that mother and child are at cross-purposes. The mother wants her child to move and to be active, as normal children are at this time of life, while the child wishes to better his orientation in his surroundings through hearing, a task which is best fulfilled in the absence of motility.

REACTION TO FOOD

An instructive example of the different reactions of blind and sighted toddlers is their behavior toward food and feeding. As the sighted toddler waits for his meal and finally sees it coming, he responds with his whole body: arms and legs wave in uncontrollable excitement. Not so the blind child: no, or little, reaction is noticeable as he listens to the noise of preparation, the clattering of dishes and pots, and the footsteps of his approaching mother. Where the sighted toddler shows excited restlessness, the blind child remains immobile, intent on listening, and therefore strikes the onlooker as lacking interest.

Perhaps we have not yet learned to discern the blind child's signs of hunger, of expectation, and of pleasure when satisfaction follows. They must be there, however different from the familiar movements of the sighted. No doubt, sight of the desired food stimulates different reactions from those aroused by the sounds connected with it. But we would still expect that the memory of satisfactory feeding has some repercussion, manifestly noticeable or otherwise, on the child's behavior. We know little about the role played in this whole sequence by the sense of smell, but we would expect that in the absence of sight this also plays a significant part.

USE OF THE MOUTH AND TONGUE

There should be no difference regarding the use of mouth and tongue between sighted and blind infants. As an erotogenic zone in the oral phase, mouth and tongue are important sources of pleasure. Due to their sensitivity they are also important tools for gaining information. New material objects are brought up to the mouth by the child, licked, played with, and investigated by means of the tongue. In the normal course of events mouth pleasure recedes in importance when the oral phase passes. Obtaining information via the mouth gives way to other methods of investigation.

In this respect the development of the blind diverges from that of the sighted. Even though mouth pleasure may recede as the oral phase of drive development passes, use of the mouth as a means of gaining information does not. In the absence of vision, the blind child learns to distinguish by mouth between the consistency, shape, and contours of objects. The mouth remains a source of knowledge which has great importance for him.

Unfortunately, this favorite approach meets with consistent maternal disapproval. Mouthing and licking, once the infantile stage is passed, are too reminiscent of animal behavior to be welcomed in the sighted world. The blind child's wish to be obedient and approved of does lead to the abandonment of a useful source of information, or at least to its abandonment in public. Privately, blind children, and occasionally even adults, cling to it, and we have seen our own nursery school children use their mouths and tongues freely when they were curious to know certain details which would further their understanding of an unfamiliar object. This is illustrated by the following examples:

1. Cassie, aged 1;10, was playing with some buttons, investigating them by putting them into her mouth. When she discovered the doorstep with her foot, she bent down and investigated the doorstep with her mouth as well.

2. Matthew, aged 3;11, was putting on his mittens. He had difficulty in finding the thumb. He put it to his mouth as if to feel the shape better.

3. Caroline, aged 4, was trying to put interlocking cubes together and did not succeed. She then put them in her mouth and obviously investigated them with her lips, and could then complete her task.

4. Matthew, aged 4;4, showed a book to a visitor. (This was a book, specially made for the blind children, in which an article, such as a toothbrush or a sponge, was stuck on each page.) He not only fingered each article but mouthed it as well. Matthew knew it thoroughly, so that touching each article with his mouth was either a confirmation of what he had learned through his fingers, or pleasurable in itself, or both.

5. Alan, aged 7;4, sandpapered a piece of wood: he then felt it with his mouth to see whether it was smooth.

MUSCULAR DEVELOPMENT

In the second year of life the blind toddler is persistently deprived of the pleasure which is normally dominant at this age. Sighted toddlers delight in developing their motility and they despair only when they are immobilized. There is no surer way of irritating such a child than to make him sit or lie when he wishes to crawl, walk, run, or jump. Motility at this age also represents one of the important pathways for discharging aggression.

While vision serves development in this area by tempting the child to move toward what he or she sees, sound does not seem to attract similar movement. When listening, the blind toddler remains still, passive insofar as muscular activity is concerned. Furthermore, after he has learned to walk and gained some confidence in this activity, this is not followed by the usual delight in increased speed and greater efficiency. Instead, what it leads to is an increased awareness of danger from the unknown and unexpected. Thus, instead of moving in ever-widening circles and becoming an active menace to his environment, the blind toddler feels threatened and makes painstaking efforts to control himself. He avoids danger by holding out his arms to protect himself; by examining the floor in front of him with his foot; by restricting the area he moves in; and by taking short steps or even running in the same place.

All these avoiding measures are self-taught and, from the blind child's point of view, they are effective. They are invaluable in combating the dangers surrounding him, but at the same time they unavoidably curtail freedom and prevent impulsive action. They also widen the gap between the developmental progress of the blind and the sighted.

It is another disadvantage that these achievements of the blind, considerable though they are, often fail to elicit praise. The mothers of the blind, even though worrying about the child's safety, sometimes excessively, still cannot help experiencing the child as slow and clumsy, potentially backward. It is seldom appreciated how far this backwardness in motility is compensated for by advances in thought processes, attention, and concentration.

It is not that the blind child cannot also experience pleasure in motor activity. As an infant, he responds well when played with actively. In the nursery school, children delighted in a game called "hello—good-bye," moving a few steps away from the teacher and running back into her arms; or jumping on the trampoline in safety. Obviously some of the pleasure in motility could be restored to the blind child if at the same time more methods or apparatus were devised to keep his activities safe (for example, the walking frame).

1. Richard, aged 3;9, would not dance with Joan, but preferred to make tiny steps by himself.

2. Matthew, aged 4;4, was running from one teacher to the other. He ran like a rabbit, not quite straight, but as if uncertain about which direction he should take. At first he ran with little steps, but as he gained confidence, he took longer steps.

3. Matthew, aged 6;4, accidentally rode into the flower bed on his tricycle. He went round and round in a circle, keeping to a small space, just as he had done when walking with small steps.

Attitudes toward the Sighted World

The blind child becomes even more isolated when he becomes aware of the difference between himself and the sighted. Where he moves slowly, they are fast; where he has to search for objects painstakingly, they can find them without difficulty. They are aware of objects, changes, and events of which he remains oblivious. Even the fact that he can make use of senses which they use much less extensively does not make up for his disadvantage in that one respect.

As far as we could observe during the nursery school years, the blind child's discovery that other people possess a faculty which he lacks does not come suddenly. It begins as a puzzle which is solved very gradually in the stages shown below.

Examples for the puzzled child:

1. The teacher asked Matthew to pull up his sock, and he asked, "How do you know my sock is down?"

2. The teacher remarked that a child's mother was at the gate. "How do you know my mother is there?" he asked.

Examples for the realization of differences:

3. Matthew, aged 4;8, asked the teacher to watch him water the flowers; when she said she would come with him, Matthew retorted, "You do not have to come with me, you can look through the glass door."

4. George, aged 5;1, said, "Look, my face is all clean now." When the teacher said she would feel it, he said, "No, you don't feel it, you look at it."

5. Joan, aged 6;5, asked a visitor how she knew that the door was open and was told that she could see. Joan said, "Then you are one of the people who can see."

6. Winnie, aged 6, asked a sighted child who was sitting next to her, "Tell me where Mrs. K. has gone to, because you can see."

For the realization that sighted people can act faster and more efficiently:

7. A little boy dropped big beads on the floor and they scattered and rolled in all directions. The teacher asked him to pick them up. He hesitated and said, "You do, you can do it so much quicker."

For the onset of disappointment and frustration:

8. A little girl sitting at a table dropped her toys on the floor. She startled, then sat absolutely still for a few moments, then left the table and walked away without a word.

9. Annette, aged 4;1, climbed into the basket and enjoyed tipping it over with herself inside it. However, when it rolled away from her after a minute or two, and she followed it in the wrong direction, and could not find it at once, she gave up and did not ask for help.

10. Peter, aged 4;2, tried the most difficult peg set, putting in the pieces wrongly. Suddenly, he wildly threw them all behind him and curled up, head on knee and hand in eye.

11. Helen, aged 13;7, said, "I hate to feel I won't be able to do this, or feel I won't manage when I grow up."

STRUGGLE FOR INDEPENDENCE

In every normally endowed infant's life, there is a period when dependence on mother's care and help comes into conflict with the child's healthy wish for independence and self-determination, a wish supported from the side of the maturing ego functions. Just as during the separation-individuation phase (Mahler, 1963) running away from the mother alternates with running toward her, so does "help me" alternate with "want to do it myself."

There is no doubt that the young blind child enters the same phase, but without the same sensory equipment, and therefore without the same ability to satisfy the second of the two wishes, "do it myself." Without vision it is extremely difficult for the child to learn to open and shut doors without assistance, to turn taps on and off, to take and collect things from the kitchen, and to return toys to their rightful places. For example, the combination of carrying an object while orientating oneself in a room and covering the necessary distance requires a degree of concentration and skill not needed by the sighted. What should be a healthy move toward independence thus becomes only too often a frustrating struggle accompanied by growing resentment of the help which is so sorely needed. On the other hand, whenever independence is accomplished, the resulting satisfaction is impressive.

1. Caroline, aged 4, asked the teacher not to hold her hand, "I like it best on my own self."

2. George, aged 5;3, said, "I want to take my dinner money to the kitchen all by myself, with nobody and nobody to watch me."

3. Alan, aged 6;11, had been helped by the teacher to fasten his belt. The whole time he was whispering, "Do it myself."

4. Caroline, aged 4;1, was helped by the teacher to hammer a drawing pin into the wall to attach Christmas decorations. Caroline said, "Don't tell me how to do it."

5. Winnie, aged 5;4, when shown how to put a screw into her puppet, asked, "And then will you let go?"

6. Joan, aged 6;2, did not want to be helped as she practiced jumping off a chair. She asked the teacher to stand by the door, then to sit on the bench which was farther away and, finally, to go into the next room, in this way proving to herself that she needed no help.

DEPENDENCY ON THE SIGHTED AS A NECESSITY, AND THEIR ACTIVE USE AS TOOLS

The blind child's limited success in achieving independence in this phase has an important bearing on the quality of his relationship to sighted peers and adults for many years to come. Turning to the sighted for assistance is only too often the only way in which the blind child can achieve his aims. While this would be regressive in the case of a sighted child, a return to early days when the mother is needed as auxiliary ego, it is normal for the blind, and in most instances needs to be appreciated as a sensible and rational device. Neither regression nor passivity are involved when a blind child engages the help of the sighted to carry out his wishes.

1. Matthew, aged 5;3, was striving for independence at this time. He had a younger sister, a toddler who accompanied him to the nursery school. As she began to move about and became interested in objects, he noticed that she could do what was impossible for him. Realizing this, he got her to bring him what he wanted, to carry out his orders. He was far from passive in relation to her, and she became his willing slave. She could see what he needed, and he could use her hands and feet as his tools.

2. The teacher was used by Joan (aged 4;7) and George (aged 5;1), who were occupied with play material, to find something on the table that they could not find themselves. It was our impression that the teacher was used more as an extension of their own bodies than as a helpful person.

It was also noticed in the nursery school that when blind and partially sighted children were together, the latter had to act for the former to the limits of their ability. (As an old German proverb says, "The one-eyed is king among the blind.")

It seems that as far as blind children are concerned, the concept of "auxiliary ego" needs to be extended to that of "auxiliary body." Blind children are apt to use the hands and feet of the sighted for the purpose of acquiring greater efficiency and ability, treating them as extensions of their own bodies, like tools temporarily under their command.

Adults often resent being used as tools. A mother of one of our blind children expressed her feelings to the therapist as follows, "It isn't that she needs me as a mother, as someone she has affection for, she only uses me for support, as if I were an extra limb." What the mother complained of in this manner was that, in place of an object relationship, she only fulfilled an ego need of the child. What the mother did not realize was that while she had to act as an auxiliary ego, she also paved the way for the child to enter into a true object relationship with her.

THE NEED FOR THE COOPERATION OF THE SIGHTED

It may well be that blind children notice the resentment of adults when they are treated in this way, and that this is the reason why they are wary of expressing negative feelings toward them. Furthermore, in order for the sighted to be willing to comply with the demands of the blind, the adults have to be kept in a loving and friendly mood.

AGGRESSION

For these and other reasons there seems to be a continuous effort on the part of blind children to avoid expressing any signs of aggression toward the sighted. Even at the toddler stage sudden shifts from love to hate are less conspicuous, or at least there is less expression of hate in muscular activity. The fear of being separated from the caring adult results in the blind child's wish to keep that person in a loving attitude toward him. Signs of dislike or annoyance might affect the helper's wish to care for the child. There is little he or she can do but give in to the wishes of the caretakers, but what is striking is the lack of annoyance or even sulkiness shown and the unquestioning compliance of such a child. That this compliance does not come easily to him and his blind playmates can be shown by the following examples:

1. Matthew, aged 3;11, had thrown beads on the floor and, when told to pick them up, said in despair, "I can't walk, I can't see, I can't do nothing."
2. Matthew, aged 5;5, had been opening and slamming doors for several days. When told this was not a good idea, he said, "This is what my mother does when she is angry." He then slammed the door with great force, opened it, and closed it again carefully, saying, "This is the way you can do it"—with a calm and satisfied expression.
Here Matthew was not only expressing his angry feelings by reproducing the mother's behavior, but was also showing at the same time that these feelings could be controlled. His pride in this ability was evident.
3. Jacob, an 8-year-old boy from an institution, was escorted to his

session by a teacher and left outside a shop. He was left standing by the wall, while the teacher went into the shop, with the warning, "Don't move." Jacob was terrified and stayed glued to the wall, but when the escort returned, he showed no resentment.

There is nothing for Jacob to do but to comply, since to show annoyance to his escort might make the latter less friendly toward Jacob, with dire consequences. Anger must be controlled for the sake of safety.

GUILT

Could it be that the exaggerated guilt shown by blind children is a result of the continuous necessity to control the anger felt toward the helpful object whom they cannot do without?

Anger is experienced on account of the lack of sight; for the inability to do what the sighted do. This is especially true at the stage of development when the blind children are struggling for their independence ("I want to do it by myself") and are thwarted by their need for help: "I want to do it on my own but have to ask for help. I don't want your help, but have to pretend I do, so that you do as I wish. Without control of my real feelings, of my anger, you would leave me, I would lose you, and I cannot do without you. How can I help feeling guilty about the anger and hate I feel continuously?" It is only possible to function lovingly, at least outwardly, when control of anger succeeds. But guilt remains for this inner and never-ending anger.

FEAR OF HURTING

This inhibition of aggression out of practical considerations, out of concern for safety, may link with an exaggerated fear of the degree to which their actions might hurt people. Such fears of hurting were often observed in our nursery school. There may be, of course, a close connection here with the repeated warnings issued by parents who try to teach their blind children to check their awkwardness, to be careful not to hurt themselves or others.

1. George, aged 5, built a tower of large bricks and asked the teacher if he should knock it down. When asked, "Why not?" he told her,

"Move right over to the chairs before I knock it down." George is clearly afraid of hurting her with the bricks.

2. Jacob, aged 8, was being taught how to play ninepins with miniature balls. An alley was created and the nine pins noisily placed in front of him. The therapist was standing beside him. His first throw was backward and it was hard to convince him that he would not hit her. Eventually he had great pleasure when he hit the nine pins and heard them fall.

Only One Person Cathected at the Same Time

It has been observed in the nursery school that children seem unable to cathect more than one person at any one time. One adult can be exchanged for another, but, once exchanged, that new person receives the child's whole attention, while the other is ignored as if nonexistent. We think that the balance between the child's ego needs for protection by his objects on the one hand and his ability to cathect them libidinally on the other is not of the usual kind. The former, that is, the ego need for protection and support, is so overwhelming that it overshadows the latter, that is, the libidinal cathexis. Consequently, the adult who assumes the role of protector appears to receive at the same time the whole of the emotional tie, much more than is really the case. Similarly, the fact that a blind child takes any stranger's hand and accompanies him to wherever he is directed may make one think that his relationships are shallow. But this is not the case. This docile behavior is dictated by the predicament caused by the blindness.

1. Matthew, aged 3, was taken by the teacher to the car to be driven home by a driver he knew well. Matthew hung on to the teacher's hand, showing clearly he did not wish to leave her. But when he got into the car, he started an animated conversation with the driver and did not respond to the teacher's friendly efforts to say good-bye to him. He ignored her completely.

2. Sylvia, aged 4, was in therapy at the time. She was being taken by her therapist to a teacher and kept saying, "Please don't tell her I do not want to go with her, she might be unhappy about it," and hung on to the therapist's hand. But when she reached the teacher, she hugged her, asked to go with her at once. It was as if the moment she

had let go of the therapist's hand, the latter ceased to exist for her.

3. Helen, aged 7, was with her therapist when she heard her teacher approaching to fetch her. She hung on to the therapist, then slammed the door, shutting the therapist out.

Here Helen was aware that the change of helpers was inevitable and actively took charge, first showing where her affection lay by hanging on to the therapist, then changing the situation so as to avoid being with two people at once. Thus she was able to give her undivided attention to the person assigned to her for the moment.

THE SEPARATE EXPERIENTIAL WORLD OF THE BLIND

In observing the children in the nursery school, we could discern two different developmental processes. One proceeds as a consequence of the interaction with and stimulation by the sighted world to which the child tries to adapt. The other pursues a different path, determined by the absence of vision and the use of the other senses and abilities at the child's disposal. It is the latter which fits the child's inner needs in the first place, and helps him to build up a sightless world in which he feels at home. There are many clashes between the experiences in this world, and the conclusions the child draws from them, and the experiences which stem from the lead given by his sighted parents or teachers. These clashes come together, more or less, and are expressed in the blind child's speech which uses the same word representations as the sighted, whereas the thing representations may have quite different meanings for the blind.

It is not easy for any sighted person to enter the special experiences of the blind child; nor do we know very fully what communication there is between blind children. We observed in the nursery school, for example, that a noise by one child at one end of the room received a response by a child at the other end, though it was not noticed by anyone else. In our film of the blind (1972), we observe that one little girl, Cassie, knows that the brick Annette is playing with represents a baby, while no one else might have recognized this. And even though we often wonder how far the children grasp the meaning of their own blindness, there is no doubt that they are aware of the others' visual defect and its degree, as the following example shows:

Alan, aged 7;2, was asked why Winnie couldn't see the sky. He answered, "Because she is all the way blind," and he added that he himself was a little blind, and Joan and Matthew "all the way blind."

Once we have grasped the fact that blind children have to respond to two separate forces that promote development, it should not be too difficult to gear their upbringing and education to that fact, and to neglect neither. In this way such children can derive the utmost profit from external stimulation on the one hand, and from the elaborate uses they make of their remaining sense impressions on the other. To omit the former would be to let the child flounder helplessly in the sighted world; not to regard the latter as essential would imply the risk of estranging the child from his own spontaneous experience and would lead to what has been called in the literature a "false self" (Winnicott, 1955).

George, aged 5;3, had a shy and pleased expression as he threaded a string of beads and showed them to his teacher. When he had finished the task, he swung the beads around himself, touching the floor with them. Finally he took them with him on the trampoline. The beads banged on various surfaces and made a noise as he jumped.

This example shows how George, using one and the same activity, responded, on the one hand, to the expectations of his sighted teacher and, on the other, satisfied his own needs for sensory experience. Like a sighted child, he experimented both with fine and coarse motor activity, was proud of his achievements, and looked for the teacher's approval. But also, as only a blind child would do, he related to the beads through the noise they made, touching the floor with them and jumping noisily onto the trampoline.

VOCABULARY

If one pays close attention to the vocabularies of blind children, it is often possible to tell whether the words they use express their own thoughts, or whether they are words taken over from the sighted.

1. Caroline, aged 4;7, after eating three lollies, said, "You can't believe your ears but I have eaten three lollies."
2. Joan, aged 7, after visiting the school she was going to attend, said, "It's the nicest school I ever heard."

3. Joan, aged 4;9, asked for "a chair with handles." (Arms would most likely make her think of her own arms.)

4. Stewart, aged 5;5, while putting on a rubber apron, said, "It's like a mac"; then added, "It's got a zip, it's like Bonna's boots." (He was remembering the feel of things previously encountered.)

5. Caroline, aged 4;3, kept speaking of the Montessori buttoning frame as "a frock," "a girl's frock."

6. Caroline, fingering the plastic press studs on her apron, said, "They are like rice crispies, they snap."

7. Caroline, aged 4;7, gently rubbing a blossom between her fingers, said, "It's like Barrie's [her baby brother's] hair."

Examples for the use of words taken from the sighted are the following:

1. Matthew, aged 4;2, played hide-and-seek in the cupboard and called out, "It's all dark in here." When asked what he meant, he answered, "Well you know, all cold and rainy."

2. A boy bent and touched Caroline's hair. Caroline, aged 4 at the time, said, "I don't want him to look at me." (Caroline uses "look" here instead of touch.)

Examples for words used but not understood:

1. When the teacher told Gillian, aged 5;11, that she, the teacher, had a headache, Gillian asked, "What did it sound like?"

2. Matthew, aged 4;8, said, when soap got into his eyes, "It stings"— and added, "They're delicate—I wonder what delicate means."

3. Matthew, aged 4;8, was opening a coconut. The teacher had told him "to examine" it. Matthew asked, "Is there a temperature inside the coconut? Will it be like when the doctor examines us?"

4. Boris, aged 7, said, during power cuts, "When the lights are put out, who will look after us?"

5. Adam, aged 4;9, was taken by the teacher to the bakery to buy some rolls. She first told him for whom the rolls were intended and described the smell of the bakery. In the shop Adam asked for the rolls, paid for them, and waited for the change. The rolls were handed to him in a paper bag and he carried them to the nursery school with both hands, holding them against his body and saying, "But they are not rolls to wipe your bottom." (The word roll had only one meaning for him, that of toilet rolls.) In spite of every effort to make the word meaningful, he remained confused. Possibly if he had felt the rolls, the two meanings of the word would have become differentiated.

6. Winnie, aged 6, was obviously searching for something and re-peatedly asked, "Where is my Hoover?" (There is no Hoover in the nursery school.) The teacher offered her whatever substitute she could think of, but to no avail. Finally Winnie came across a small dinky

car. She at once said, "You see, here is my Hoover," and proceeded to push it on the floor and then hold it to her ear. The noise reminded her of the similar noise of the Hoover.

The following are examples of the children's use of expressions such as "you look lovely," and "I am so happy." Even though such phrases are picked up from the sighted, they illustrate the use of these phrases to express affect:

1. George, aged 5;5, was attracted by Katherine's new plastic raincoat. He asked, "What have you got?" Katherine explained. George said, "I want to see it." He felt the coat and fingered the buttons, clearly enjoying the sensations. He then said with genuine admiration, "You do look lovely."

2. When Judy was 6;8, the teacher ran on the grass with her until both of them were out of breath. Judy was obviously enjoying herself. She kept repeating to herself, "Lovely, lovely, lovely." When asked what was lovely, she answered, "She was a lovely girl."

STRUGGLE FOR AWARENESS OF SPACE AND DISTANCE

To gauge the dimensions of space and distance, so important for orientation, is easy for the sighted. It is, however, an extremely difficult task for the blind.

1. Richard, aged 4;10, had demonstrated in many ways how this ability could be achieved. By measuring with his hands the distance of a rope from the ground, he was then able to keep this distance in his mind and to jump accurately over the rope. He had picked up the necessary clues of how the sighted jump from a standing position and land on the other side.

2. Joan, aged 6, while in her treatment room, heard the sound of a horse going down the street and asked what the sound was. When told it was a horse, she asked to have it brought into the room, probably imagining a horse the size of a toy, or the rocking horse in the nursery school that she had handled.
The following example demonstrates how objects should be handed to a blind child.

3. When Joan was 4;6, a partially sighted child tried to hand her a cup. The teacher intervened and told her to put the cup in Joan's hand. Joan knew better and told her to "put it on the table." There she could hear the sound of the cup as it was placed on the table, and then could pick it up appropriately.

REACTIONS TO MISTAKES

The difficulties encountered when judging space and distance are only part of the reasons for the constant mistakes blind children make. Unavoidable as these mistakes are in the absence of vision, they are not taken for granted by the children; on the contrary, they are deeply resented by them and make them feel humiliated.

1. Richard, aged 4;10, was pleased that he had been able to build a village. He could recognize a church with a steeple, but when he picked up the figure of a little man, he thought it was a tree. When this was brought to his attention, he was disappointed. He continued with his efforts to identify the figures, but he now dropped the ones he could not recognize. He was ashamed of his difficulty and wished to hide it from the sighted.

2. Matthew, aged 5, was playing with clay; he had made a cup and wanted to make a saucer to fit it. Inadvertently, he used the cup he had just made to make the saucer. When told of his mistake, he acted as if he had done this on purpose, since this would not have been such a blow to his self-esteem. He felt he should have remembered where he had placed the finished cup.

To safeguard a blind child against the innumerable hazards to which he is exposed needs constant watchfulness on the part of the parents, who may also repeatedly warn him "to be careful." In the eyes of the children, this is the reason why "to be careful" assumes the status of a major moral issue, and "to be careless" means a lapse from this standard, that is, a form of wrongdoing. It is easy for the observer to notice that warnings issued by the parents not only are heeded but are truly internalized, becoming part of the child's superego. In the very young it is of course not always easy to decide whether a child blames himself for an accident, or whether, in simply repeating the parents' words, he is self-critical in the true sense of the phrase. It must not be forgotten, however, that the parents not only admonish the child: they repeatedly feel forced to apologize for their blind child's awkwardness to the sighted people around them.

1. Joan, aged 5, was transferring beans from one container to another, and accidentally dropped them on the floor. She said to herself, "Not on the floor, Joan."

2. Peter, aged 5;4, was going up and down a cement path and came to some steps. At first he would fall on the steps, then he would stop before reaching them. Later, when he nearly tripped on the steps again, he said, "I shouldn't have done that."

In the nursery school the children were continually heard to say "sorry, sorry," when they unexpectedly bumped into a person or an object. One sometimes had the feeling that this was an automatic reaction taken over from the parents and not a real feeling for the other person. The children also said sorry when they accidentally hit themselves, as the following examples show:

1. Adam, aged 4, bumped into the climbing frame, hurting himself, and said, "Sorry, sorry."
2. Winnie, aged 5;2, in the sandbox, hit her hand with a spade and exclaimed, "Sooo sorry."
3. Joan, aged 4;5, bumped into the chair on which the teacher was sitting. The teacher excused herself for being in the way and said, "I'm sorry, Joan." Joan reacted to this remark by hitting her left arm with her right hand and said to herself, "Say sorry, Joan."

In fact, since all the accidents described are more or less unavoidable and occur only too frequently, the children react much of the time with guilt feelings about their shortcomings. This shows in the remark of a child to the teacher, "It is very hard to be good all the time. Do I have to clean it up and say 'I'm sorry'?" It is almost a relief for the onlooker to find a blind child blaming someone else and not himself, and trying to distinguish between accident and action on purpose:

1. Joan, aged 4;7, bumped into a bench, which had been moved from its accustomed position in the nursery school. She was upset and angry and acted as if the bench had been naughty. (Turning the anger against the bench may also have hidden a feeling that if she had been more careful, she need not have run into the bench.)
2. Matthew, aged 5;11, spilled a glass of water and apologized to the teacher and said it was an accident. He then asked the teacher whether she would be cross if he spilled anything again, explaining that his mother says that if it happens again, it is not an accident. (Was Matthew worried over the various effects produced by his actions? For him, a faulty action was an unhappy event which brought the reflection that perhaps he could have been more careful, while a purposeful action was one of which he could be proud and even boast about.)

On the other hand, the demands for self-reliance and self-protection which the children make on themselves must also be taken as a sign that they are outgrowing their complete dependency on parental help and protection, even if this development occurs through processes of imitation, identification, and introjection. After all, there are many occasions when it is brought home to the children that the parents are not infallible and all-powerful; that they are unable to give them what normal children have; that they are unable to understand them; and that they make irrational demands on them. Any disappointment of this kind can be matched by an increase in independence and reliance on their own judgment. Unluckily, as described above, it also leads to an increase of self-blame and guilt. This blame for faulty actions goes to extraordinary lengths, as shown in the following examples:

1. An adolescent boy on a station platform, under the supervision of a teacher, walked off the platform and fell onto the track. When rescued, his reaction was: "If I had been more careful, this wouldn't have happened."
2. A blind teacher on his way to his school fell into a manhole which had been left uncovered. His immediate reaction was to blame himself for not having been more careful.

Guilt over accidents is balanced by the justifiable pride and raised self-esteem which follow the successful solving of difficult problems and the handling of dangerous situations. By achieving the latter and by learning to safeguard themselves, blind children develop the skill to make the fullest use of their own abilities and talents.

GUILT OVER BROKEN OBJECTS

In psychoanalytic child psychology it is a well-known fact that during the phallic period of development, children experience intense anxiety concerning the intactness of their bodies. Boys show concern about the safety of their male organs, while girls become acutely conscious of their lack of a penis and cannot help wondering about the reasons for it. It is only logical that all children with actual physical handicaps not merely share these fears with their sighted peers, but, because of the real reason for feeling damaged, display them to an intensified degree. This process extends over various phases of their development.

The reluctance to touch broken and damaged objects, found in all children, is, for the above reasons, quite especially noticeable in the blind. This fear is also linked with their assumption that everything that happens is their fault. Since it is impossible for them to know whether an object which has been dropped has remained intact or has been damaged or broken, the children only too often assume that it is irretrievably damaged and that it is they themselves who have to be blamed for the disaster—"I did it."

1. Albert, aged 4;11, became upset when an egg broke, although his younger sighted brother, to whom the egg belonged, did not mind. His mother reported that if something was not perfect, Albert thought the fault was his, and that other people did not make mistakes.

2. Joan, aged 5;7, although warned by her therapist that the toilet chain was broken, came out of the toilet panic-stricken, screaming, "I don't like it, don't lock me in." She was convinced she had broken the chain herself.

3. Boris, aged 7, took several weeks to learn that wrinkles in bed clothes could be smoothed out. Once he had learned this he was quite satisfied that "now we can sit on the bed," that is, it can be mended.

As with sighted children, imperfect and damaged objects are feared and avoided. For the blind to handle them is especially distressing.

1. Richard, aged 4;1, was offered a biscuit. The one he took had a small piece broken off. When he felt it, he said, "I don't want it, I want a mended one."

2. Richard, aged 3;9, was walking with his teacher when he suggested that they cross to the other side of the street because there was a broken wall which might be interesting for him to feel. Richard resisted crossing the road and in a tearful voice said, "I don't like the broken wall, I don't want to feel the broken wall."

Pleasure is shown when objects are mended and can be used as before. However, this does not diminish the children's feeling of responsibility.

1. Joan, aged 5;9, showed great pleasure when the trampoline was returned to the Nursery after being repaired. The teacher heard her saying to herself, "I won't break it again." When it was explained to her that no one had broken it, and that the trampoline had only been damaged through fair wear and tear, through so much use, Joan still repeated, "I won't break it again."

2. Joan was aged 5;7 when a door had been removed for repair. The empty space shocked her. When the door was replaced, Joan was delighted.

Since the blind child cannot actually watch what is happening, any kind of breakage is experienced as a sudden noise, a shock. Time and reflection are needed to remove the uncertainty from the situation. But even then the uncertainty remains; is experienced as frightening, and the worst is imagined. With some children this may lead to experiments:

Richard, aged 3;9, accidentally dropped a china bowl on the floor. The bowl did not break. Immediately afterward, seemingly on purpose, he dropped another bowl, which did break in two pieces. The teacher picked up the pieces and explained that china broke and wanted Richard to feel the two pieces. He became frightened, cried, and cringed away, refusing to touch them.

When made to touch a broken object, blind children sometimes become panic-stricken. Obviously at such a moment the feared mistake, the feeling of responsibility in general, and the specific castration fear and castration guilt reinforce each other so that anxiety rises to a pitch which overwhelms the child.

It would be a mistake to think that their lack of sight makes blind children less aware of the difference between the sexes. Evidently they gather the relevant information from sitting on their mothers' or fathers' laps, from listening to noises in the toilet, and so forth. Joan's development, which has been followed in detail, may serve as an illustration in this respect.

Joan's younger brother was born when she was 2. Her mother allowed her to feel his body and to help bath him. When aged 5;7, she started therapy and in her first session showed her concern over the differences between the sexes. She asked of every toy, doll or animal, "Is he a little girl?" "Is he a boy?" She showed her envy of her brother by continually pushing him away from wherever she wished to sit. She wanted everything her brother possessed, and this wish extended, in the usual way, to the children in the nursery school, from whom she would take possession of everything they were playing with. When bathing her doll, she washed it repeatedly between its legs, saying, "I wash his winky." "Isn't he a lovely boy?" The mother reported how, when the children had gone to the toilet together, they had returned giggling excitedly, the brother remarking, "Joan has a hole." Guilt over her sexual involvement and jealousy also showed; when building a house for her brother, she immediately destroyed it, but then tried to build it again.

It must be kept in mind, of course, that in the case of a blind child, the girl's normal envy of the boy's different physical equipment is reinforced by the envy of his being sighted.

INTERACTION WITH THE SIGHTED WORLD

In a discussion of the interaction of the blind with the sighted world, some repetition of former statements is inevitable.

For sighted people, vision is such an essential part of their experience that misconceptions and misunderstandings of the reactions of the blind are the order of the day. Sighted parents of blind children usually have the greatest difficulty in identifying with them and are frequently unable to understand the cues which the children give as indications of their needs. The same is true, almost inevitably, of most sighted adults who work with the blind; although they are most helpful in their intentions, their familiarity with normal child development does nothing to prevent their undervaluation of the children's endowment; and only too often they experience them as more defective than they really are. They fail to appreciate the progressive nature of the child's developmental moves, different as these are from those of the sighted. It is not unusual for parents of blind children to make denigrating remarks about them, even in their presence. When one observes such events, it is not difficult to grasp the ways in which an understandable parental disappointment becomes transformed in the mind of the child into a feeling of worthlessness. Many parental demands and prohibitions usually are based on sighted norms and are therefore quite inappropriate for the blind child and impossible for him to comply with.

As previously stated, the realization of blindness is probably the most distressing and poignant in the child's life. It is questionable whether blind individuals, either in childhood or later on, can ever fully come to terms with the limitations imposed on them. In fact, once this important step has been taken by the child and blindness has become a fact for him, an urgent and increasing wish to see and to become the same as the sighted is fully established and persists. Interaction with the sighted now takes place more consciously and develops in a number of stages.

In the first of these stages, as described before, there is a basic trust in the sighted and an overvaluation of their powers and capacities. This is not unlike the normal infantile overvaluation of the supposedly all-powerful adult. While this lasts, the child actively seeks the proximity of the sighted parent, teacher, or peer. However, it does not take long before this trusting attitude comes into conflict with the child's normal struggle and wish for independence.

Independence for the blind is hard to achieve and is constantly thwarted by their needs for help, guidance, and protection. This does not mean that independence is in any way less desired.

A next phase is ushered in by the developing use of those functions of the blind which are intact—their understanding of the world through listening; their experiences gained by touch; and their intellectual functions of reason, judgment, and memory. As we watch the children grow, we also observe the ways they face reality, the ways in which they become aware of their own increasing capacities and simultaneously evolve a more realistic appreciation of the abilities of the sighted. Like all children who outgrow their unquestioned idealization of their parents as all-powerful beings, the blind also begin to realize that there are tasks beyond the possibility of the sighted; that the sighted are not infallible; and that they too can make mistakes and erroneous judgments. What they say and do cannot always be relied upon; and the blind child's basic trust can be shattered. The children learn very gradually, at least to some degree, to rely on their own opinions, values, and decisions.

Watching the children, we feel that they gradually realize that their own interests and experiences do not always coincide with those of the sighted; that they are attracted by different matters, moved by different needs, and react to similar situations in dissimilar ways. Parallel with the need to depend on the sighted, the blind develop a growing desire to follow their own inclinations and to go their separate ways. This move is essentially a progressive one. As indicated before, we see the child advance, from the position of using the sighted as tools with which to enlarge his own knowledge of the world through the others' sight, to the point of envying them and wishing to be like them; and from there again, to the urgent desire to share in their lives, to take part in their experiences, and to be accepted by them as an equal human being, in spite of blindness and the differences which stem from it.

We learned something about the growing attraction of the sighted world when we contacted some of our nursery school children at a later stage. We learned that, for the growing blind children, it is not so much the actual advantage of vision which attracts them so much as a certain ambience which, according to their feeling, surrounds the sighted who are active and spontaneous, who move unhindered from place to place, who are able to get what they want without any of the constraints and restrictions which dominate the life of the blind. Their expression of emotion, pleasure, pain, surprise, sadness, shock, and anger is more spontaneous than that of the blind; and laughter as a sign of enjoyment seems especially attractive. We have seen blind children join in the laughter of the sighted, even though they are ignorant of its reason:

A blind child told, in great excitement, about a visit to the zoo and how he had liked best the monkeys. "One monkey chased another one and bit it until he bled." When questioned how he could know this, he admitted that he could not have seen it—"Someone told me." It is evident that the dramatic scene in the monkey house attracted the sighted children who were standing around and watching. The blind child heard the exclamations and their laughter and was caught up in the emotional excitement and was excited as well.

Conversations which are overheard by the blind, especially those expressing emotions, are also enjoyed vicariously. It would be wrong to say that listening of this kind merely serves the intellectual purpose of gaining information about the world. An equally important purpose seems to be the fulfillment of emotional needs in order to make up for the comparative poverty of their own experience. One wonders whether it is the continual strain of maintaining orientation and solving problems which deprive the blind of much opportunity for enjoyment, so that in this respect as well, the contact with the sighted is used to make up for what they miss.

The wish to share the life of the sighted was expressed by all blind children known to us. Follow-ups after they had finished their education in school show how gratified they are when they come in contact with the sighted, whether in college, in social functions, or in work.

1. Caroline, aged 18, and Joan, aged 17, attended Mormon groups separately, and each expressed her pleasure in being the only blind person there with sighted people. Caroline said that she felt at ease, that no one felt sorry for her or fussed. She was accepted. Joan told how much happier she felt since she was with the sighted.

2. Matthew, aged 21, after graduating from school with high marks, was accepted at a college for the blind. He was very unhappy in his segregation and he left before finishing the course. He then told how he himself searched for and found what he was looking for and was accepted at a music college, and for the first time mixed with all sorts of young people and felt accepted and happy.

3. Helen, aged 24, expressed the same general pleasure and well-being: "I am a changed person; I am happy, I have friends, sighted friends."

Talking to these adolescents (or young adults) gives one the feeling that the segregation of the blind during their schooling, advisable though it may be in some respects, nevertheless represents an added hardship through limiting the interaction with the sighted which, in certain developmental phases, seems of such importance.

BIBLIOGRAPHY

BURLINGHAM, D. (1972), *Psychoanalytic Studies of the Sighted and the Blind.*
New York: Int. Univ. Press.
———— YORKE, C., & FREUD, A. (1972), *Growing Up Without Vision,* a film
photographed and directed by Peter Hylton Cleaver. London: Hampstead
Child-Therapy Clinic.
MAHLER, M. S. (1963), Thoughts about Development and Individuation. *This
Annual,* 18:307–324.
WINNICOTT, D. W. (1955), Metapsychological and Clinical Aspects of Regres-
sion within the Psycho-Analytical Set-up. *Int. J. Psycho-Anal.,* 41:585–595.

"The Ordinary Devoted Mother" and Her Blind Baby

DORIS M. WILLS

"THE ORDINARY DEVOTED MOTHER AND HER BABY" WAS THE TITLE of a series of talks broadcast in 1949, by D. W. Winnicott. Its implication, that ordinary mothers *are,* for the most part, devoted placed a welcome stress on the positive factors in mothering at a time when professional workers, in their attempts to understand early handling problems, had perhaps become too preoccupied with the negative factors. However, when the baby is blind, "ordinary devotion" in the mother is often not assumed to be probable or perhaps even possible, and the mother is frequently blamed for things that go wrong with the child's development. Yet, the majority of mothers of blind children also become devoted, especially when they are given some degree of support and insight during the vicissitudes of the child's development. For the mothers of sighted children, such support and insight are more easily available.

This paper is based on work with the mothers of blind children, mainly under 3 years of age, during visits to and observa-

The work with blind children is part of the Educational Unit of the Hampstead Child-Therapy Course and Clinic and as such was maintained by the Grant Foundation, Inc., New York. The research work with the blind was assisted further by the National Institute of Mental Health, Bethesda, Maryland.

The research has been directed since its inception by Dorothy Burlingham. I am deeply indebted to her for ongoing help with the work on which this paper is based, and my thanks are also due for many helpful comments on the paper itself to A. Curson and A.-M. Sandler.

tions in the home. My aim was to study, together with the mother, the baby's development for two reasons. The first was, naturally, to support her through her depression, and to help her understanding of her child. The second was, with the aid of her observation, to build up more understanding of all blind children's early development. Visits generally were made weekly or fortnightly. Preferably they were started at the time the blindness was diagnosed, and they continued until the child went to nursery school and in some cases to ordinary school at 5 years. This paper does not concern itself with the classification of parental reactions to blindness; these have been described, e.g., by Lairy and Harrison-Covello (1973). Instead, it attempts to focus attention on the need for immediate support for parents of these children, and on the importance of providing them with relevant information about development.

Naturally, all handicaps cause anxiety, concern, and sometimes revulsion, but blindness occupies a special place. It is particularly incapacitating and it has a strong link with ideas of punishment. Some people, for example, still assume that blindness is caused by venereal disease, even though the routine antenatal care available in Britain today effectively prevents this. However, an unconscious link between blindness and the fantasy of punishment by castration certainly remains.

That a parent reacts with grief, anger, and depression, and perhaps with some revulsion to the birth of a blind baby, is of course natural.[1] But it is too simplistic to assume that the grief, anger, guilt, and depression will *necessarily* lead to withdrawal and understimulation of the baby, resulting sometimes in his rejection on the one hand, or his excessive protection on the other. A mother will respond to the catastrophe in terms of her psychological makeup, with its strengths and weaknesses, and will be influenced by the help that is given by the family and others. As to the question of a mother's revulsion at caring for an obviously blind baby, it has to be remembered not only that she may blame

1. This is sometimes considered a good reason for delaying the diagnosis of blindness. Late diagnosis, however, also has its dangers since the blind infant needs more handling and contact of all kinds to compensate for the loss of visual interaction.

herself, but that during pregnancy many women fear having an abnormal child. How far a mother can cope with this confirmation of her fear will depend on her personality. Fortunately, as Mac Keith (1973) points out, any revulsion is usually accompanied by a wish to protect the helpless baby. Mac Keith makes the interesting point that parents "fall in love" with a normal baby so that the child is felt as part of them whatever happens to him; but if a handicap is evident at birth, there is no time for this to happen (p. 524). In my experience, most parents do "fall in love" with their blind babies to a greater or lesser extent, but it may take them longer to do so. Of course, the degree to which the handicap affects the baby's appearance will influence the parents', and particularly the mother's, reaction. When the baby's eyes look more or less normal, a loving relationship is facilitated; when they are absent and only sunken eyelids meet her gaze until artificial eyes can be fitted, it will be impeded. (The blind children discussed in this paper had no additional major handicaps. All were within or above the average range of intelligence by 5 years.)

Nicholas was a premature child,[2] blind because of retrolental fibroplasia; he weighed 1 lb. 15 oz. at birth, and was the survivor of twins. He remained in the hospital for 6 months, during which time the parents had little contact with him. When he came home, he was sedated because he cried so much. A few months later, after a holiday when he slept in the parents' room (instead of alone), he settled down. When I first visited, the mother was expecting a second baby, and Nicholas was 11 months old. The parents had grown very fond of him and the father wanted my fortnightly visits arranged when he too could be present. Both parents proved exceptionally sensitive to Nicholas's needs, which made considerable demands on them. His speech was late in developing so that this sensitivity was of vital importance.

Here we have a healthy family coping with a blind baby, who because of the long hospitalization was almost a stranger, and learning to love him in spite of difficulties. Some parents find this task very much harder and may even resent the fact that the child was allowed to survive. Others no doubt manage to cope with this unaided, but professional help can provide support through the

2. Lairy and Harrison-Covello (1973) remark that premature blind children are often overprotected, but this was not the case with these parents.

difficult early phase when the calamity is first confronted. In addition, the worker's interest in the baby, at a time when the mother finds it hard to become attached to him, does something to hold the mother's interest until she feels better able to relate to him, and so learns to love him.

The impact of a blind baby on the parents is greater when the child is the firstborn. It may be less traumatic when the child comes later in the family. If the blind child is the firstborn, the subsequent birth of a normal child often reassures and comforts the parents, though their children's rather different needs may put heavy demands on them. Lairy and Harrison-Covello (1973) report that further pregnancies occurred most frequently in families where the blind child had been satisfactorily accepted (but it cannot be assumed that the avoidance of further pregnancies is linked with nonacceptance of the blind baby).

All parents greet their new infant, whether normal or handicapped, with a range of reactions, and it is true that blindness often exacerbates tendencies to overprotection or rejection. Overprotection is often based on a limited knowledge about the blind child's capabilities, though it may cover an unconscious wish to reject such a puzzling and apparently unrewarding child. Overt protection usually has complicated roots. To judge from our work, a very high proportion of parents can establish a meaningful and rewarding interaction with their blind child, and adapt their handling on the basis of this, *provided they are given the immediate and ongoing support and information* for which they frequently ask, but which, at present, is in such short supply. Where resources are limited, it is my impression that the most concentrated visiting should be in the first 18 months, at least weekly or fortnightly. During this period the parents have to make major adjustments. Moreover, after the birth of a baby, many women are emotionally very accessible. When help is delayed until the child is 3 years or so, some mothers will already have settled for methods of handling which are as unsuitable as they are difficult to modify. Such methods often were adopted under stress and became the standard means of coping with the anxieties and conflicts aroused by the child's development. To re-examine them may make the mother feel that her previous

handling was unwise and reopen the whole conflictual situation—
a course which many mothers naturally resist:

Nancy (blind because of retrolental fibroplasia) was referred to our
nursery school at 4;3, where she remained for 2 years. The mother
would never use the word "blind" in speaking of Nancy. She insisted
that Nancy should do everything like a sighted child, constantly teaching her verbally. The positive effect of this was that she encouraged
the child to be active; the negative, that the child naturally failed to
function like a sighted child and the mother insisted she was stupid.
The mother's attitude was not easy to modify.

It is true that not all mothers need the same amount of support
and help, since this depends both on their other resources and the
problems the blind child presents.

While some blind children develop normally, others arrive at
school with personality distortions that express themselves in a
variety of ways, ranging from unruly behavior to poor orientation,
parroting, excessive anxiety, withdrawal, and autoerotic habits.
These problems may largely disappear as the child grows older. It
is sometimes thought that, in some children, these features are
linked with brain damage of a kind that cannot be identified; but
more often many of them are attributed by teachers and medical
officers to the mother's early mishandling.

Since vision plays the main role in organizing experience in the
sighted, how does the blind infant circumvent this deficiency? Perhaps we handicap ourselves by concentrating on children whose
late development appears deviant, and would be wise to pay equal,
if not greater, attention to the well-developing blind child, to the
way the mother of such a child manages to follow his interests and
needs and so make up to some extent for the constant lack of
visual feedback. Rather than expecting the lines of development
in blind children to progress like those of sighted children (even if
they lag a little), we should expect greater unevenness between
the lines. For instance, in assessing a blind child of 3 years, I would
look for: his ability to relate to, and discriminate between, people;
the growth of his curiosity about the world around him; and his
ability to move and communicate. I would not be unduly concerned with everyday skills at this stage. Desirable as these are,
they are useless without the former accomplishments.

MOTHER AND CHILD IN THE FIRST YEAR

Most mothers are sufficiently stable to use the support and insights offered by the worker, especially if she arrives as soon as the blindness is diagnosed. Nevertheless it is often difficult for the mother (and indeed the father) to keep a reasonable balance between the claims of the handicapped child and the claims of the other children. There is a danger of swinging too far in one direction or another, of showing too much or too little concern for the blind child's special needs. Families have very different ways of coping, both with the handicap itself and their grief about it. These should be respected and indeed studied in their own right.

The mother of a visually impaired, backward little girl was asked by the hospital pediatrician to describe how she felt about the treatment she had received during her visits. She wrote:

> I am always aware that any remarks that I make, even replies to routine questions, are being automatically weighed to see if they are really concealing hidden meanings, and I used to feel considerable resentment that my views were not accepted at their face value.

Some mothers feel that they are watched by professional workers to see if they have "come to terms" with the handicap, which is always a lengthy and ongoing process. How it is dealt with depends on the mother's personality and on the support she receives from her husband and others. Indeed, the grief involved may never be expressed directly to the worker, who nevertheless indicates by her attitude and availability that she is there if the mother needs her. She has to be flexible and adaptable, since different mothers will use the worker differently.

If the worker arrives shortly after the diagnosis of blindness, the family may be in a state of crisis. The parents may wish to discuss the diagnosis and its implications, which they have sometimes been too shocked to take in properly during the hospital consultation where time limits discussion. The parents may think that they have not been told everything, and, with the worker acting as a liaison, obscurities can usually be clarified. Of course, it is sometimes the case that the diagnosis at an early age can only be vague.

Parents, feeling perhaps that they know so little about a blind child's development, may want immediate information about education so as to see the way ahead for their child. They are often angry, at this stage and later, with various members of the "establishment": doctors, local authority visitors, and the worker herself. They are often angry about the paucity of nursery school and school provision. Some of this anger may be warranted, since services for the preschool and school-age blind are in a state of flux; but some, no doubt, is a very natural way of avoiding sadness. However, after the early stages, most mothers want to report and demonstrate all the child's latest achievements, however small. Some mothers like to hear of similar experiences in the development of other blind children; others simply prefer to talk of their own children. Some mothers wish to meet others who are in a similar situation, others do not. But if the worker can offer support and help in whatever area the need is felt and, if necessary, even accompany mother and child to the hospital, it will do something to relieve the inevitable and continuous stress on the family.

A mother's love, whatever its admixtures, for her sighted baby develops and is cemented by the pleasurable interaction between herself and the child, a process in which visual interchange plays a very great part. The mother can understand the child on the basis of her own sensory experience and so is soon responding to him meaningfully; this gives her not only pleasure in the relationship but a feeling of value as a mother. The mother of the blind child, however, at a time when she is sad and disappointed, is confronted by a passive baby whose responses to her overtures are by no means obvious. For example, he may become still and silent when she comes to pick him up in order to *listen* to her approach. He does not smile and coo like a sighted infant who can *see* her approach (Burlingham, 1964):

Sarah was blind because of retinitis pigmentosa. During her first 6 months she became silent not only at her mother's approach, but also when her mother left the room, even if she were crying at the time.

A mother is relieved and interested when she is alerted to the reason for this behavior. She cannot understand the child easily on the basis of her own experience, and it will be a little time before she learns to interpret the small cues the baby offers, and

so to respond to him in a way which furthers an enjoyable interaction between them.

The situation is often made worse by relatives and friends who
pity and thereby further depress the mother, nor is it helped by
the advice, still given to some mothers, that the child will have
to be taken away and "trained" at 3 years. This advice not only
may sap the mother's self-confidence but also may make her avoid
too deep an involvement with the child because of the prospect
of losing him to a nursery boarding school at 3 years.

During this early period the worker must help the mother onto
the blind child's wavelength by stressing the need to make up for
the child's loss of vision by close contact in other ways, and by
pointing out the degree to which the child's cathexis of the world
around will be mediated by her:

On my first visit to Cynthia (blind from retinitis pigmentosa) at 9
months she sat in her mother's arms with her hands held up and fisted
like a younger child. I commented on this late fisting of the hands
and suggested the mother should play with them. A fortnight later, on
my second visit, Cynthia was beginning to open her hands as she held
them in the air, at times touching her mother, who said all this had
started after my last visit.

The worker can also help the mother by asking questions about
the meaning of their joint observations. This gives more background and insight to both. The worker can suggest other goals
toward which the mother can aim during the first year. The
benefit from such a contact is by no means onesided. As the
mother comes to understand her child, the worker is also learning
from her, building a picture of the early natural history of these
children, about which all too little is known with certainty. The
mother can be told this, and that she is helping the worker with
insights that can be recorded and used by other mothers. Once
alerted to a general point, for example, that a blind child takes an
important step when he first reaches for an object on a sound cue
alone, a mother may be able to think of some clever way of interesting her child in carrying out the activity:

Cynthia in her second year loved playing with mother's hands as she
sat on her lap. The mother used this to get her to reach on a sound
cue. She faced the child toward her on her knee. She clapped her hands

in various positions around the child, encouraging Cynthia to reach out for them.

Again, Sheila (blind from retrolental fibroplasia), a backward blind girl, at 3 years had regressed from walking freely. When the mother was alerted to the need for Sheila to explore her environment, she took to carrying her around the sitting room, always clockwise, always entering by the same door (out of 3), meanwhile naming objects to Sheila as she reached them.

This kind of incident does something to restore the mother's confidence in herself and furthers her pleasure in handling the child. It also is a useful learning experience for the worker.

At the beginning of the first year the worker can tell the mother that the baby will smile about the normal age, but in response to her voice, since he cannot see the mother's face. But voice will not regularly elicit the smile, the most reliable stimulus being "gross tactile or kinaesthetic stimulation" (Fraiberg, 1971b, p. 115). Mothers work very hard to obtain these early smiles which make them feel in better contact with their baby. Indeed, the main task in the first year is for the mother to establish a strong relationship between herself and her blind baby, so that the child begins to make the move from preoccupation with himself and his own body (his most available source of pleasure) to interest in his mother and her body and so to the objects with which she supplies him:

When Boris [3] was very small, his mother tied noise-making toys on each side of his carry-cot, and by 6 weeks said she knew which he preferred. By 2½ months the mother was taking Boris along in his carry-cot as she moved about the flat working; when she had to leave the room, she would kiss him on coming back. In spite of his having been born without eyes, she established a very positive relationship with him. One day when he was 11 months old, he was rocking with great pleasure on his little horse and his mother tickled his ear from behind. He stopped rocking and turned, smiled, and put out his hand to catch hers. The fact that Boris turned from rocking himself to touching his mother showed that he had made the first move from interest in himself and his own body to his mother. This meant that she could continually widen his experience.

3. Boris and his mother are described in greater detail in this volume (pp. 95–105).

Fraiberg (1971a), who intensively studied a small number of intact blind infants,[4] suggests that parents be alerted to the various little indications of attachment which the blind infant shows. She points out that the early smiling is already selective, and is given in response to the *parents'* voices, not the worker's; that around 5 months the blind infant shows a preference for the mother's arms, but squirms when the worker picks him up; and that between 8 and 12 months stranger anxiety begins to develop, thus indicating an important step in the child's attachment to the mother.

As for motor development in the first and the early part of the second year, the *postural* achievements of the blind child are essentially similar to those of the sighted. Sitting, stepping movements with hands held, and standing unsupported may all be expected to appear around the usual time. But *self-initiated* mobility is delayed. Attempts to lift himself by his arms when prone, to raise himself to a sitting posture, to pull himself up to a standing position, and to walk by himself—all these achievements will require motivation supplied by the mother (Adelson and Fraiberg, 1974).[5]

There are few standardized norms of development available for young blind children, but the worker can turn to the Maxfield and Buchholz Social Maturity Scale for Blind Pre-School Children (1957), and to the Norris et al. (1957) breakdown of a very similar scale, the Maxfield-Fjeld.[6] Despite the obvious significance of the mother-child relationship, however, these scales do not adequately cover it; instead they concentrate on the child-*toy* interaction, which well beyond the first year is of lesser significance. It is probably unwise to link any behavior too closely with age levels, because blind children who ultimately do well often show, at earlier stages, developmental lags in one area or another.

4. Fraiberg's group had the advantage of her and her colleague's support.

5. This paper was written prior to the publication of Fraiberg's book (1977) in which she slightly modified some of the median ages she gave in her earlier papers.

6. Dr. Joan Reynell at the Wolfson Clinic, London, is in the process of publishing a Developmental Scale for the Blind Children which should prove very useful (Reynell, 1978).

MOTHER AND CHILD IN THE SECOND AND THIRD YEARS

Most mothers look forward to the time when the blind child will be able to walk a few steps alone, realizing how important it is for him to explore the environment he cannot see. But since this is a self-initiated activity, it is delayed in many blind children. Norris et al. (1957) report it at 21 months; Adelson and Fraiberg (1974) report it at 15¼ months. It has to be borne in mind that, without sight, standing upright considerably diminishes the child's contact with the environment since contact by touch with his surroundings is suddenly reduced to the soles of his feet. Some children panic in this position, and refuse to relinquish support from the mother's finger or from a pushcart. Others may suddenly give up the few free steps they have learned to take because of some upsetting experience in another area of their lives.

If the first year has gone reasonably well, and the child is starting to move about by crawling or hitching, the mother usually anticipates that now in the second year he will begin to play with toys or household objects. Here she may suffer a further disappointment if she expects him to enjoy the constructive and manipulative type of play typical of the sighted child. The blind child remains centered on people. His interest moves only very slowly from people, who are to him so much more meaningful in terms of sound, touch, smell, and movement, than the inanimate world around him (Burlingham, 1967). Moreover, it is difficult to find toys and activities that are suitable for a blind child.

Sarah, at 15 months, certainly enjoyed handling combs and other everyday objects. The mother was in despair about her inability to find suitable toys. Sarah tended to sit and throw all her playthings—a plastic telephone, dolls, ring towers, rattles, cotton reels—over her shoulder. She was not yet able to imitate the noises mother made with pots and pans. We therefore discussed letting her do some of the "naughty" things children love at this age, and 2 months later she was, for instance, tearing up at least one newspaper a day. Such an activity allows the child gross hand movements; moreover, she gets a satisfying feedback, the rustle of the paper and the effect she has had on it since it is now in bits!

Sometimes the play of blind children looks repetitive and meaningless, but they need more time than the sighted to build on the basis of cumulative experiences.

Edward (blind from unknown causes) was 2 years when his mother said that he played with toys for only some 10 minutes each day. Mostly he walked around in the room where his mother was or went with her as she did her work: downstairs for the ironing, upstairs to "help" with the beds. He was allowed to open certain drawers, to fling the contents out, describing each as he did so (his speech was advanced). He and his younger brother played a little with the contents before his mother put them back. While this gives the mother little respite, the child is all the time learning to understand what goes on in his world.

The mother now waits hopefully for speech to develop, but here again the expectation of speech is somewhat different at this age for the blind child. The Vineland, a scale standardized on sighted children, places the item "Uses names of familiar objects" in the second year (Doll, 1947), while the Maxfield and Buchholz Scale (1957), standardized on blind children, places this item a year later, a placement which Norris et al.'s study (1957) supports.[7] Since this is a norm, some children are in advance of it; but some, who eventually develop normal speech, lag far behind and continue to echo what the mother says or to name the object only when it is present. It therefore is essential for parents to support the child's understanding by keeping their language simple and meaningful, by playing little body games with him where he can respond to simple instructions, and by showing him, through their own responses, that words can *get* him things. Moreover, parents need to provide ongoing mouth pleasure through such activities as blowing bubbles or "raspberries." They need to make language fun, and not to let it become an issue between them and the child.[8]

Some blind children vocalize very little in the first year, even though they are well-mothered. Other children, also well-mothered, may show a speech delay which is part of a general backwardness,

7. Fraiberg's recent book (1977) places "uses words to make wants known" in the second year for her advantaged group (p. 225).

8. Since the speech development of blind children is described in detail in this volume, it will not be taken up here.

and which may be linked with damage other than blindness. The extent of this may be difficult to assess until 3 or 4 years. In both cases the parents not only have to suffer disappointment at this lag in development, but at times may even be blamed for it. All too often the assumption is made that the child has not been adequately stimulated. In fact, many concepts used by the sighted are at first difficult to grasp for the congenitally blind child. For instance, he is presented with a variety of sensory cues concerning an object such as a "table" when only sight or long experience can bind these into a whole. Again, while sighted people frequently speak of what they are *seeing,* the blind child's main experience may be of what he is *hearing,* to which, often, they make no reference. Older children may give us insights into this:

Sam (blind from retinitis pigmentosa) was 5½ years when I heard a taped record of one of my sessions with him and realized that his bringing birds into his play was linked with the birds singing and twittering in the garden outside. I was habituated to this and so had ignored it. We all still have much to learn about how the blind organize and make sense of their world.

In the second year, there may be problems in the feeding area. For example, many blind children cling to the bottle. This seems to be due to a tie to the familiar rather than an arrest in development. The children cannot see others eat normally and lack encouragement from this experience in terms of rivalry or a wish to imitate. The mother may have to exercise considerable ingenuity if she is to help the child through this phase without a head-on collision or without winning compliance at the price of a reaction in some other area of development.

Many normally developing blind children suffer from a prolonged period of separation anxiety (Fraiberg, 1968). This may partly be due to their unavoidable dependence on the mother who has to act not only as a love object but also as an auxiliary ego in supporting their activities. These children probably take longer to achieve a stable idea of the mother's continuing existence and to be sure of her ultimate return whenever she is absent, since they are without a *visual* image to assist their recall of her. The anxiety reaction is often not easily understood:

Cynthia (2 years) became clinging and uncooperative after visits to the Welfare Centre accompanied by her mother. She showed the same response after being taken by her mother and left to stay the night with the very familiar grandmother. The mother thought that this was a reaction to a change in routine since Cynthia did not immediately come to her when she came to collect her. I suggested that Cynthia was reacting to the separation. The mother concurred in this after the next joint visit to the grandmother when she observed that Cynthia was unwilling to leave the room where the mother was in order to play in the garden. Following a day spent alone with her grandmother, Cynthia continued to stay close to her mother for some time.

A blind child who cannot glance at the mother on her arrival to collect him or her probably misleads the mother (and later on his teachers) more easily than does the sighted child, whose reactions are easier to observe and interpret. The following anxiety reactions show some protraction:

Edward (2;1 years) was taken to visit a local nursery by his parents, and, with his agreement, was left in a large group in the care of an adult who played with him for 10 minutes. On his return home, about 11 A.M., he demanded a bottle and to be put to bed, where he stayed for ¾ hour. That night, an hour after he had been put to sleep, he screamed nonstop for 5 minutes. The mother understood this behavior as reactive to the brief separation. He showed a similar but more intense reaction a month later to a further separation from his mother.[9]

Here we see the blind child's overcompliance, his subsequent response, withdrawal, and belated expression of the affect in anxiety and rage. Helped by his advanced speech, the mother was in very good contact with this child and so understood the reactions, which could well have been missed in a less verbal child since they did not occur in the context of the event itself. Such a belated reaction can sometimes be avoided by reminding the child *before* the next separation that he did not like his mother leaving him last time. This intervention enabled Edward to cope better on subsequent occasions. Even if such a comment provokes an outburst, this is better for the child's development.

9. Fraiberg (1968) describes a somewhat similar case of a younger child, Jack, who reacted with long screaming fits after a longer separation from his mother.

The Step to Day Nursery School in the Third Year

When the child is about 3 years old, the mother may look for a small day nursery school group to relieve her of the constant task of supporting the child's understanding and of widening his experiences and contacts. Since there are so few blind children, she is unlikely to have a specialized school in her locality and may try a sighted group where the teacher is sympathetic. Some teachers do not want the mother to stay with the child until he is able to let her go, and the child not only has to undergo sudden separation, but, if there are many children, the noise will confuse him and he may well become overwhelmed by the new experience. However, the mother may be fortunate in finding a smaller and more suitable group and the transition may go more easily.

We were able to make arrangements of this kind for Cassie:

When she was 20 months old, Cassie lost her sight (due to retinoblastoma) and her mother brought her to our nursery school every week for some months in order to watch the teacher's handling of other blind children. As the journey was some distance, the teacher continued the contact by visiting once a fortnight. At 3 years (the usual age for intake) Cassie asked to come to the school again. She came twice with her mother and then came with the escort only, telling her mother to stay at home.

Some home visits by the teacher before the child starts probably are the ideal arrangement in that the child gets to know her, and the teacher gets a better picture of the child and his or her background. Some schools do manage to arrange this and find other suitable ways of introducing the child to school,[10] and of appropriately handling the child's separation anxiety before it becomes acute.

When it is difficult to find the right nursery group, the mother, and sometimes the worker, may be tempted to make arrangements for the child to attend two different groups during the week. For the blind child in particular this is not a good idea. Since without sight it is so much more difficult to make sense of his surroundings, the blind child needs to be in *one small* group where he can gradually learn to relate to known adults and a few children.

10. For an example, see Curson in this volume.

As we come to understand better what the blind child is facing when he starts in a day nursery group, we may be able to make more adequate provisions for his first experiences away from home. Quite apart from the mother's need for some relief from providing the constant support that the blind child must have, his tie to his mother must slowly be loosened as it must be with the sighted child. Both blind and sighted children do not develop well without a strong relationship with the mother or her substitute; but both need to make some move toward a measure of independence. The child without sight, which does so much to make the world attractive, is less strongly motivated than the sighted. However, it is crucial for his further development how his strong tie is loosened when he starts in a day nursery group, especially if his speech is not well developed. If the separation is sudden, it is liable to be traumatic, and while some children may make a spurt in some areas of development in order to master the situation, others become confused and regress.

It is outside the scope of this paper to discuss the traumatic impact of placement, whether gradual or sudden, in weekly boarding school at 5 years (and sometimes younger), but here again the children frequently regress in such a way that teachers find it difficult to believe when mothers tell them that the child performs better at home. While these schools offer many benefits, including teaching geared to the child's somewhat different and delayed understanding of the world, they cannot but be disorientating for a blind child. In Britain greater variety of provision is badly needed (Vernon et al., 1972).

CONCLUSION

In this paper I have attempted to highlight the difficulties the mother may have to contend with in bringing up a blind child, in order to demonstrate that it may not be her ability in mothering which is at fault, but rather that too little support and knowledge are made available to her. If her blind child develops well, we can probably assume that she is a *more* than ordinarily devoted mother.

Workers offering such support need training in child development of both sighted and blind, and a willingness to follow and get to know the children in their homes. I did not regard my task as psychotherapeutic in the strict sense; rather, I worked with the mother in an attempt to support her and to understand the child with her help.

Why, when there is such a wealth of careful research on school-age blind children, has so little attention been paid to the preschool years, especially since it is known that by the time they are 5 many children show deviant development? The first reason is probably a practical one. Since there are very few blind children in Western cultures where workers are available, they are geographically very scattered, and keeping regular contact weekly or fortnightly requires much traveling. A second reason may be that such children distress us, perhaps more than those with any other handicap. All of this may have led to the wish to equate the blind with the sighted. As a result, even when careful work *is* done, certain basic questions are not asked. There is a tendency to describe the blind child as a sighted child lacking only one sensory modality, and while this tendency certainly lays stress on his need for normal childhood experiences, it can be used to deflect attention from his somewhat different course of development, and from a proper understanding of the ways he can use to circumvent his lack of vision.

We still have much to learn from blind children themselves. The range of sensory input on which they must rely is in all the rest of us largely dominated and organized by vision. They show very little facial expression, which hinders our observations. For these reasons we have to make a very special effort to empathize with their experience of their inner and outer world.

BIBLIOGRAPHY

ADELSON, E. & FRAIBERG, S. (1974), Gross Motor Development in Infants Blind from Birth. *Child Develpm.*, 45:114–126.

BURLINGHAM, D. (1964), Hearing and Its Role in the Development of the Blind. *This Annual*, 19:121–145.

——— (1967), Developmental Considerations in the Occupations of the Blind. *This Annual*, 22:187–198.

COLONNA, A. B. (1968), A Blind Child Goes to the Hospital. *This Annual,* 23:391–422.

DOLL, E. A. (1947), *Vineland Social Maturity Scale.* Minneapolis: Educational Test Bureau.

FRAIBERG, S. (1954), Counselling for the Parents of the Very Young Child. *Soc. Casewk,* 35:47–57.

———— (1968), Parallel and Divergent Patterns in Blind and Sighted Infants. *This Annual,* 23:264–300.

———— (1971a), Intervention in Infancy. *J. Amer. Acad. Child Psychiat.,* 10:381–405.

———— (1971b), Smiling and Stranger Reaction in Blind Infants. In: *The Exceptional Infant,* ed. J. Hellmuth. London: Butterworths, pp. 110–127.

———— (1977), *Insights from the Blind.* New York: Basic Books.

———— & FREEDMAN, D. A. (1964), Studies in the Ego Development of the Congenitally Blind Child. *This Annual,* 19:113–169.

FREEDMAN, D. G. (1964), Smiling in Blind Infants and the Issue of Innate vs. Acquired. *J. Child Psychol. Psychiat.,* 5:171–184.

HEWITT, S. (1970), *The Family and the Handicapped Child.* London: Allen & Unwin.

LAIRY, G. C. & HARRISON-COVELLO, A. (1973), The Blind Child and His Parents. *Res. Bull. Amer. Foundation for the Blind,* 25:1–24.

MAC KEITH, R. (1973), Feelings and Behaviour of Parents of Handicapped Children. *Develpm. Med. Child Neurol.,* 15:524–527.

MAXFIELD, K. E. & BUCHHOLZ, S. (1957), *A Social Maturity Scale for Blind Pre-School Children.* New York: American Foundation for the Blind.

NORRIS, M., SPAULDING, P., & BRODIE, F. (1957), *Blindness in Children.* Chicago: Univ. Chicago Press.

REYNELL, J. (1978), Developmental Patterns of Visually Handicapped Children. *Child: Care, Hlth & Develpm.* (Oxford), 4:291–303.

SANDLER, A.-M. (1963), Aspects of Passivity and Ego Development in the Blind Infant. *This Annual,* 18:343–360.

———— & WILLS, D. M. (1965), Preliminary Notes on Play and Mastery in the Blind Child. *J. Child Psychother.,* 1:7–19.

SHERIDAN, M. D. (1960), *The Developmental Progress of Infants and Young Children,* London: H. M. Stationery Office.

VERNON, M. ET AL. (1972), *The Report of the Vernon Committee on the Education of the Visually Handicapped.* London: H. M. Stationery Office.

WILLS, D. M. (1968), Problems of Play and Mastery in the Blind Child. *Brit. J. Med. Psychol.,* 41:213–222. Also In: *Readings on the Exceptional Child,* ed. E. P. Trapp & P. Himelstein. New York: Meredith Corporation, 1972, 335–349.

———— (1970), Vulnerable Periods in the Early Development of Blind Children. *This Annual,* 25:461–479.

———— (1978), Entry into Boarding School and After. In: *Readings on the*

Visually Handicapped Child, ed. P. F. Portwood & R. T. Williams. Leicester: British Psychological Society, 2(2):39–44.

WINNICOTT, D. W. (1949), *The Ordinary Devoted Mother and Her Baby.* London: Tavistock, 1959.

The Blind Nursery School Child

ANNEMARIE CURSON

THE NURSERY SCHOOL FOR BLIND CHILDREN, ATTACHED TO THE HAMP-
stead Child-Therapy Clinic, was established to meet the specific
needs of young blind children and to give their mothers relief and
support. At times, children who had some sight attended the nursery school; but these children were classified as "blind" for educational purposes because they would have to learn Braille. They
were visually handicapped and needed much help. However small
their amount of vision, however blurred or blunted it may have
been, they nevertheless had visual experiences and their development differed from that of the child who grows up without any
visual awareness.

This account concerns itself only with children who were totally
blind from birth. It does not deal with children who become blind
later, because I have been convinced by my work with young blind
children that even the very primitive visual awareness which a
baby experiences in the first months of life has a lasting impact
and influence on him. It seems that some recollection, however
dim, of a visually perceived world remains with the child who
loses his sight even in babyhood. In our group it was clear that
such children were more adventurous, more lively, more socially
expressive, more animated, more assertive in their postures than
those who were blind from birth. As Helen Keller (1903) says in
her autobiography:

Headteacher, Nursery School for the Blind, Hampstead Child-Therapy
Course and Clinic, London, which was maintained by the Grant Foundation,
Inc., New York, and by the National Institute for Mental Health, Bethesda,
Maryland.

... during the first nineteen months of my life, I had caught glimpses of broad green fields, a luminous sky, trees and flowers, which the darkness that followed could not wholly blot out. If we have once seen, "the day is ours and what the day has shown" [p. 8].

Nursery school is intended to be an extension of the home, not a substitute for it; it aims to encourage curiosity, to give children meaningful group experiences, to help fulfill the individual needs of each child, and to develop fully whatever potential there may be.

The Hampstead Nursery School for the Blind is housed in a large, prefabricated hut in a pleasant garden. It is self-contained with its own front door and another door leading from a small veranda straight into the garden. There is a hallway, which is used as a cloakroom, with an adjoining lavatory and washroom. The main room is large, bright, and cheerful. At first glance it may appear like any nice nursery school, but subtle differences soon reveal themselves. Some areas of the wooden floor are covered with lino, some are carpeted, and some are covered only by occasional rugs made from various materials such as wool, cotton, and velvet. The different surfaces help the children to orientate themselves and supply them with information about the geography of the room. This kind of information, which a sighted child takes in at a glance, is gained by the blind child through laborious exploration with his hands, arms, feet, and legs. Very often his whole body is used, and his bottom plays an important role.

The pictures on the wall of our classroom are "feeling pictures": dried leaves, shells, various shapes of wood, cork, and corrugated cardboard. In the cloakroom and by the washbasins the hooks for the children's coats and towels are marked by symbols in different materials: a felt triangle, a tin square, a corduroy circle.

Our work with blind children began before the hut was built, in a large room of the main clinic. Thus we had the opportunity to explore the process of construction with a group of children. (Our group never consisted of more than six children with two teachers.) They could feel and listen as floorboards were nailed down, and they could feel the walls as they were built. One little boy examined a drainpipe very carefully, touching it, pressing it, tapping it. In the end he asked, "May I smell and taste it?" Gerald (age 4½) wanted to know how the water ran into the lavatory cisterns when he flushed the toilets. For many weeks after they were installed, he would put his ear to the pipe and with intense concentration listen to water trickle into the cistern on the roof. When the walls had been painted, Carrie (4) gently ran her hands over them and said, "It's all lovely and smooth."

Being involved in the building of their nursery school was a valuable experience for these children. It has helped them to form concepts of the work and materials needed. All too often the blind child has to struggle with words, concepts, and situations which to him are totally meaningless. Adam, now a teenager, and one of our nursery school children, revealed that until recently he had thought all roofs were plastic sheets, a larger version of the plastic sheet we used to cover up the sandbox to protect the sand from rain, snow, and falling leaves.

A WELL-FUNCTIONING BLIND CHILD

Adam first came to the nursery school when he was 3 years old. He was born prematurely and weighed less than 4 lbs. He was in an incubator for some time, and his blindness was due to retrolental fibroplasia.

Before Adam's birth his mother had several miscarriages and later she had a stillbirth. Adam's parents have a second son, 2½ years younger than Adam, a healthy, normal child. Adam's father is a motor mechanic. The mother worked as a cook before her marriage. She came from Spain, where she and her 12 brothers and sisters were brought up on a farm in an atmosphere in which babies and children were taken for granted. This unselfconscious acceptance of children included handicapped children. Adam's blindness therefore did not involve the intense strain seen in more sophisticated families.

Adam's mother recalled that when she was first told of his blindness, she was "very sad and happy too because I had a baby at last." His father "got drunk and felt like killing somebody." In spite of the very natural shock and grief, these parents instinctively found ways of furthering their child's development and gaining pleasure from it.

Adam's mother had confidence in herself as a mother. She enjoyed handling her baby and realized that a blind baby needed more physical contact, more picking up, more playing with, and more talking to than a sighted infant. In this she was well supported by her husband. From early on the parents encouraged exploration and whatever Adam touched, they described and put into words. They did not offer him toys until he was over 2 years old since they felt that he must first become familiar with everyday things and with his immediate environment. At every vital stage they stimulated, shared, welcomed, and praised the child's natural curiosity and his desire to cope in his own way.

Before a child entered the nursery school group, we always arranged to see him, and whenever possible both parents, at a time when the other children were not present. In this way he could acquaint himself with the room and the teacher before facing the new and strange environment. These individual visits continued until the child was familiar with the new environment and seemed to be at ease.

Adam, holding his father's hand, impressed us as a well-developed, dark-haired little boy with deep-set eyes. His mother carried the baby. Adam's posture and movements were freer and better coordinated than those of many blind children, but, compared to a sighted child of 3, they were awkward, slow, hesitant, and lacked the boisterous and lively spontaneity so typical of that age.

In a way, the slow, careful movements of a blind child represent an achievement—he has sensibly learned to protect himself, to control and repress his natural wish for quick motion. To walk, to keep his balance, to avoid obstacles are, without vision, difficult, dangerous tasks. They need concentrated energy.

On entering the room, Adam stood silently, motionless for a few minutes, his head bent down, listening to his parents chatting to each other and to me, perhaps taking in the new smells and sounds of the room. My immediate reaction was to take his hand, to lead him around the room, and to introduce him to toys and equipment; but, instead, I just said, "Hello Adam," and lightly touched his hand.

The sighted child, on meeting a stranger, often turns his head away and at first avoids eye-to-eye contact. Slowly, carefully, he will let his eyes turn toward the new person, slowly look at her until eventually their eyes meet in a smile. It seemed that Adam was doing the same thing. He listened to me talking to his parents; and he let himself become familiar with my voice before he allowed direct contact by saying, "Hello, you lady."

Every nursery school teacher tries to make the schoolroom as bright, welcoming, and stimulating as possible; but in a nursery school for blind children this atmosphere has to be conveyed by the teacher's voice and attitude to the child. Just as the mother of a blind baby has to find ways of eliciting his first smile because he cannot imitatively respond to her smiling face, the teacher of young blind children has to find ways of making contact with her small pupil by means other than the usual glances of encouragement and praise. While the sighted child will respond to a reassuring nod, an applauding gesture, a smile of approval, the blind child needs to be touched, to be talked to directly, to be addressed by name each time in order to receive the same message. The practical necessity for physical closeness naturally creates a more intimate mother-substitute relationship than is usual in nursery school work with the sighted.

Unable to see the brightly colored toys, the inviting trampoline, the slide or the swing, Adam followed my voice and footsteps as he began to explore the new environment. At first he limited the area which he could encompass to a small one, stepping forward by himself and going back to where his mother's voice could be heard.

He began with unsure, tentative steps, his hands stretched out toward the wall, cautiously negotiating around a corner. Stumbling on a step between the main room and the small veranda, he immediately knelt down to feel it, with his hand and foot simultaneously, in a most awkward position. Standing up, he felt it again with his foot, stood on it, stamped on it, stepped over it, and ran his foot along it, as if to make a mental picture. He then sat down on it with his bottom, seeming to receive physical pleasure from sliding backward and forward across it, while smiling to himself. After he had built up an image of the step in this way, he could go further and his exploration became more assured. On hearing me fill a kettle with water, he came to the sink and touched it all over. He patted it outside and inside; he knelt down and with his lips explored the entire rim of the sink before investigating the supporting wooden part with his hands. He then kicked it gently with his foot. When he had discovered all he wanted to know about the sink, he moved on to chairs and table. He was not satisfied with just feeling each little chair. To a blind child the small nursery chair is a new and strange object; only vision can link it with the adult chair with which such children are familiar at home. Several times, in his exploration, Adam put his cheek or lips to the wooden seat. He lifted up one of the chairs and then sat on it for a brief moment. Adam did all this silently and by himself. Once or twice he called out, "Mum," and his mother very quietly answered, "Yes, I am here." In fact, this contact between mother and child was really a "verbal glance."

Adam used his whole body to explore and find out about his world; other blind children employ different means. Mary (3;3 years) needed her mother to be close by her before she would be active and explorative. The mother had to give her constant verbal encouragement and confirmation. For example, when she came across a small chest of drawers and asked, "What is it?" I told her, "It's a small chest of drawers, let us feel it." But Mary ignored this and, pulling at her mother, asked again, "Mum, what is it?" After the mother's confirmation, Mary could go ahead, pull each drawer out, listen to the sounds she produced by opening and shutting them, and at the mother's invitation feel inside them. Holding her hand, Mary walked around the table. Her mother said, "They have little chairs here." Mary felt each one, saying, "It's a chair, a little chair, it's not like Mummy's chair"; or she would ask, "Is it a chair, Mum?" Then she would sit on it or climb on it and ask her mother to do the same before passing on to the next chair.

On the other hand, Stewart (4;2 years) gave the impression of a passive child on entry into nursery school. Although he could walk well, he spent almost the whole of his first term sitting on the floor in the middle of the room. He sometimes smiled and he responded in a friendly, preoccupied manner to the teacher's efforts to interest him. We slowly learned that Stewart was indeed preoccupied in a most constructive way. He listened to all that went on in the room, to the sounds and echoes, to the teachers' and the children's voices, to things which were fetched and put away, to the taps turned on and off, to the doors being opened and closed. He used this intensive listening-memorizing experience to make sense of the world around him.

As a teacher one may be tempted to persuade a child who sits motionless on the floor for long periods of time to become involved—to be "active." But in Stewart's case, this would have been an interference with a very important learning process and would have broken the concentration needed for acute hearing. Stewart was, in fact, active. Once he had taken in, and sorted out, all the acoustic information necessary for his confidence, he moved about the room freely and was well oriented. Subsequently, however, when Stewart was unwell or upset in any way, his good orientation easily disintegrated. In circumstances in which sighted children merely become grumpy and disagreeable, blind children become disoriented and are unable to find their way about even in the most familiar circumstances.

On his preliminary visits, Adam stayed for about two hours; and he progressed from exploring, in great detail, individual areas of the room, to activities which appeared more like play. For instance, he no longer explored the sink, but approached it directly and confidently and turned on the taps, wanted to wash up, and obviously imitated his mother with remarks such as, "Oh dear! Where is the towel?" or "Dear me! What a mess!" When Adam felt at ease in the room and with me, he started to attend the nursery school, though only with his mother. "Gradual entry" is the accepted practice of most nursery schools; and mothers of new entrants are not expected to abandon their 3-year-olds at the nursery school door, as they once did.

Children vary a great deal in their ability to separate from the mother and to adjust to group life (however small the group), but on the whole it takes the blind child longer to reach the stage in his development where he can separate from the mother and accept some group life without undue distress. It seems to be a complicated task to establish, without the help of a visual image, the firm, stable idea of mother's presence—somewhere. It is a difficult lesson to learn that she will be close again, even if she is absent and cannot be touched, heard, or smelled for a moment. The mother is, to the blind child, not only his love, but an auxiliary ego, a perpetual interpreter and classifier of the world. She acts as his eyes in that she protects and guards him from danger or accident in situations where vision centers both on warning and protection. Thus, the mother encourages, albeit unconsciously, the child's total dependence and curbs his curiosity. It is therefore particularly painful for him to feel that she is not there.

The blind child rarely screams, kicks, or protests like his sighted peers when separation is attempted before he is ready for it. By his overcompliant, accepting behavior, he plays into the tendency of the environment to deny that he could be upset, frightened, or unhappy. Certain everyday phrases take on a special significance when used about blind children. "He goes happily with anyone. He takes so well to you [and anyone]. He loves to be in the nursery and does not mind if I [mother] am there or not."

Blind children are often treated like inanimate objects, picked up by well-meaning, pitying strangers, carried about, and put down like parcels. By the time they entered nursery school, most of our children had been in hospitals at least once and frequently more often. These experiences could well account for their resigned compliance, since the latter serves as a protection against further indignity and possible pain.

We considered it most important for the mothers to stay in the building with their children until the latter really felt secure. The close tie to the mother was therefore loosened gradually and smoothly; but this was not always an easy process.

Susi was 3;9 years when she joined our nursery school. Her mother attended with her for three months; and would then go into the waiting room for short periods. Susi seemed not to mind when her mother left, but always wet herself during her mother's absences, even though she had been reliably dry and clean from the age of 2½. We suggested to her that she could cry and say that she missed and wanted her Mummy. She did cry, and soon regained bladder control.

Boris (3 years) started nursery school twice weekly, accompanied by his mother. At the end of three weeks, his mother slipped out for half an hour after telling him she was about to do so and would shortly return. He said good-bye to her quite cheerfully. A few minutes after she had left, he called for her and seemed puzzled and confused when reminded that his mother had gone out shopping. During her short absence he needed repeated explanations of where she was and much reassurance about her return. He did not seek or accept physical comfort from the nursery school staff. He listened to a favorite record, sitting very erect on his chair, occasionally stretching himself, sucking his lower lip, and repeatedly putting both hands on his genitals for brief periods. His mother returned while he was still listening. On hearing her voice, he burst into tears. He was quickly comforted by her cuddle and loving request to be "a good boy"; following this incident, however, his mother reported that at home he was very clinging for a few days and difficult about going to bed in the evenings. Afterward, at our suggestion, his mother did not attempt any separation for several weeks, and when she did, she only went to the waiting room. Boris was always taken to her before he got upset or confused. He soon accepted her short absences, and these were gradually increased in length. Nonetheless, the separation was still difficult for him and for several months he insisted on waiting for his mother to take him to the toilet.[1]

In Lisa (4;3) and several other children, separation anxiety seemed to express itself through displacement to a new person. The mother was ignored and the teacher gained attention; the teacher was ignored in turn as the escort was cathected; and interest in the escort was lost as soon as the child met the driver. This did not mean that Lisa was not deeply attached to her mother; rather, children like Lisa have learned by experience how dependent they are on the protective presence of any sighted person. They are aware that they cannot cope on their own; by clinging to the new person, they do not risk being left alone.

During their first weeks, or sometimes months, in nursery school, many of the children were preoccupied with the doors, and kept opening and closing them. Assuming that these activities represented, in some way, the children's separation from their mothers, we turned them into games in which "Hallo" and "Good-bye" were said to teachers and other children, and finding each other led to expressions of surprise and delight. The activity of opening

1. Boris's early development is described in detail in this volume (pp. 95–115).

and shutting doors is itself pleasurable. The child is in control; he produces noises and vibrations by his action; he can feel and thereby comprehend the end results of his efforts. In fact, it is an activity which does not require vision for complete satisfaction and pleasure.

As most of the children had to travel a long distance from their homes, the local Health and Welfare Service provided the transport and the escorts. Consequently, the day-to-day contact with the mothers—so much a part of normal nursery school life—was missing once the children were settled. However, the periods during which the mother stayed with their children in the nursery school gave the teacher an opportunity to establish an easy, friendly relationship with the mother. As a result, information was gained about the child's early development and the child-rearing methods used by each mother. The mothers were encouraged by these contacts to discuss their problems at any time they wished, by telephone or even during home visits. Mothers of blind children need relief and support. They need to share the strenuous effort, as well as the pleasure and pride in the slow progress, the ups and downs, involved in bringing up a handicapped child.

Adam's mother stayed with him for about six weeks until one day he declared that now he was "a big boy" and wanted to come by himself. An escort was found for him, a kindly elderly lady, who managed to make the long car rides meaningful for Adam by singing to him, telling him simple stories, and talking with him about the traffic noises they encountered.

During the first few terms in nursery school, Adam's main pleasure was in physical activity involving the use of large muscles. He had to be sure he was safe; that is, to trust and have confidence in the teacher to provide danger-free conditions, before he could allow himself to relax his motor restraint and fully enjoy free movement. A habit common to many blind children is to remain on one spot and carry out all the motions of running, thus remaining safe, while at the same time enjoying bodily movements as though they were gaining ground. But this pleasure is not of the same order as that which the child experiences when he can run freely between two teachers or jump alone off a box—a pleasure that can clearly be seen in the children's postures and facial expressions when they change from subdued, dull-looking children to energetic, lively, bright ones. Adam discovered the joys of swinging, sliding, using the trampoline and climbing frames. But without vision, obtaining even these simple joys requires complicated learning processes, great effort, persistence, and the active involvement of the teacher. The swing had to be felt, the ropes holding it investigated by standing on a chair, the wooden seat tapped and knocked for audible information. After slow, careful exploration of the swing, Adam then gently pushed it to and fro, at first not letting go of it, but gradually pushing harder and harder. He listened to the faint sounds made by it and turned his head from side to side to feel the current of air as it brushed against his face. He experimented in this way for several days and became so absorbed in the actual pushing motion that he lost the original aim of the activity.

Frequently a blind child is held up in his investigations by sound, smell, or tactile sensations, and will not be able to advance his understanding or further his achievement. For example, Joan, when threading beads, became so interested in the fact that one of the beads was scratched that she could not go on with the threading, but repeatedly fingered the scratched bead. Or, as Peter stepped on the first bar of the climbing frame, his rubber-soled shoe made a squeaking noise. Further climbing was abandoned, in favor of the repetitive squeaking movement of his foot against the iron bar.

Adam, Joan, and Peter could be helped back to the initial purpose of their activities. For example, the teacher sat on the swing while Adam pushed her. He had to experience again and again the teacher's feet touching the ground and, most importantly, he had to hear her verbal expressions of pleasure in swinging before he could enjoy it himself. Joan needed the teacher to sit next to her, to feel her necklace, to be encouraged to make one for her mother, before she gained pleasure from undertaking and completing the task. Peter regained interest in the climbing frame when his ability to produce a squeaking noise on its first bar was acknowledged and praised. He was encouraged to go further by comments on the different noises that could be heard as he climbed from one bar to the next.

Constant, gentle activity by the teacher and a close relationship with the child are not only necessary for his progress, but essential in the prevention of feelings of isolation.

In Ann, the inhibition of free movement was severe and the effects of her very restricted and cramped home life were obvious. Her loving, but overprotective parents had not given her opportunity for exploration. When she first came to nursery school, Ann would sit apathetically for long periods on a favorite little basket chair, her back bowed, her head almost on her chest, her eyelids all but closed. It was soon apparent that Ann, like so many blind children, liked listening to music. Indeed, at home she spent hours listening to records, to the TV, and to the radio, which her mother put on "to keep the child happy." We used Ann's pleasure in music to propel her gently toward action. The teacher, playing the piano, would improvise little songs, such as "Ann is sitting in her chair, listening to the piano, come and clap your hands Ann, clap, clap, clap." It took some time before Ann would clap in response; the teacher had to do it first and take Ann's limp hands into hers while clapping. But by holding hands during dancing or musical movements, Ann slowly loosened up and began to move with ease. However, when left on her own, she quickly reverted to spinning in circles on the spot.

It is not surprising that many blind children find pleasure in rhythmic, repetitive movements like spinning, rocking, jumping up and down, with hands flapping a little, and head shaking. These odd-looking mannerisms, commonly referred to as "blindisms," are safe, effortless, natural outlets for the child's physical energy. After all, running, jumping, kicking, and throwing a ball are exertions and struggles associated with danger to oneself or others. While the sighted toddler is always on the move, "into everything," never still, the blind toddler resorts to these rhythmic movements, which may also express anger, frustration, and boredom.

Generally, blind children are unaggressive. It is as though they cannot afford angry feelings for fear of losing the favor and love of the people on whom they are so dependent. Normal expression of aggression is inhibited further for practical reasons: hitting, pushing mother (the usual target for a young child's aggression) is difficult, if not impossible, unless the child can locate her with certainty and aim his attack correctly.

For the sighted child, unless he is asleep, there is always something to do—that is, there is always something to be seen. Even so, he is bored at times, but it is not the same kind of boredom, not the flat emptiness, not the blank void, which the total absence of vision imposes. Blindisms offer an escape from this boredom. They often indicate, by their very intensity, a blind child's withdrawal into himself; that is, he seeks and gains interest and satisfaction from his own body and its sensations, instead of from the world around him. To counteract this tendency, he needs close involvement with the caring adult to make the world more attractive and meaningful for him, to arouse his interest, and to motivate the moves from preoccupation with his own body to constructive games.

When, for example, a child started rocking, he was taken on the teacher's lap for a rocking-horse game. But, after brief rocking, this was turned into a "naming body parts" game. Blind children do not automatically know that everybody has a face, arms, legs, and all the other body parts. How can they know what only vision conveys so clearly and undeniably? We also used body games to help the children conceptualize numbers. The great advantage of learning concepts with parts of the body is that fingers and toes do not disappear, as so many other things do once they are out of the child's reach.

For the baby, his own body and the body of his mother are his first toys. He plays with his hands and with his mother's hands; he pulls her hair; she touches his toes; she tickles his tummy; he feels her face; he pokes his finger into her mouth. Through this mutual pleasure in touching, the infant gains knowledge of, and confidence in, his own body. He learns to value and use his body. For the blind child, equally, this is of crucial importance; and yet, in many cases, his mother is too sad, too preoccupied with her grief and disappointment in his blindness, to gain pleasure from playing with her baby and letting him play with her spontaneously.

Adam had had this valuable experience in early infancy. His case illustrates that the ability to use one's body for exploration and imitation of what has been comprehended has a great deal to do with the growth of independence and curiosity. At 4 years, he wanted to know and to find out everything for himself. What size are birds and will he be able to feel one? (We managed to find a dead bird, which Adam examined carefully, before burying it in the garden.) He asked about trees, "Where do they end?" And of the sun, "Can we switch it on like the electric heater?"

Engaged in rhythmic musical activities, Adam asked anxiously if the movements he was making resembled what he was trying to imitate—an animal, an aeroplane, or a workman. Flapping his arms, he would ask, "Is this really how a bird flies?"

Conversely, it was Adam's very curiosity, his wish for mastery, his drive for independence, that needed and demanded the close and supporting tie to the teacher. He used it for enlarging his understanding of, and therefore, his control over, his environment. In many blind children, curiosity and the drive behind it, so essential for learning, are sadly lacking. It is as if all their energies are concentrated on taking in and organizing auditory impressions. Their attention is focused on understanding and making sense of the immediate environment. Incidents which demand a blind child's full attention are often very ordinary happenings in a sighted world: somebody enters a room or a chair is moved. Their comprehension almost always occasions anxiety; and the blind child's confusion does not leave him much strength to seek new experiences. Consequently, curiosity and the driving force behind it often lie dormant.

Boris was such a child: a rigid, unadventurous little boy, fearful of anything new, clinging to routine and familiar activities. For many weeks after coming to the nursery school, his activities were limited to using the swing and pushing a doll's pram to and fro—activities that were always initiated by his mother. She carried Boris, $3\frac{1}{2}$ at the time, into the nursery school; she took off his coat and asked, "What do you want to do?" Boris stood silently listening to the sounds, voices, and noises around him. The mother asked again. Boris echoed her question. She then took him to the swing, where he stood stiffly, passively waiting for her to put him onto it and push him.

Before Boris could progress in his development we had to evoke in him the wish to widen his narrow world—to infuse him with the will to venture forth. We did this by expressing our own pleasure and enthusiasm in shared experiences rather than by superimposing our ideas, by picking up and following the small clues that Boris supplied. For example, when he pushed the pram which kept him occupied and gave the impression of activity, but lacked purpose and vitality, we pushed another vehicle, giving a running commentary in very simple words about who was pushing faster or slower; and we varied the game as Boris responded. This was taken a step further to the earliest form of fantasy play, something usually observed in sighted children at about the age of 2. For instance, mummy and daddy (Boris and teacher) push baby in the pram to the park and go shopping.

The teaching of these young blind children differs in many respects from that of other children, for example, in the balance between activities chosen by the children on the one hand, and those suggested, organized, and directed by the teacher on the other. Blind children naturally need more stimulation, more detailed information, more help and support than sighted children do. Almost every action that a sighted child "picks up" by coping has to be "taught" to the blind child.

All of us who deal with children, whether as mothers, nurses, or teachers, have, whatever our practical or academic training, one supreme qualification—we have all been children ourselves. We know what it feels like to be a child. But we do not know what it feels like to be a blind child. We understand the sighted child's play, his mode of expressing emotions and fantasy because we played, because our children played, because children all over the world play in much the same way.

The blind child represents his initiative and imagination in ways which are difficult, if not impossible, for those of us who function by vision to understand and follow. His play looks so different from what we expect play to look like, so odd, strange, even bizarre, that we may be inclined to direct it toward "normal"-looking, reality-oriented activities. This was demonstrated very vividly by Adam after a train ride. Real life experiences such as train and bus rides, visits to the zoo or a fire station, shopping expeditions—all much part of the regular nursery school program—helped to further and widen the children's knowledge of the world.

Adam had enjoyed the outing. He had enjoyed buying his own ticket, counting the change, and the excitement of waiting for and boarding the train. On returning to the nursery school, he wanted to play "going on the train." He was offered a big, wooden toy engine. He felt it briefly with his hands and then wandered away, his facial expression and posture indicating puzzlement, bewilderment, and dejection. The following day, Adam was on the rocking horse. He was pushing it and shaking it violently and although the activity looked almost manic, Adam looked relaxed and cheerful. Adam was playing trains and the noises, sounds, motions, and vibrations he produced by shaking the rocking horse were indeed very much like those of a train. To Adam, the suggestion that what to him was after all just a piece of wood with four wheels should be a train with all its strange noises and sensations must have seemed "crazy" and left him feeling lonely and confused. The blind child must often sense this "craziness" in the environment and feel the loneliness of not being understood, of an ingenuity unnoticed and lacking appreciation. Adam's play looked very far removed from that of a sighted child's play; but once his teacher understood his actions and his fantasy, it became quite clear that his play made very good sense.

Adam needed the close presence of his teacher in order to enjoy his activities. Some of the children played with bricks or manipulative toys in a seemingly primitive way, knocking them together to produce noises or merely enjoying the crash as they tumbled onto the floor. Adam, on the other hand, wanted not only to construct buildings, bridges, roads, and tunnels, but also to understand their construction. This was often discouraging and frustrating for him, because the relationship between a model and the reality it represents demands an awareness of scale and space which stretches the blind child's capabilities to the limit. Adam could be taught to build—to put one block on top of the other; to join several of them in a straight row; to make high, low, square, or oblong buildings—and in so doing, to increase his tactile skills. But he could not reproduce them from his imagination since he had no visual images to guide him. Sight enables a child to look at his own work and the result of his labors. He can check and correct himself. Without it, the pleasure of re-creating from fantasy or experience is defective. Adam enjoyed the teacher's praise when he managed to pile up five or six blocks without in the process accidentally knocking them over; and although the achievement boosted his self-esteem, the building activity was a difficult learning experience—hard work rather than spontaneous play.

Similar considerations apply to the use of conventional toys designed by sighted people for sighted children. Miniature models are meaningless to the blind child. The sighted child loves playing with toy farm animals, houses, cars, people, because they look like the real things, and, because they are small, can be manipulated to give him the satisfying feeling of power to control and master his world; but for Adam, a rubber duck was just a bit of rubber—he could squeeze it, even produce a sound when he pressed hard enough, and it had an interesting smell. He learned by demonstration that this piece of rubber would float on water and not sink, and he got pleasure from experimenting with it. While the toy as such was not very interesting, the play with water—washing up, filling, and emptying cups, pots, and jugs— playing with real things was. Adam could feel the rubber floating, and he could feel when a cup was full, half full, or completely empty. He knew when he had splashed water onto the floor. Through his available senses, he knew when he had been successful; and, like a sighted child, such awareness gave him pride and satisfaction.

We found that Adam's wish to construct things was better met by using large, real-life props. For example, in encouraging the children to use the slide, trampoline, chairs, and climbing frame, we held up the two planks of the slide by the climbing frames, thus turning them into a bridge. Adam could climb onto the bridge and walk on or under it. He could run toy cars (which to him were four wheels, called "dinkies") over the planks and, by their sounds, assess and judge distances. He played this "game" over a long period until he had developed and mastered the concept of a bridge. Another very popular "game" involved the use of an upturned table, covered by a cotton tablecloth, which made quite a reasonable tent. The children held tea parties in it and put themselves, the teachers, and each other to bed on the floor. The game was suggested when one of the children returned from a camping holiday and Adam asked, "Is the tent made from wood or bricks?" The tent game led Adam to wonder if he could touch the ceiling of the room, as he had touched the roof of the tent. We helped him pile up chairs, tables, and boxes, so that he could climb onto them to reach and touch the ceiling. After that he became interested in heights. By marking heights with wooden pegs on the wall, we tried to help him relate his own size to that of other objects. This interest was furthered in other directions by measuring the rooms and garden with ropes, wire, and yardsticks.

Adam, like his sighted peers, was keenly interested in cars. He shared this interest with his father, who had taught him a great deal about the mechanism of cars. To satisfy his very natural wish to find out how things work, we frequently took Adam (and the other boys at his level of development) to the front seat of my stationary car and allowed him to turn the switches and operate the knobs. Adam knew which lever made the windshield wiper work, which pedal had to be pressed to brake, and how to operate the indicators. He chatted with great excitement about horsepower, speed, and petrol consumption. When being driven, Adam appreciated every gear change, and he was very aware of corners as the car turned around them and of hills as they were climbed. During a walk, when waiting to cross the road, Adam was able to distinguish passing vehicles by their sounds and to differentiate between a lorry, a bus, a taxi, a minicar, and a motorbike. He even recognized some makes of car by their sound and could accurately detect his father's car by its sound.

Yet, this impressive knowledge, acquired through identification as well as through his acute hearing and memorizing capacity, was deficient in detail. The kind of detail, which any sighted boy of 3 or 4 can pick up by visual observation was missing for him. For instance, riding the tricycle in the garden was a source of great pleasure to Adam. He learned to steer it around the nursery school building with considerable speed, and he rarely bumped into things. He, as most of the children, seemed to know and remark on every crack, rise, or decline on the grass and concrete. While for a considerable time this activity was mainly practical and geared to reality, his skill in manipulating the tricycle increased to the point at which he turned it into a fantasy game of driving a car. Sitting on the seat, he made appropriate movements and sounds as if to close a car door. Then with his whole body involved, he rattled and shook the tricycle, imitating the vibrating sensation of a car starting to move forward. Riding along, he called out from time to time that he was approaching a traffic light and had to stop or that a big lorry was coming the other way and he had to drive very slowly. Presently he left the tricycle and appeared to be searching for something. He went into the classroom, found a shopping basket, and said, "Come on now, we have to buy some petrol." This intelligent boy, fascinated by cars, with plenty of information about them, did not know that petrol is put directly into a car. He had heard people say "we must buy petrol," but the word "buy" was associated with going into a shop and using a shopping basket. A neighborhood garage was helpfully cooperative in filling this gap in Adam's knowledge. In many cases, however, these gaps remain open, but are obscured by the blind child's ability to remember and repeat words, terms, and phrases. Thus pretence takes the place of real understanding.

While language obviously helped Adam in his struggle to understand the world—he used speech to orientate himself, to collect information and clues, to make and maintain contact with people—it was also an area of great difficulty for him, confusing, conflicting, and puzzling.

All children learn to talk by imitation; they imitate the language of their mothers, a language expressing their shared impressions and experiences, largely based on visual perceptions and concepts. The blind child too imitates his mother's language and the language of those around him, but without sharing the experiential basis of that language. We constantly talk of what we see and do, but we do not talk in the same natural way of what we touch, hear, or smell. By our facial expressions, which the blind child cannot see and imitate, we convey diverse feelings—shyness, embarrassment, doubt, worry, pleasure, anger—but we do not normally put them into words with the same facility.

Adam's speech (like that of many blind children of nursery school age) was fluent and he had a large vocabulary. Yet, many of his words remained meaningless for him, and his efforts to compose a language expressing his own sensory perceptions were often discouraged, unappreciated, and corrected by an environment peopled by those who want the blind child to conform to the sighted world—to be like a sighted child. For example, Adam referred to the table legs as "them wooden sticks." When it was pointed out to him that they were called "table legs" and he was helped to investigate where they joined the table top, he felt up and down his own legs, then touched the teacher's legs, and murmured to himself, "Legsticks, legsticks." Adam was clever in describing the table legs as "sticks" because, on the floor, they felt and sounded much more like sticks than human legs.

Blind children have to adapt to the sighted world and to speak the language of the sighted, but I believe they need to learn to do so gradually as part of their own psychological growth as individuals.

An objective of our nursery school was to follow and facilitate the children's own way of thinking and forming concepts. This does not mean that all visual terms were avoided in the day-to-day contact with the children. Such an avoidance would have been artificial. However, it was important to verbalize what was happening as it happened, and to say what children were doing, touching, smelling, or hearing. We listened to and responded meaningfully—on the child's level—to their interpretations of the speech of the sighted.

Adam (on the way to the toilet): "I don't want to go in there by myself, it's all dark." Teacher: "What do you mean?" Adam: "Well, all cold and horrible."

Susan: "My hands are not dirty—they are not sticky." It was suggested she wash her hands all the same to "make them smell nice." Susan: "Are they clean when they smell nice?"

Anne was complimented by a visitor on her "pretty pink dress." She answered rather indignantly, "It's not pink, it's cotton, my Mummy made it, it has a pocket," and she put her hand into her dress pocket to confirm that she and the visitor were talking about the same item.

Adam, like all the children, said "see" when he meant hear, smell, or feel. In the shops he would turn his face toward the fruit counter and say, "I can see grapefruits over there." Hearing the familiar steps and sounds of the milkman, he called out, "Look, I can see the milkman coming." His explorations and investigations were accompanied by remarks such as: "I see your boots have a zip; I will look for the ball; I saw a big tree in the garden; I saw an aeroplane in the sky."

Although, in this example, Adam was using "sighted" words, he did so to convey his own experience. He borrowed and adapted the words to his own needs. (It is interesting and relevant that to some extent we all do this. "See" can mean "I understand, it is clear to me, I have perceived"—not necessarily through vision.)

Adam's usage of "I see" was in one way a denial of his blindness. He did not want to appear silly; and if he talked like everybody else, he was like everybody else. But it was also a logical response to our repeated explanations that his way of "seeing" is by touch, hearing, smell, and taste.

Adam first showed his growing awareness of what blindness meant when he was about 4 years old. This coincided with, and was triggered by, the period when his younger brother developed from a placid, undemanding, rather passive infant into an active, boisterous toddler. He became a threatening rival for the mother's attention and affection, a competitor who soon outshone Adam in many of his performances. He could move faster, find things more easily, fetch and carry for mother more efficiently. For Adam's mother, it had been a triumph and joy when she finally produced a normal baby and had succeeded in dealing wisely with Adam's reaction to the birth. She found the next step more difficult. With her increasing delight and pride in the very attractive sighted child, she became more aware of Adam's defectiveness and at times impatient with him for being so much slower than his younger brother. Adam reacted by becoming more demanding and very negative. We were able to help the mother realize how much Adam needed her admiration and appreciation of his person. Through our support, the relationship between Adam and his mother remained a close, satisfying one, and he could talk about his blindness at home as well as in nursery school.

Some mothers found it extremely distressing to discuss the subject of blindness with their children. Several mothers said to me, "You talk to him; it makes me cry to talk about it." Others denied their children's handicap, like the mother who stated emphatically, "My Joan does not know she is different from anyone else—she is never going to know it." Another mother firmly declared, "The word 'blind' is never mentioned in my house—a pair of hands are as good as a pair of eyes." These attitudes, which no doubt can be understood as stemming from the parents' inability to accept their child's blindness, add to his difficulty in understanding and adjusting to his reality.

Talking freely about blindness seemed a great relief to the children. We found that they did not talk readily about it until they had been in nursery school for some time and had a firm trusting relationship with the teacher. Even then their first references were cautious, as if they were testing the adult's reaction. One meets this cautious testing when sighted nursery school children tentatively mention sexual matters or other "forbidden" subjects. In the first phase of realizing that they lacked something, many of the children equated growing up with acquiring this mysterious something. Adam, at this stage, always asked, "Will I be able to drive a car when I am as big as my daddy?" Ann thought she would learn to see when she went to the big school.

Subsequently, Adam's awareness seemed to pass through a phase in which the painful knowledge that there were many things he would never be able to do, even when he was grown up and as big as his daddy, led to depression and sadness. These feelings were reflected in his temporary inability to concentrate and strive toward achievement; and he showed both fearfulness and clinging dependence.

We dealt with this by verbalizing his sadness, sympathizing with it, and stressing his positive qualities. The passing of this phase was marked by Adam saying, "Blind people cannot drive. I am all blind, I can only ride the bicycle," and he began to talk about the future when he would learn to read with his fingers, have a guide dog, and go about by himself. He would go to work, have a wife and children, just like his daddy. It seems likely that Adam will realize these ambitions and lead a full, satisfying life within the limits of blindness. He is intelligent; and his very good early mothering allowed him to grow up under favorable conditions as the valued member of a close, warm family circle.

In the nursery school, it was the teacher's task to build on this firm foundation and to foster Adam's progressive development by providing age-adequate activities.

A RETARDED BLIND CHILD

Children who, in addition to being blind, were also mentally retarded needed help to make up, as far as possible, for stages of development missed out at the appropriate age. Working with these children involved the kindling of any flicker of interest they might have, and trying to find ways of communicating and making contact with them. Tim was one of these children—a slim, fair little boy, good-looking, but rather frail. Like Adam's, his blindness was due to retrolental fibroplasia and diagnosed when he was about 4 months old. At this time, his mother became concerned when she noticed that he was not looking at her or responding to her as she had expected him to do.

Tim was born prematurely. His birth weight was 3 lbs. 10 ozs. The parents did not expect him to survive, and he was given oxygen in order to do so. He remained in the hospital until he was 12 weeks old. His mother did not handle him at all before he was 6 weeks old. She told us that during her daily visits to him in the hospital he was usually asleep and she just looked at him. The parents also have a second son, 14 months younger than Tim. Their marriage, always precarious, ended in divorce when Tim was about 4 years old. The father was in the export business and traveled abroad a great deal. His wife, while enjoying his financial success, resented being left alone so often with the children, and attributed the failure of their marriage to this. A contributory factor, no doubt, was the strain put on the relationship by their severely handicapped child.

Tim's mother appeared lively, gay, and friendly, but this bright façade hid a rather lonely, disturbed personality. She coped with any feelings of bitterness or sadness by completely denying them. In relation to Tim and the severity of his handicap, she seemed to escape from too close an involvement with him into never-ending social activities.

Tim was referred to the nursery school by the local medical authority officer at 2 years. He was too young for daily attendances, and for some months he visited once a week with his mother and baby brother. The mother welcomed this arrangement, because she found observing other blind children and the teacher helpful to her own handling of Tim.

At this stage Tim's motor development seemed advanced for a blind child. He walked freely and confidently, and was well orientated. He rushed around, tumbled over, picked himself up, jumped and kicked. He climbed on chairs and tables, fearlessly unconcerned about his safety. He was totally absorbed and tensely involved in motility to a degree which perhaps did not leave him enough energy to learn to vocalize.

In contrast with the children described above, for whom the mother, or mother substitute, was essential as an auxiliary ego, Tim's constant activity, his explorativeness, and his energy appeared quite independent of the mother's presence. When the mother cheerfully bade him good-bye and left him, there was no visible reaction to her departure. When she returned and greeted him with cuddles, no pleasure, relief, or anger could be detected. His face remained expressionless, blank, and vacant. While his younger brother would gurgle and babble with delight and stretch out his arms to be lifted and held by his mother, Tim wandered off, silently. Indeed, Tim remained largely silent until he was well over 4 years old and had attended the nursery school daily for 18 months. He looked like a toddler, but he was oddly unchildlike, moving in a world of his own, contented and quite oblivious of other human beings. His comprehension was very limited. For example, like a puppy dog, whenever the words "walk" or "garden" were uttered, Tim rushed to the door; but he seemed unable to understand concepts like "later," "it's raining," or "it's too cold for a walk."

The teacher's attempts to form a relationship with Tim as a possible basis for further development met with no response for well over a year. He was busy moving about freely and manipulating inanimate objects, but was strangely detached from human contact and excluded people from his activities at all times. His attitude seemed to say: "Leave me alone, I am busy and I am alright on my own." For example, in the garden he heard sounds from the kitchen and managed quite by himself to climb through an open window, feeling for a drainpipe, wall, and windowsill with his feet, hands, and bottom. He did all this patiently, with an air of intense concentration, aloof from the adult by his side, and ignoring her running commentary on what he was doing.

We tried in this and many other ways to make him feel our presence as enjoyable. For instance, when he moved about on a toy car, the teacher made sounds like a car; when he rocked on the rocking horse, she praised his skill and patted his back, head, or knees; when he lay down on his tummy, face on his folded arm, in a posture suggesting withdrawal but perhaps listening intently to what was going on around him, his teacher would sit close by him, on the floor, and would gently stroke and whisper to him, "It's alright Tim, I am here too—I like being with you." Or, "I think I can hear what you're listening to." In reality, she was just trying to breach his isolation. Very gradually a change occurred: Tim, of whom at 3 it was said, "He is not cuddlesome and never seeks physical comfort and closeness," began climbing onto the teacher's lap, enjoyed being cuddled, and played "ride-a-cock-horse" and similar primitive mother-baby games. Holding him, one felt he could not get enough of the warmth and closeness of this contact in which he found so much contentment, as if he were trying to make up for something he had missed. It was in this situation that Tim responded verbally for the first time. We were playing his favorite rocking game, and when I stopped singing and rocking he said, "Ah-booh." I said, "Do you mean 'again'?" and Tim answered, "Ah-booh." That same week, he said "Bo-bo" when he heard a dog (the family dog was called Bob), and "Ga-ga" when he handled a gate. Up to this point "ma" was the only word-like sound Tim made, but it was not linked to his mother; it became so only when Tim was 4;7 years old. He used "ma" in many different circumstances and managed to put varying expressions into this one sound. Tim occasionally squealed for what he wanted, but more commonly expressed his wishes in very definite non-verbal ways. For example, he would tug determinedly at the teacher's hand to get her to go with him when he wanted to get something. If the teacher did not respond immediately, Tim would scream or grizzle or even butt the teacher with his head.

Unlike many blind children, Tim was not interested in music and did not respond to it. His interest in the record player was determined by the pleasure of turning the knobs and of hearing the result of his activity with a sense of control. When he was frustrated or angry, attempts were made to verbalize this, but he was inclined to withdraw. He would give up and drift away, rubbing his eyes with his fists without muttering even a single sound. The teacher therefore decided to change her approach. She dropped the emphasis on talking and instead encouraged pleasurable mouth activity. For example, she provided a large plastic bottle which Tim used in numerous ways. He would suck it, put his tongue in and out of it, feel the rim with his lips and finger, and fill it with water. He also tried to control the flow of liquid from the bottle by tipping it from different angles. The teacher made different sounds to accompany each activity and encouraged Tim to feel her mouth and lips, as she did so, touching his at the same time. As a result of this different approach and handling, Tim made progress and was able to make appropriate sound-object connections—"ah-booh" for again, "bo-bo" for Bob, and "ga-ga" for gate—showing, at the same time, pleasure in physical contact. However, there was little evidence that he related to the teachers as persons. Any lap or pair of arms would do, and although he used "ah-booh" when he meant again or more, this did not last. For many weeks he also used the phrase meaninglessly and undifferentiatedly. Eventually he dropped it altogether. During the following few months, all efforts to elicit further sounds or words from Tim met with no success. The minute gains he had made were transitory. Even his motility diminished. He often flopped about listlessly, and what had appeared lively exploration, activity, and even curiosity at the age of 3 years, was at 4½ aimless movement for movement's sake, lacking in any purpose. At that time, he suffered from a chronic rhinitis and diarrhea, and he frequently looked physically neglected. Tim presented the picture not only of a defective blind child, but of a depressed one.

These changes were, perhaps, not surprising in view of the disturbing events in his life at that time. The family had moved to a new house; there were frequent changes of escorts and multiple baby-sitters; his mother was worried and preoccupied with her marital problems; and, as a final bid to save the marriage, she joined her husband for three weeks abroad, leaving the children in the care of a young friend. This was a difficult time for Tim and those who were involved with him. Yet, the teacher saw his depression almost as a hopeful sign. This child could feel, could react, could be sad; and he was perhaps reacting in this way to the many separations and to his mother's likely, but undiagnosed depression. As mentioned earlier, Tim did not at that stage differentiate between the adults in the school. However, as a new assistant teacher started to work in the nursery school, something happened which gave the first glimmer of a developing relationship between Tim and myself. The new teacher took Tim's hand to take him to the toilet. At the door, Tim pulled away from her, made his way across the room to me, stood by my side, waiting for me to take him. This sign, which could so easily have been overlooked, showed that the rudiments of an emotional tie to me were present, but that Tim needed my active help in fostering it.

I therefore made myself Tim's exclusive mother substitute, something usually avoided in a nursery school setting. I insisted on taking Tim to the toilet even if he was willing to go with somebody else. I expressed the wish to sit next to him at snack time, and I held his hand when we were out walking. When he put up his arms to be lifted by an adult, I stepped in, lifted him up, and cuddled him. With this approach, which aimed at conveying to Tim that he was valued and respected, his attachment to me slowly increased. The following term, it was observed that whenever I returned to the room after the briefest absences, Tim stopped whatever he was doing and walked toward me, smiling faintly. He became aware of the other children as rivals for my attention, and he either pushed them away or else withdrew. When I was away for two days with a cold, Tim reacted by going to sleep on the floor both mornings, something he had never done previously. He also showed richer affect in relation to his mother and for the first time cried when leaving her in the mornings. She was able to see this as a positive step forward, and it made her feel more "in touch" with her little son. Instead of pulling away or wandering off when she attempted to cuddle or kiss him, he now tolerated and even enjoyed her affection, though in a rather passive, submissive way. At about this time Tim, on prompting, produced the sound "ss" for "yes," and within two weeks it turned into a clear, meaningful "yes." He began to copy many words and named some things himself without prompting—cup, ball, nose, foot, and knee. Since he gained much pleasure from physical activity, it was most helpful to name the activity while he was engaged in it—pushing, pulling, sitting, running. These words had a definite meaning for him, and he learned them and used them appropriately. Sitting on the swing, he would try to say "push,"—making an enormous effort; and when he managed to do so, he blew out his cheeks, pursed his lips, and worked hard at producing the correct sound. Other words came with ease and were well enunciated; "seesaw" was one of these, and he said it clearly, smiling delightedly, after using the seesaw. He also used speech in relation to food, which he enjoyed. It satisfied him, it was meaningful to him, and it made the learning process worthwhile for him. He could say "biscuit, banana, crisps, tea," daily adding new words to his vocabulary. For example, Tim and his teacher visited the kitchen and the cook offered him a cracker. He felt it and then passed it back to her saying clearly, "Butter." In nursery school, he usually had butter on the sort of biscuit he was offered. Thus, he was able to communicate to the cook that that was what he expected and wanted.

The ability to express and communicate his wishes verbally emerged clearly when Tim was 5;2 years old, and at that point the family moved to another part of the country, where the mother had friends and relations. Follow-up contacts with this mother indicate that Tim has maintained his progress.

In Tim's case it was not known, and detailed neurological tests did not reveal, to what extent his defectiveness was due to inherent organic abnormality (other than blindness) or to environmental factors. Tim certainly went through enough traumatic experiences in his young life to account for at least part of the retardation. These were: separations from his mother, for which there was no preparation; unfamiliar and frequently changing baby-sitters; his father's total disappearance from his life after violent rows between the parents; and, perhaps most importantly, during the first 12 weeks of his life, Tim missed out on warm, lively interactions with his mother.

The work of the Hampstead Clinic with blind infants and their mothers has made it clear that mothers often need skillful help during the first few months of the child's life to establish a good, pleasurable relationship with the child. This is not easy without the important eye contact, but vital for the child's future development. No such supportive help was available to Tim's mother, and it is doubtful whether a firm, secure relationship was established between her and Tim before the birth of the second child—the healthy, sighted, perfect son whom Tim's mother had always wanted.

In the nursery school the teacher attempted to give Tim something of what he had missed; and although his progress was slow and relatively small, it was nevertheless evidence that he had potentiality for further development.

THE GROUP

Work in a nursery school for blind children is in many respects similar to work with sighted toddlers. It will already have become evident that all young blind children, whether of normal intelligence or retarded, need patient, individual help and teaching, and do not readily interact with each other. They function best in a one-to-one relationship with an adult. Normally, the sighted 3½-year-old, presenting himself for entry into nursery school, has reached a stage in his development at which he will profit from some community life. He can relate to other children as playmates and eventually as partners. This is not the case with blind children. Each child felt that the others disturbed and interfered with his intimate relationship to the teacher. They related to each other more as inanimate objects. This attitude is illustrated by the following examples:

1. To help Anne move more freely, the teacher "sang" Anne's name. Anne responded well, enjoyed the game after a slow, careful beginning, and would run toward the teacher. But as soon as Mary also wanted to play, Anne grew stiff and was unable to maintain the contact.

2. Mary played happily with the Lego. She told the teacher she was building a house, but when the teacher, who was sitting next to Mary, paid verbal attention to Ronny, Mary slowly and deliberately dropped the Lego pieces on the floor.

3. Stewart had learned to wash and dry his own hands and enjoyed the praise with which the teacher responded. He grew sullen and could

not find the towel when Susi came into the bathroom and she, too, was praised for some achievement.

4. Ronny, on hearing the music box, went up to Adam and took it from him like one takes something off a table or shelf. His facial expression as Adam protested was one of puzzlement, as if surprised that the music box produced these different sounds. He seemed totally unaware of Adam as another child with feelings.

5. Susan wanted to use the slide, but was told to wait because Sandra was on it. She said, "Take that child away," in much the same way that she asked for an obstacle to be removed when it hindered her free movement.

Whereas in most nursery schools one is met by a group of friendly 3- to 5-year-olds interacting with pleasure and enjoyment, in a nursery school for the blind the children play on their own, ignoring, as if they did not notice, the noisy presence and activities of the other members of the group. But in reality they are listening all the time and comment in a matter-of-fact way on what they have heard—sometimes days or weeks later. Thus, they reveal to the teacher that they have an intimate knowledge of each other. They seldom address each other directly, but use the adult as a go-between. For example, although Anne sat right next to Susan, she asked the teacher if Susan had brought her doll to school that day. When reminded that she could ask Susan herself, Anne felt rebuffed and said, "I don't feel like it."

Typically, in our nursery school one could observe one little boy calling "ice cream, ice cream"; another child, sitting on the floor turning the wheels of a toy lorry (in investigation); a girl, sitting by herself at the table threading beads; and yet another child playing alone at the sink. All this may give the impression of sad, withdrawn children, but close observation and knowledge of each child in the group proved otherwise. Like much younger sighted children who play contentedly at their mother's feet, not needing other companions, these blind children were quite happy on their own and not yet ready for group activities. When these were attempted, for instance, in the form of a simple musical game, as soon as the teacher tried to join two children's hands, the ring disintegrated. When she stopped dancing or singing to explain a point to one child, the other children drifted away.

Music in various forms played a most important part in the nursery school. Most of the children could be reached by music and reacted positively to it. At times, with all the children gathered around the piano, one had the impression of a group activity; but rarely was there a feeling of group participation in the sense that the children derived pleasure from producing music together. Mary, as so many blind children, had an excellent sense of rhythm and pitch. By tapping on one or several percussion instruments with great abandon and exuberance, she frequently initiated music-making, but she would not join in spontaneously when a singsong was suggested. The words, content, or melody of the song were of less importance to her than simple rhythmic expression. She was happiest when "the group" consisted of the teacher at the piano and herself. As soon as the group widened, she was inclined to lose interest and sit with her fingers held to her eyes, listening passively with a preoccupied and troubled look on her face. Bill, too, loved playing the drum and did so in perfect time, but so loudly that it drowned the sounds of the other instruments. He became very upset when this was explained to him or whenever another child wanted the drum. Other children repeatedly interrupted the playing or singing to ask questions, either to clarify the content of a song or, more often, to keep in contact with the teacher. If one cannot see, an answering voice is assurance that one is not forgotten and that all is well.

Celebrations, such as birthdays, Christmas, or Easter are the highlights of the year in all nursery schools and an opportunity for bringing about group cohesion. Naturally it is difficult to make a Christmas tree or Easter egg, even a birthday cake, meaningful to children who cannot see them, but decorations can appeal to senses other than vision. For example, we decorated a Christmas tree with mobiles which fluttered in the breeze and tinkled, and with tinsel paper which made a nice sound when gently touched. Candles on a birthday cake could be smelled and their fleeting warmth felt from a safe distance. Easter eggs were wrapped in different-textured materials, pleasant and interesting to the touch. At the same time it was important that everything associated with a party—with a celebration—felt especially nice. Blind children in general are far more attuned than sighted children to the feelings generated by their immediate environments. A festive atmosphere could be conveyed to the blind children by the mother's and the teacher's aesthetic pleasure in such things as pretty party dresses, attractively laid tables, and so on. If the important adults in their lives enjoyed themselves, the children "caught" the general excitement and pleasure of celebrating a special occasion together. In the day-to-day life of the nursery school, snack time was experienced as the only real group activity. Not only did all the children take part in it and sit around the table together, but food and eating seemed to provide them with a common basis from which they could interact. It was at snack time that some sort of community spirit prevailed. For instance, Anne and Mary would actively help in the preparations, grating apples, putting biscuits on plates, and reminding the teacher what kind of food each child liked. One little boy, when offered a Coke, asked, "Are you going to give one to Adam? He likes Coke." Susi, on hearing Ronny feed himself for the first time, commented, "Clever boy," as if proud of his achievement.

Another child insisted on wrapping up and keeping a chocolate biscuit for a boy who was absent, because "they are his favorites." When one child learned to pour out his own orange juice or to eat with a fork, it spurred others on to do likewise. A child's noisy, pleasurable crunching of potato chips could evoke delighted responses from the whole group and be copied and improved on by all its members. This led the teachers to improvise a game in which each child guessed by sound what the others were eating; each child, on his own level, participated in this game with great pleasure.

Gradually, the game was extended and the children were in-involved in conversation about what they had for dinner at home, what their mothers and fathers liked to eat, where one buys food, how it grows, and so on. It was in this situation, when physically safe and secure, that the children first expressed concern and respect for the feelings and wishes of their peers on a purely verbal basis.

Education strives toward independence. Growing up without sight limits this goal. However, the ability to relate to people, to feel concern and respect for others, equips the blind child to face life as an individual with all his weaknesses and with all his strengths.

BIBLIOGRAPHY

KELLER, H. (1903), *The Story of My Life.* Garden City, N.Y.: Doubleday, Doran, 1931.

Early Speech Development
in Blind Children

DORIS M. WILLS

MANY BLIND CHILDREN HAVE A WIDE VOCABULARY AND GOOD VERBAL ability, but relatively little attention has been paid to how they acquire it. The language of the sighted child is closely related to an experience of the world which is largely organized in visual terms. Can we share the blind child's experience of the world sufficiently to understand the way he copes with the learning of a language not altogether suited to his needs? We would expect that each phase in the early speech development of sighted children will occur *at some stage* in that of the blind child who acquires speech. However, in the blind some phases may occur later, for example, original phrase or sentence construction; while others may occur earlier, for example, precise mimicry. Phases which are fleeting in the sighted child's speech development may be more extended in that of the blind. An example of this would be the repetition, unchanged, of a sentence in circumstances which call for its modification.

The work with blind children is part of the Educational Unit of the Hampstead Child-Therapy Course and Clinic and as such was maintained by the Grant Foundation, Inc., New York. The research work with the blind was assisted further by the National Institute of Mental Health, Bethesda, Maryland.

The research has been directed since its inception by Dorothy Burlingham. I am deeply indebted to her for ongoing help with the work on which this paper is based, and to Karen Marschke for help in tackling the extensive background literature on speech and relating it to blind children. My thanks are also due for many helpful comments on the paper itself to Anne-Marie Sandler.

During our work over two decades with blind infants and nursery school children at the Hampstead Child-Therapy Clinic we have been impressed by the high incidence of echolalia in children who later develop normally and do well in school. Warren (1933) defines echolalia as "relatively automatic reiteration of words or phrases, often of what is spoken to the patient." I use the term more broadly and include, for example, children who repeat, with no apparent relevance, what they overhear in the same room as well as children who repeat what they have heard on television or radio on earlier occasions. Elsewhere we have described various reasons for this kind of recall (Sandler and Wills, 1965). This imitation appears to cover an attempt at some kind of mastery. Sometimes the child seems to have little understanding of the meaning of the words he repeats, as in the repetition of what he hears on television, at other times the child's understanding seems less incomplete. It is clear that the blind child's language is to some extent "freewheeling" and not *closely* linked with meaning. Observing some younger children who were slow developers but who acquired language with some delay, we have also been struck by how difficult it was to get these children to appreciate that they could use their mothers as agents. These children tend to name objects only when they come across them. Blind children appear to take longer to understand that they can *act on the environment* by the use of words alone. A sighted child will point to something that attracts him and urgently name it so that his mother fully understands his wish and can give it to him or respond in some meaningful way. Blind children may well recall something from the past and name it, but with little sense of urgency. One child said "tea" at an unexpected hour in the morning, and his mother thought this unimportant and ignored it. Such a mother may well be right when she thinks he is merely referring to some previous experience and is not making a request; but she would be wise to try to respond, if possible, to *any* word that might convey a request, since in this way the child will learn that communications are worth making. It appears that there is a crucial step, peculiar to the speech development of the blind child, which some have difficulty in taking. To begin with, all children, blind and sighted alike, vocalize to get an *unspecific* response from the mother—the mother vocalizes back, touches a cheek, and so on. Then, without the aid of sight, the blind child has to learn that he can get a *specific* response from the mother, and it is the mother who has to show him this by giving his words meaning.

While at Hampstead we have largely confined our studies to blind children without other concomitant damage, we inevitably have followed some where the damage did not become apparent until they were older. In this way we have come to know children whose mothering was adequate, who persisted in using situational words and phrases, and who resorted to meaningful direct speech only rarely—to get food, or to get a cuddle. Such children give the impression that the task is beyond them and that their language would certainly be more adequate if they could see, since it would greatly ease their learning of it.

Observations such as these have prompted these further comments on the blind child's way of learning language. Meaningful speech is probably the most vital skill a blind child must acquire, and greater understanding of the child's needs on the part of both parents and workers will increasingly enable them to foster its development more effectively.

With this in mind, I shall first compare the development of speech and its precursors in sighted and blind children. This is followed by detailed observations of two blind children who eventually achieved normal speech. Study of the way they learned may help us in our work with other blind children. We tend to correct blind children's speech in terms of the expectations we would have of sighted children. More understanding of the blind child's speech development in its own right would enable us to support him in solving *in his own way* the tasks it presents.

Medical expertise has fortunately greatly reduced the number of children born blind, or who become blind soon after birth. This means that there is a very small population from which to draw a group of blind children who are otherwise normal. Some children, in the course of development, do prove to have other damage which was not apparent in the first year, while others develop a very little sight. In these ways, the homogeneity of the group is further reduced. Since the problem brooks no delay, this paper is based on the studies we have available.[1]

COMMUNICATION IN THE FIRST YEAR OF LIFE

By the end of the first year of life the sighted baby is described as:

> babbling loudly, tunefully and incessantly, imitating the adult's playful vocalizations with gleeful enthusiasm . . . [and as] turning round in response to his own name, understanding several words in their usual context and comprehending simple commands associated with gesture [Sheridan, 1960, p. 7].

Sheridan's description suggests that vocalization has for the sighted child, his mother, and his family become a pleasurable activity, which is slowly gathering meaning. This pleasurable mother-child interaction appears to be a precursor of speech. The child begins *to wish to communicate* (and to be developing a tool for this purpose).

Fraiberg (1968) reports that of the well-supported blind children she studied, 7 out of 8 "followed language norms for sighted children throughout the first year of life" (p. 276). However, we have followed several children who eventually developed normal speech but had been very silent in the first year in spite of our intervention.

What is the history behind this? What role has vision played in the sighted child's developing language, and how can we help the blind child to compensate for its lack? For some time we have been aware of the importance of the visual contact between mother and child in the first year. We know that the child gazes up at the mother's face at 6 weeks if she looks at him when feeding (Gough, 1962), that he smiles responsively at about the same time, and that both derive much pleasure from visual exchange. We also know that stranger anxiety begins to develop around 8 months and that it is an indicator of the child's specific relationship to the mother.

---

1. All children cited were educationally blind, unless otherwise indicated; all proved eventually to have an intelligence which fell within the average to superior range.

The blind baby's experience is mediated by senses other than vision. He too begins to smile, in response to voice and touch, at about 6 weeks, and a mother works very hard to obtain this first smile. If she keeps the child near her, talks to him, and plays with him, she can create a pleasurable bond in spite of the absence of visual interchange.

When we advise a mother not to leave her blind baby alone, we do so because we know how easily these children can feel alone in situations which would not spell solitude for a sighted child. The moment the mother of a blind child is out of *bodily* contact with the child *and* silent, he feels alone. Blind children appear to profit from being carried on the mother's body; and we have observed a kind of symbiotic hunger in them. The child "comes alive" on the mother; and the child who rocks may stop if offered some slight bodily contact at an age when we would offer the sighted child some other diversion.

If the mother can meet both her own and her blind baby's needs for various forms of contact, a tie can be established in spite of the lack of vision. Fraiberg (1971) describes blind children's differential reactions to being held by mother and stranger as early as 5 months, with stranger anxiety proper developing between 8 and 12 months.[2] In the first year, mother and sighted child also communicate more specifically via the wide range of facial expression available to both. Having no knowledge of the mother's expression and lacking visual reinforcement, the blind child's expression varies little, apart from somewhat fleeting smiles. As Fraiberg (1971) put it, "the blind baby appears to have no modulated vocabulary for expressing need or wish before speech appears" (p. 387). None of the interchange of expression and glance which enables the mother and sighted child to keep in touch with each other's needs and wishes is open to such a couple. Even in optimal circumstances, mother and blind child repeatedly get on different wavelengths, resulting in a failure in interaction.

Other recent work has underlined a further aspect of visual interchange which has a bearing on speech development. In the

2. This paper was written prior to the publication of Fraiberg's book (1977) in which she slightly modified some of the median ages she gave in her earlier papers.

second month the sighted infant can imitate a mouth movement
of the mother or the protrusion of her tongue (Trevarthen, 1974,
p. 231). This is more or less concurrent with the appearance of
early smiling. The mother at this time often mimics the baby's
expression and vice versa.

Vocal imitation can to some extent substitute for visual imitation, and the blind child seems to take great pleasure in his
mother's imitation of *his* vocalizations. This is probably one of
the few areas in which he is aware that she is imitating him,
giving him the feeling that he is able to act on her in a very immediate way (in contrast to screaming for her to come).

Sarah (a blind child of 24 weeks) had started to laugh. Her mother
reported that one day Sarah had coughed; the mother had imitated
this; and the child laughed and coughed again. The mother copied her
and went on coughing. Sarah did not again repeat the cough, but became so excited laughing that her mother had to stop.

Finding other substitutes for the early visual interchange is not
easy, but mothers intuitively help to establish alternative interactions:

During the first year Sarah, while taking her bottle on her mother's
lap, would lie with arms outstretched, fingering her mother's skirt with
one hand and holding the other on her mother's throat where she felt
vibrations as the mother talked. These vibrations acquired a strong
cathexis. She often held my throat or neck while in my arms. By 1 year,
she was sometimes holding her own throat when she vocalized. (Indeed,
soon after Sarah's first birthday, the mother reported that she would
find Sarah holding the washing machine when it was running, with
a look of "pure pleasure" on her face.) It may in fact be useful if the
mother encourages her blind infant to feel her throat and mouth while
she is talking.

So far I have only described the manner in which vision furthers contact with, and imitation of, the mother during the first
year, and discussed some of the ways of circumventing its deficiency.
But there is also the variety of visual experience that the sighted
child and mother *share* which gives a basis for their prevocal and
vocal interchange. The sighted child acquires a body image fairly
early and learns that other people are distinct but similar. In the

blind child, this achievement is delayed, a fact that may be reflected in his not using correct pronouns freely until later. Sight is the great organizer of perception: without it many sense impressions, in the first instance of the mother, are sequential and not easily organized into a whole. Many small events occurring in a home at a distance from the child cannot be understood merely by listening. In fact, it takes the blind child longer to understand his world, and to do so he will need insightful support from his mother. Nothing gives an event as much background—framework—as the visual experience of the setting.

To summarize: in the first year the mother of the blind infant is faced with two main tasks at a time when she is inevitably depressed. She needs to make a full and mutually pleasurable contact with the child in the absence of visual interchange; and she needs to get sufficiently onto his wavelength to share his interests and difficulties. In this way he too will have a prevocal and early vocal experience of a meaningful kind, and one that will make him *wish* to continue to communicate with the loved partner.

COMMUNICATION IN THE SECOND AND THIRD YEARS

It is after the first year of life that the speech development of blind children diverges more obviously from that of sighted children. There may be delay, deterioration, or other anomalies.

One must always bear in mind that parents frequently react to having a blind child with depression and withdrawal, which may become manifest at different stages of the child's development. Marcy (1975) reports that between 16 and 20 months, many blind infants stop using words they have previously learned and do not add new ones because the parents have become more aware of the child's handicap, and the mother in particular has become depressed. The child's language progresses again when the parents are helped with their depression. While sighted children may also react to a depressed mother with a deterioration of speech, they are not so dependent on it for interacting with her, nor do they need its help to the same extent for the understanding of their experience. They can fall back on vision, and their development is not so greatly endangered.

Most workers who have intensively studied blind children's
speech agree that there is some delay in its acquisition. Fraiberg
(1968) reported some delay in naming in the second year. More recently she has reported a delay in the free use of "I," in contrast
to the syncretic use of it ("I wanna") because of a difficulty in the
development of the self representation (Fraiberg and Adelson,
1973). Norris et al. (1957) attributed any speech delay in their
66 educationally blind children to some failure in the parents.
They place in the third year items such as naming familiar objects
and talking in short sentences, which we would expect in the second year of a sighted child. Their findings are supported by the
Maxfield and Buchholz Scale (1957), which is based on some 500
blind children.

It is inevitable that blind children should have some difficulties
since so much of our language deals with the visual aspects of objects (color, shape). Again, so much language has single words for
objects which can be experienced only sequentially by touch, the
obvious alternative sense for the blind child. For example, he must
feel his way around a car; he cannot at once perceive it as a whole.

We have followed blind children who eventually achieved normal direct speech and whose speech development took a fairly
normal course. Some of these, though by no means all, were children who had had some sight in the first 2 years or who, while
educationally blind, had a little residual vision. But most of the
blind showed *some* anomalies, such as occasional repetition of
what they heard outside a meaningful context or of "situational
phrases"—that is, phrases not fully appropriate to the context in
which they are used but which the children associate with it. For
example, a child said, "Turn the record over," when in fact no
record had been played (this phrase appeared to carry a request
that a record *be* played). Some of our children suffered from a
plethora of such anomalies, with a delay in the development of
direct speech.

Smith (1971) contends that "the child is not learning words and
finding meanings for them, instead he is acquiring or inventing
words, which may or may not have a close relation to adult language, to meet his own particular requirements and represent
meaning which he needs to express" (p. 52). This statement is

based on the assumption that the sighted child needs words for interacting in the *current* situation, to communicate his needs and wishes often for things he can see, to express his current feelings, and to share in current events with mother and family. We take it for granted that he understands his *past* experience reasonably well, has assimilated it with the help of vision, and thus has a secure basis for present interactions.

We approach the blind child with the same expectation—that his aim in using speech will be to express *his* feelings and wishes in the *current* situation. But, for a child who cannot *see,* the current environment, apart from people, is not inviting and carries little cathexis in these early years. He cannot easily share in many family events; and he is slow in realizing how to express his own wishes or feelings. Observations of our children's speech suggest that the blind child tends to recall earlier cathected experiences which he has already heard described, such as family visits and outings. He also may be prompted by something in the current situation to recall and repeat verbal exchanges in which he has been involved, or has overheard, in the past. He constantly appears to use the past to explain the present situation in the attempt to collate them because so much of what is happening is incomprehensible to him until it has been talked about. Such children need help in organizing their experiences. They also need help in expressing their feelings and wishes in the current situation (Lopez, 1974).

We should not be surprised by this if we think of other aspects of the blind child's early development. Some children are greatly tied to routine, to the extent that they ask the adult to repeat familiar phrases and sounds of the home. For example, Sam, during his fourth year, sometimes said to his teacher, "Tell him to go to the toilet," and then would go.

During the preschool years the play of blind children is often an exact repetition of some event: reversal of roles or some small change of wording is not allowed. Such observations support the hypothesis that these children have problems in mastering their experiences, and that harking back, whether it takes the form of echolalia or situational phrases, is an attempt to do just this—to work over the past to help with the present. It is a stratagem useful to them and one which we should try to further rather than correct.

While sighted children also are tied to language routines and tend to hark back to earlier situations, blind children appear to have a much stronger tie to previously cathected experiences because of their difficulties in comprehension and generalization (Wills, 1965).

Whenever Caroline (4;4) felt a stone in the book [3] about the garden, she said, "It's a bit of wall." Caroline's mother said that near their home was a flint wall which Caroline frequently felt. (A sighted child of this age would see stones almost daily and be able to say "a stone.") Once we understand such a difficulty, we can help with the generalization: for example, by recalling to the child her other experiences with stones.

Language plays a major part in the ability to generalize and categorize which is basic to the organization of experience. Luria (1961, p. 10) states that sighted children between 1 and 2½ years recalled the correct colored box in which a sweet was always hidden much more easily when the color was named for them; that the learning did not easily extinguish; and that it transferred to other objects such as cups or bricks, which they would start to classify in a similar manner. This finding underlines the way in which speech and intelligence constantly interact and further one another. It follows that this kind of teaching, occurring almost automatically with sighted children, should be given to blind children in terms of *their* experience. We should try to apply simple meaningful adjectives to things we name for a blind child, for instance, *soft* hair, *hard* nails, enabling him to group his experiences and to lay a basis for further categorization. The blind child's body is one of his surest points of reference. He also uses sound for purposes of categorization. All this is a challenge to our ingenuity as parents and teachers.

The following records of the speech development of two blind children are similar in illustrating the role of the mother in sustaining their development and making language meaningful; they

3. Our nursery school had special "books" in which an actual object is attached to each page.

are dissimilar in that Boris was a slow learner, while Cynthia in many ways learned quickly but showed some unusual features, especially in comparison with sighted children.

Case 1: Slow Speech Development

Boris was born, somewhat postmaturely, without eyes. His brother Philip, 4 years older, had a problem in enunciating words until he was over 5, but it was not thought necessary to offer him speech therapy.

FIRST YEAR

I first saw Boris when he was 3 weeks old, and continued to make weekly home visits until the age of 3 years when he started to attend the Clinic's nursery school. At first the mother was naturally very shocked. Boris's eyelids were sunken and mostly closed (though otherwise he looked normal). He was bottle-fed and was not a cuddlesome child. For the first 3 months, he frequently showed the tonic neck reflex as he sat on his mother's lap. He would lean away over her arm and sometimes fall asleep in this position. Most mothers hold the child closely at this stage. Lack of eyes in a child imposes a serious extra strain on the mother (and family). She cannot for a moment forget the child's blindness. This mother's behavior reflected a very natural difficulty in initiating a relationship with this disappointing baby.

It was often difficult to know whether Boris was asleep or awake. Soon, however, the mother could tell that he was asleep by the cessation of his sucking movements or his having spat out the pacifier. She was delighted with his first smiling response to her voice and touch at 6 weeks. She kept him with her while she moved about the flat, talked to him a great deal, and by 2½ months said, "I always kiss him when I come into the room where he is." Despite the gradual buildup of a pleasurable interchange between mother and child, Boris vocalized hardly at all.

The mother said he enjoyed music, even at 2 months; he was quietened by it and sometimes laughed to it. (We encourage mothers to use music in moderation to give the child an extra interest, and to use records or tapes rather than radio because of the confusion caused by hearing many different voices in the same program.) At the same time, Boris not only was startled by loud noises, but it could be observed that fleeting frowns crossed his face when his brother made a good deal of noise. The mother reported that she had to move Boris out of the kitchen when the clothes washer was running because the noise upset him.

During the second quarter of the first year Boris became more rewarding to his mother. She could make him smile a little by kissing him on the mouth or by tickling his face; he laughed when she put his toe in his mouth, which in turn delighted her (by 7 months he was able to complete this action for himself), and at last, she said, he liked being cuddled to sleep.

After a visit to the hospital for two nights for an eye examination at 5 months, he showed a very marked reaction to a stranger's lap, sitting quite still for about five minutes, apparently listening and taking in the new situation.[4] The mother also reported that he had screamed when she was outside the flat for a few minutes talking to a neighbor. It seemed as if his hospital experience had made him more aware of separation and sharpened his discrimination of people.

Boris also screamed when his mother put him down unexpectedly or kept him waiting for his bottle. At 6 months, the mother reported that he fed better if she talked to him; hitherto she had remained silent to allow him to concentrate.

In spite of the growing strength of the mother-child relationship and Boris's general awareness of sound, he still vocalized very little. Some single sounds emerged by 6 months; for example, the mother reported that he was "gargling" at times. But he certainly did not vocalize tunefully, using single syllables, which Sheridan (1960) puts at 6 months. In the absence of glances and facial expressions, Boris had only somewhat unspecific modes of communication, smiling and laughter, or grizzling and crying, screaming and stiffening. Sometimes the reason for his pleasure was obvious, so that the mother could repeat the stimulus which made him smile; but during the day, he often got bored and fretful, and she did not

4. Fraiberg's (1968, 1971) 8 intact blind infants also showed differential reactions to handling at 5 months.

know what he wanted. On one occasion when he was 5½ months, he was grizzling in his swing; the mother removed him, put him on his feet, which he loved; laid him on the floor on his back, which he disliked; and on his tummy, which he liked better. Without the child's glance to help her, she sometimes inevitably offered him an activity he did not want, and he would fret for a period.

By the time Boris was 6 months, his mother was showing genuine pleasure in his small achievements. His motor development was advanced (holding an adult's hands, he walked at 8 months). At 7 months he was again hospitalized, which perhaps further accentuated his ability to differentiate mother from strangers. When she visited him, he greeted her with shrieks of excitement. "He knew my voice," she said with pleasure. During the second half year, in spite of two further hospitalizations, he demonstrated his closer relationship with her in a number of ways. He sometimes bounced and vocalized when she reentered the room and spoke to him, and he more obviously became still when she left. She could now more easily pacify him when he was upset.

Around 6 months he took to squealing, sometimes, it seemed, for fun, sometimes for food. He began to say "baba" and "haha," in this way copying his brother. At 9½ months he vocalized while biting a toy, and it was tempting to think that his new teeth (he had four at this age), which he ground at times, were increasing the cathexis of his mouth.

His mother talked to him constantly, played little body games with him, and let him listen to music. Toward the end of the year he was delighted when she imitated any sound he made vocally, and he would immediately repeat it.

At the same time as the sounds of his mother and family gained importance for Boris, he was becoming interested in the sounds made by inanimate objects, but his behavior with them was often hard to understand. For example, at 7 months he would sit on the floor with a soft toy between his legs and press his hands on it. We did not know why. This soft toy had a bell, but it remained silent under this treatment. A little later, because he pressed his hands on other toys which *squeaked,* we realized that he had hoped to obtain that sound from the toy with the bell. Soon he became very fond of a metal rocking horse, partly because of the squeak it made. At 9 months he took to banging things against each other—a table spoon and the pacifier he was biting, or a spoon and his zip. He also banged things on the carpet or a table. This child, with his meager vocalizations, seemed to prefer making a noise in this way. It could be argued that he learned more about his environment by listening to its resonance than by vocalizing himself, a process which *interferes* with input in the blind child. (The sighted child can talk *and* look; the blind child cannot talk and listen.)

In addition to his interest in noises and his links with his family, his pleasure in gross bodily activity stimulated his vocalizing. For example, he had a bouncer for a short period at 6 months. He vocalized and smiled much more in it than he did ordinarily; he would work himself up to a little screech at the end of a few bounces and then pause. According to his mother, he enjoyed this activity so much that after it he would accept nothing but play on her lap.

By 12 months his mother said she was sure, from his responses, that Boris understood the words "cuddle," "kiss," and "clap your hands" ("till daddy comes home," which was part of a game), and she could demonstrate this. She reported that he could say "dada," "mamma," and "hullo," and during interviews occasional syllables resembling these words could be discerned. For the most part, however, he was still remarkably silent, and emitted what can only be described as noises. He certainly did not imitate speech patterns, as other blind children do at 1 year; nor did he exhibit simple acts upon a familiar command (Maxfield and Buchholz, 1957). His motor development was advanced, and he could pull himself up to a standing position and walk sideways holding on to the furniture. His enjoyment of bodily activity helped to induce his sporadic vocalizations, and gave him an area of interest and mastery when he was alone.

SECOND YEAR

In the first part of the second year Boris was still in many ways an unrewarding child for his mother. He had a growing wish for independence, which was held up by the fact that he never crawled and did not walk independently until the age of 21 months, although he walked around the flat before that, supporting himself on furniture and bars that the father had fixed for him. When his curiosity and explorations brought him into conflict with his mother, he could not easily turn away to something of equal interest, as a sighted child might have done. Nor did he have enough language to communicate clearly what he wanted. Like other blind children of this age, he did not play with toys for long, nor did his play look meaningful. It was therefore difficult to encourage him to extend it. All this, as well as the fact that he was teething and was having frequent colds, meant that he was often fretful. However, his relationship with his mother, both in its loving and aggressive aspects, was becoming of great significance to him; and his wish to communicate with her increased:

At 1 year, the mother sat him on the table facing her, then on her lap where he rocked a little. It was noticeable that he vocalized more when he was near her. She repeatedly said to him gently, "Give me a kiss," and kissed him on the mouth. When he sat on the floor, Boris began to lift his face up in readiness for these kisses. Indeed, we thought it helped to make him hold his head up.

One month later, his mother took Boris on her lap. He smiled when she kissed him. He kept holding up his face, and she kissed him on the cheek. He cuddled close to her in a way I had not seen before. His mother said that he had done this during the previous week. She was pleased because he had not behaved in this way since his return from the hospital at 9½ months. She said that one day when she was playing with him on the big bed and was kissing him, she was distracted by the boiling kettle and did not respond again to his lifted face. For the rest of the day he would neither kiss her nor do little things at her request.

During his second year Boris got into other clashes with his mother. He was slapped and put in another room for misbehaving during dinner. After crying for about half an hour, he was brought back and ate properly. However, he continued to let himself be cuddled to sleep on his mother's lap, so he was learning to reconcile mother's loving and angry aspects. Boris's slow but meaningful speech development during this second year has to be understood in the context of these vicissitudes in the mother-child relationship.

Throughout this year, when Boris began to use words, he pronounced them so poorly that I often found them incomprehensible. There may have been a congenital difficulty in Boris's case, but his failure to babble in the first year must also have played its part. While the mother talked a good deal to him, frequently naming things, she may have used sentences rather than single words. This may have been one reason why Boris also imitated his brother, whose language, though poorly enunciated, was simpler.

Between 12 and 18 months Boris showed much pleasure in mouth activity, such as blowing bubbles. He also vocalized more, and began to repeat words he had heard. Gradually, this repetition of words became more persistent. For example, his mother would wait for certain words in a nursery rhyme she usually sang to him, and Boris would fill them in. He began to use words and phrases in situations in which he had heard them, though not always appropriately, thus showing that he did not fully understand them. For instance, at 15 months he would say "more" after a drink, though in fact he did not want more; by 18 months, however, he knew that "more" would get him something. Gradually, he began to use other words to obtain things, a most important step for a blind child. He used "ishoo, down" at his mother's knee to get her to play ring-a-roses, and "(s)ee(s)aw" to be rocked foot to foot as he stood beside her. One day when he was passing a bakery, he said "bun" and his mother immediately bought him one, thereby establishing a precedent.

By 17 months "no" was becoming meaningful, and Boris used it when he did not want to do what mother wanted. "Aya" (hello) continued to be used a good deal when his mother and I were talking and Boris was, for example, playing with a toy on the floor. Apparently, it meant: "Look what I'm doing!" We continued to respond and Boris would resume his play. Thus pleasure in vocalizing and communicating was slowly becoming established.

Between 18 and 24 months words continued to be poorly pronounced, but he sometimes improved the pronunciation when his mother repeated the word slowly for him. When he was nearly 2 years old, his mother started to teach him bits of the alphabet. We had the impression that he pronounced some of these new words better than those he had learned earlier.

He continued to use words or phrases in situations in which he had heard them, often fairly appropriately. For example, at 19 months he said, "Dow(n) up" as he jumped at mother's knee; less appropriate were " 'Ere y'are" when he was given a tricycle; "Done, done" ("What have you done?") when he had hurt himself. With great pleasure he adopted words Philip used in play; for example, "Brrm" as Boris rode his tricycle; or "Ready, steady, char(ge)" when he went down the slide.

He could name many parts of his body, used more words to obtain things, and understood a number of simple instructions. Yet, the growth of his understanding was uneven. In response to his mother's warning, "Mind out or you'll bang your head," he *felt* his head. Echoing of the last word of phrases and sentences persisted, but at 21 months there sometimes occurred a vocal interchange of single words with his mother. However, they were still poorly pronounced and usually unfinished.

In the latter part of the second year "no" was heard frequently, a word far more often used by mothers, sometimes with considerable feeling, than yes. Boris slowly began to show his agreement to play with a toy suggested to him not merely by silence, but by echoing its name.

By the end of the year, however, Boris's wish for independence was expressed in his constantly saying "no." His mother often prevented him from persisting in his refusal by helping him turn somersaults or playing "I'm coming." It took him much longer to use "yes" consistently.

Records and tapes were his great pleasure at this time and nearly always quietened him. At 2 years he would ask for his favorite, "Pinky and Perky." He generally knew when a familiar record was about to stop, and would ask for "more."

Boris certainly had the "two or more meaningful words" expected by Maxfield and Buchholz (1957) at 2 years, but his level of development in comprehension and speech presented problems, even though his mother provided much meaningful experience for him.

THIRD YEAR

Throughout Boris's life there had been many discussions about the fitting of prostheses (artificial eyes) to improve his appearance, and during this third year the mother expected him to be hospitalized for examination and subsequent fitting. For various reasons the examination was delayed until shortly before his third birthday when the mother was told that prostheses would require a major operation. She decided to postpone this until he was "old enough to understand" at 7 years.

During this year he had measles, flu, many colds, and was often fretful. His mother remarked that Philip could be diverted when he was fractious, but if Boris refused his breakfast, he was upset the whole day. During my interviews, the reverse also seemed to be true. When he was in a good mood, his cheerfulness persisted and often outlasted my visit, which perhaps cheered the mother.

Stranger anxiety became somewhat modified; for example, he accepted less familiar baby-sitters. But even at the end of the third year he was still apt to cry if a neighbor spoke to him when he was out in his pram with his mother. The mother continued to reassure him and keep him with her as much as possible.

By 2;10 years he was toilet-trained, but this had never been an area of struggle. He usually ate very well, but his sleep was often disturbed, and he still had a bottle when he woke during the night.

Between 2 and 2½ he began to be able to ask for more things and activities he enjoyed: "Dinkie" (drink), the trampoline, a ball, games with his mother and body play, "tickle me back," and "piamp," which proved to mean "pick me up." He had also learned to ask for toast, and continued to ask for a bun when they were out.

Boris often named things only as he came across them. One day on his horse, he said "Silver" (the horse's name); on another occasion he climbed on the table and said "books" as he touched them. This naming appeared to coincide with the recognition of the object and to correspond to the silent visual recognition of sighted children. It was not accompanied by the excitement that is usually associated with naming in sighted children. However, Boris did not consistently name things he came across, though we frequently named objects and activities, and verbalized positive and negative feelings for him.

The following example shows his reaction to a familiar situation, feeding, which he always enjoyed. He was preoccupied with recognition and eating his dinner at the same time. He did nothing to inaugurate a social contact. After the mother had fetched his dinner, she talked to Boris (25 months) about it. He echoed a bit of what she said, "Bib on." In between the mouthfuls, he said, " 'ner." He also echoed "meat" and volunteered "bib on" again. The mother asked him if he'd like a drink. "Ya." In a cup? "No" (he wanted it in a bottle).

Boris often repeated words or phrases his mother had used in a particular situation when it recurred. Sometimes such words and phrases suggested that he was recalling her in her admonitory or comforting roles:

Boris (25 months) dropped a clock he had been playing with near me and said, "Sorry" as he picked it up. Later in the same interview he was fussing about his knee. His mother rubbed it, and he said, "Never mind."

Throughout this period he learned to repeat or finish little rhymes his mother taught him and not merely to fill in one word (his speech was so slurred that his mother often had to translate for me). Sometimes he made his own additions, for example, in repeating Jack and Jill after his mother: "Jack fell down, *I said it* . . . Jack and Jill, water, *I said it.*"

At about 2¾ years, his interest in bodily movement seemed to lessen a little and he became more interested in people. He now greeted my arrival with "Miss Wills, say hello." When sweets were handed out, he said, "One for Miss Wills." Occasionally he brought some toys for me to admire, usually naming them more or less intelligibly.

At the same time he at last learned to say "Mummy" and even said, "Mum, I want you," possibly in imitation of Philip. Just before he was 3 he would raise his voice if he did not get her attention at once. He also did this to me. In fact, he became very insistent on getting attention. He also was much more capable of expressing his own wishes. On one occasion (33 months) his mother suggested that he tell a story to me. Boris replied, "To Mummy." At other times he asked me for special toys and games. His direct speech, however, was still interlaced with situational phrases which recall the past:

His mother got out a 2-foot-high bouncer for Boris. He said, "Bouncer Miss Wills," adding a moment later, "Show me then." I think he meant, "I'll show you," a frequent saying of his mother.

Perhaps because he was learning so much by imitation, his use of "I" was somewhat unpredictable, though "I do it by myself" remained a favorite phrase. Echoing words or part of sentences continued, but he began to be able to describe what he was doing by short phrases such as, "Up the step, down the step"; "got a bus." These phrases might have been his own construction. But when he used longer sentences, they were always, at this stage, exact replicas of what he had heard, usually in a cathected situation, and they were learned as wholes since they were well beyond his powers of construction. He did not omit parts of speech which he had not mastered, as does the sighted child, though he might omit the beginning of the sentence. He often used such sentences appropriately. His mother reported that he said, "Are you going or not?" to his brother after dinner, when his brother had to go back to school, and sometimes to his father when the latter went to work. During the same period he continued to admonish himself at times, "Don't touch it or I'll smack you." And he now understood many of mother's simple requests.

His enjoyment of taped nursery rhymes and music, of which the mother had acquired a considerable supply, was enormous. He preferred sentimental music, which his mother in fact disliked; he would get a cushion and lie down on the floor to listen to it.

Compared to sighted norms, Boris's speech was very backward, but he also was below the Maxfield and Buchholz norms for the blind. Boris was only beginning to be able to fetch or carry in response to a verbal request. He used names of many familiar objects, but did not "talk in short sentences" (expected by 3 years). Yet, he was learning in his own way, on the basis largely of imitation of words and sentences, particularly of those used with emotional emphasis.

It will be apparent how essential it is to keep such a child in close contact with his family, not only because he needs time to make sense of his experiences at home, but also because communication there is strongly motivated by his tie to its members.

From 3 to 5 years Boris came to our Nursery School for Blind Children. At 5 years he went to a day school for partially sighted children, and a year later to a weekly boarding school for blind children, a separation he took remarkably well.[5] There his school progress was so good that the headmaster had difficulty in believing that Boris had always been blind!

CASE 2: SPEECH DEVELOPMENT WITH UNUSUAL FEATURES

Cynthia was a very intelligent child who developed a very little sight during her fourth year. The reason for her blindness was not known until much later when the diagnosis of retinitis pigmentosa was made. She was fortunate in that she was hospitalized briefly only on two occasions. She showed no light perception on an EEG at 1 year, but by 2½ years it was becoming more and more apparent that she had some light perception. During the fourth year she could also perceive color and some form when the object was close to her, but she continued to feel for objects, and up to this fourth year her behavior was that of a blind child.

Later, when she went to school, she could, on "good days," orientate herself in well-lit surroundings. For the purpose of reading, she had to learn Braille. It is of course possible that during her second and third years, a small degree of sight was developing and becoming organized. However, if she had been totally blind, we might have expected her to have had *more* rather than *less* difficulty in learning speech. The strategies she employed and the uses to which she put language are reminiscent of phases in the language development of some fully blind children. They are un-

5. Weekly boarding school at 5 years is the standard provision for blind children in the United Kingdom. There is currently a very slow movement toward day provision for those parents who wish it.

usual only by comparison with sighted children. Cynthia has now been in school for 7 years and is doing very well.

Cynthia was born full-term. She had a sister, Helga, 2 years older, and a brother, Simon, 4½ years older. The mother therefore had the reassurance of two older, well-functioning children. Cynthia was breast-fed for 2 months. She was referred to us at 9½ months when her blindness was diagnosed. Prior to this, her mother had thought that she had a squint.

The mother said she wished she had known earlier that the child was blind, because she felt she had left Cynthia too much on her own in the earlier part of the first year. This probably accounted for a tendency Cynthia showed throughout the second year: when she grew fretful, often on her mother's lap, she was most easily soothed by being put in her cot. After age 2 years, Cynthia no longer withdrew in this way; in fact, the mother then knew when Cynthia felt troubled by how often she came to mother instead of playing on her own.

These occasional withdrawals from the mother to the cot went hand in hand with behavior indicating Cynthia's growing dependence on her. Stranger and separation anxiety developed after Cynthia's second and last visit to the hospital at 12 months. In the second year she sometimes cried when mother left the room; and she clung to her after brief separations. During the 2¾ years under review, there certainly had developed a strong tie between mother and child, which was not upset by occasional scoldings or smacks.

In the first year Cynthia had a feeding difficulty; she could not be persuaded to take food from a spoon until she was 18 months. This was not due to any inhibition of biting: she bit her siblings hard from time to time. For blind children feeding is even more closely lodged in the mother-child relationship than it is for the sighted. The blind apparently experience *any* change in the feeding arrangements as a change in the mother, so that this frequently becomes a battle area. For example, at 2 years, when Cynthia was persuaded to sit on a little seat rather than a lap to be spoon-fed, she insisted for 2 to 3 months on being cuddled on mother's lap afterward. Upsets due to brief separation often led to regression in eating habits.

Toilet training was not fully reliable until 3½ years, but, as seems to be the case with many blind children, it was never an area of battle.

Since I started my fortnightly visits to the home only when Cynthia was 9½ months, soon after the blindness was diagnosed, little is known about her earlier development. She was a large and beautiful child, somewhat lacking in muscle tone; her hands were usually kept closed, even in response to her mother's request to play "pat-a-cake." She had preferred lying on her stomach much of the time she was in her cot, which may have played its part in her failure to open her hands sooner. In this last quarter of the first year it became apparent that Cynthia's deep interest in sound was linked with her bodily inactivity. The radio was nearly always on softly, and the mother used it to comfort Cynthia when the family went to another room in the flat to eat. Cynthia sometimes whimpered when the music was turned off, and later showed her displeasure when the music gave way to voices. Clearly, she could discriminate between the radio and family noises. She was much interested in these, and would stop manipulating a toy to listen, for example, to her mother talking to her sister and me.

By 1 year Cynthia was said to call her father and sometimes her mother. She was vocalizing and was beginning to reiterate names she recognized in her mother's conversation. She would fill in her own name in a nursery rhyme if the mother paused at the appropriate moment.

Cynthia's advancing motor development provided her with more sensorimotor experiences of her unseen world. She soon crawled forward and walked sideways around the furniture. She orientated herself largely by sound: by 16 months she walked unsupported between the parents and soon thereafter she could walk to them if they called to her from their chairs. When they moved, however, she would try another chair rather than follow them. When the mother was out of the room, Cynthia would crawl around and hold conversations in jargon with her mother's or father's chair; later she held conversations with the table where the family ate, even when they were not present. Toward the end of the year she ventured outside the door into the hall for the first time, and clapped her hands, retreating at once, perhaps because the echo of her clapping was different. Soon she not only clapped her hands but clicked her tongue (resembling her budgerigar's clicking noise) and sometimes sang in the hall, no doubt in order to experience the different resonance. All this movement enabled her to go to her family anywhere in the flat.

Her speech was mostly centered on three themes: people, the body and bodily activity, and, to a much lesser extent, a favorite toy. It was often very difficult to categorize her speech in Brown's (1973) terms of "nomination" and "recurrence" because without a glance or a pointed finger it was almost impossible to tell whether she was naming something in recognition, or asking for a repetition of something that had happened. The mother had to play an enormous role in discovering what Cynthia meant because she mostly used single words. Whether the mother always interpreted Cynthia's utterances correctly may be queried.

In the early part of the year Cynthia appeared to use names of familiar people experimentally on strangers. To begin with they were greeted, as I was, as "Dada," to which mother would of course reply, "It's not Dada, it's so and so." Sometimes Cynthia appeared to acquire new words by the association of sound. By 16 months I heard her shout *Dididi* (which resembles dada) each time I rang the doorbell. ("Didi, the name of a favorite soft toy, was one of her first words.) "Sissy," the name of an aunt, then became her greeting to strangers and to me. On one of my visits (16 months) the mother came to the door with Cynthia, who said "Sissy!" and then, when we were all indoors, "Daddy!" as if to try another alternative. The mother, of course, responded to both appropriately. "Sissy" was probably linked by sound with "see-saw," another of Cynthia's early words. Indeed, this was the first word the mother was sure Cynthia understood, because she had made it meaningful by rocking the child on her lap only when Cynthia said it, and the child would ask for it. (It soon came to include rocking foot to foot at mother's knee.)

Since people make more varied sensory impressions on the blind child than inanimate objects, it is natural that they are highly cathected. Around 1¼ years, Cynthia was showing her tie to past object-related situations and perhaps also her hope that these would recur. She often named, with some emphasis, relatives whom the family visited regularly, to which her mother would reply, "Yes, we saw so and so last Sunday." Obviously, people, even though absent, were becoming very significant for her. (This naming of absent *people* can often be noted in backward blind children.)

Cynthia also began to greet familiar people with certain additional words: "tee" to father, with whose tie she played; "pat-a-cake" to her maternal grandmother because she played this game with her, and often "seesaw" to mother. This "labeling," no doubt an attempt to differentiate people, continues in some blind children long after they have stopped wishing to return to the activity connected with it.

Sometimes, at this age, Cynthia reeled off some of her words. Once, at her mother's knee, she said "Sissy, Dada, Nana, seesaw," whereupon her mother picked her up. Five months later Cynthia stood in the room, saying, "Sorry, toes, shoes," and added her brother's name. All these words were gathering meaning for her. Less obviously meaningful were jargonlike sentences, only occasional words of which were recognizable. She "talked" in this way more when she was alone in the room. Her intonation resembled Helga's (the paternal grandmother could not tell the children's voices apart), which may have been partly motivated by rivalry. Cynthia was very jealous of Helga and around 20 months produced jargon-type sentences when Helga spoke to mother. There is no doubt that her siblings' speech provided a great stimulus to Cynthia.

The mother said that Cynthia loved listening to stories read to the other children and repeated words that she knew. Toward the end of the second year she was echoing the last word of whatever we said to her, and her jargon-type sentences were increasingly composed of recognizable words. She gave the impression that she had been practicing the various sounds, something the sighted child usually does earlier. She had trouble pronouncing Ms, but learning to kiss, a skill she acquired only about this time, seemed to improve that. (The eruption of her teeth made the pronunciation of Ms difficult; M turned into N or R, as she tended to talk with her mouth open.) Other mispronunciations, such as "fingern" for finger, soon disappeared. During her third year, she could pronounce certain new names that her older siblings still mispronounced.

While "no" and "yes" were well established by the end of the year, they were not much in evidence during interviews. Cynthia did not usually get into battles with her mother unless something she disliked was demanded of her. Then she would resist bodily rather than verbally.

Cynthia certainly had the two or more meaningful words expected of 2-year-old blind children. She was beginning to name familiar objects (expected in the third year), but it was difficult to be certain how meaningful all these words were. Some of her phrases were based on imitation, but she sometimes used them inappropriately. While there are many similarities between Cynthia's speech development and that of a sighted child, there are also important differences. Her speech was often *not closely tied to meaning* but "freewheeled," as it were, alongside it. This difficulty, together with her imperfect comprehension of what was said to her, must have been due to failures in understanding some of her experiences without the help of vision.

THIRD YEAR

Some features of Cynthia's speech development are commonly found in sighted children; others, such as playing with words, are not, certainly not to the same extent; nor are her attempts to understand phrases and sentences on the basis of the words and constructions they have in common. These points are most easily illustrated by an observation I recorded when she was 2 years old.

During the course of this interaction Cynthia was standing by her mother's knee or playing with the toy telephone on the seat of the chair:

Cynthia: Hello [to me; then silence].
Mother: What would you like to play with?

Cynthia: Baa baa black sheep.
Mother: What would you like to play with?
Cynthia: Baa baa black sheep. [She repeated this hopefully on and
            off throughout the whole hour.]
  Helga brought the telephone to her.
Cynthia: Hello telephone.
Mother: You telephone Uncle Bill.
Cynthia: Ring, ring—ring-a-ring a roses.
[Mother said something.] Get Daddy.

Cynthia manipulated the telephone. At this point the budgerigar made a noise. Cynthia immediately said, "Birdie."

Helga fetched the toy that made animal sounds; and mother pulled the strings to operate these. Cynthia was not interested, and she pushed the telephone away. Mother told Helga to go away from the telephone. Cynthia said, "No, no telephone."

In the ensuing episode Cynthia did not react directly to Helga. She was quite capable of giving Helga a shove, but she recalled an earlier situation when someone was smacked. When offered the trampoline, she did not start toward it. Instead, she recalled what happened on it, by jumping and saying, "Whoopsy, whoopsy."

Helga went away and started counting pennies. Cynthia echoed, "Two." As Cynthia was not doing much with the telephone, her mother offered her a tambourine. Helga again offered the toy that made the animal noises. Mother said, "Leave it" to Helga.
Cynthia: Leave it or she'll smack you. [She dropped the receiver, say-
            ing] What did you do with the telephone?
Mother: Drop on Cynthia's foot?
Cynthia: No!

The mother picked it up, saying, "Here we are," which Cynthia echoed. As it kept dropping, the mother asked, "Where is the trampoline?" and Cynthia began to say, "Whoopsy, whoopsy" (which the mother often said to her) and started to jump. The mother leant over and tickled Cynthia's tummy, saying, "Did I tickle it?" Cynthia echoed, "Tickle it," but in a moment or two said, "Finish, FINISH!"

I understood what motivated Cynthia's speech in this interchange only after I had studied this passage several times. It appeared that Cynthia wanted her mother to sing "Baa, Baa, Black Sheep," but her mother wanted her to play with toys. Cynthia did not comply, nor did she pretend to telephone Uncle Bill as suggested. She wanted a *verbal* response from the mother. When the mother would not do this, she played with words by

herself. In the end the mother gave up and suggested the trampoline, and then tickled Cynthia, perhaps to make up.

Later during this visit Cynthia showed how she was trying to
sort out phrases on the basis of similar sounds *and meanings*. The
mother said, "Who is mother's girl?" to which Cynthia replied,
"Who is a clever girl?" Mother said she would put Cynthia's hair
band on. Cynthia: "Gloves on." She repeatedly did this in the
course of that year.

While a sighted child would respond with obvious pleasure to
"Who is mother's girl?" Cynthia rather played with words during
this interchange. Throughout the first half of her third year,
Cynthia for the most part named things only when she came
across them. She was often unable to explain her needs and largely
depended on her mother's correct verbalization of them.

Although Cynthia knew her first name, she was far from "talks
intelligibly at play," and using "I," "me," and "you" consistently,
as is expected of sighted 2½-year-old children (Sheridan, 1960).

During a visit at that time, Cynthia climbed all over her mother
while chatting, "I'm a Miss Wills. I'm a mummy. I'm a mummy's girl.
Mummy's girl. Miss Wills's girl [if the visitor was Miss Smith, she
would say "Miss Smith's girl"]. Big big precious girl [someone had
said this the day before]. I'm a big girl."

Cynthia then talked unintelligibly and her mother said, "You're talking scribble."

Cynthia: Scrib—bul. I'm going to fall off. All fall down. I want sing
           a song of sixpence. Green green couple a tea. [She appeared
           to be experimenting with cup and couple.]
Mother: You're a cheeky girl.
Cynthia: You're a cheeky mummy. . . . This is too short and this is
           too long. Clarey Mary Clarey.
Mother: What's your name?
Cynthia: [teasing]: Mummy. Get down [and she did].

This playing with simple phrases was an extension of the association of words with similar sounds that she had shown in her
second year ("dada—Didi"). It appeared that she was recapitulating and matching phrases on the basis of similar sounds, in a
playful interchange with her mother. Several of the phrases recalled affectionate interchanges from the past.

Two weeks later I observed Cynthia going to her mother, who

thought she wanted to be picked up, but Cynthia just wanted to half-lie across her lap from time to time as she stood and talked by her mother's knee. I recorded the following:

Mother: You're talking scribble. . . .
Cynthia: Mummy [followed by jargon]. Is that talking scribble? [Mother thinks she formulated this sentence herself.]
Mother: Yes.
Cynthia: Mummy Pummy, is that talking scribble?
Mother: No, that's a song [meaning a rhyme].

Cynthia then moved off into the middle of the room and turned around and around, fingering her hands and talking nonsense in blank verse.

Cynthia continued to use "scribble talk" until she went to school, when it was slowly modified into playful speech with words, but speech of which the associations were sometimes impossible to follow. However, normal direct speech was developing alongside it.

Cynthia's turning around, her talking "scribble" to herself, and playing with her hands always gave the impression that she was pretending to play with her siblings—blind children are often left out by other children. When she was 6 years old, some of her play was very reminiscent of this and, when asked, she confirmed that she had been pretending to be playing with other children, adding, "I still do, I make up all their voices."

Toward the end of the third year, Cynthia still uttered phrases and sentences which echoed what had been said to her, but several of these were often not fully meaningful. When Cynthia was approaching 3, she kept saying, "I want a bath" as she was sitting in it, and continued to do this when her mother wanted her to come out. We thought it meant, "I want to stay in the bath." Afterward she would not let her mother dress her, and played around in her vest, clapping and talking "scribble," some of which was unintelligible, but she also said, "Got my vest off [she had it on]. Talk to Helga. Simon talks to Helga. Shoes talk to Cynthia." Then, when her mother and I were talking about walks, Cynthia said, "She wants to have walks," which prompted her mother to comment that Cynthia was recapitulating recent or earlier conversations.

Cynthia was struggling with phrases such as "not now" and

"not yet," which she generally, though not always, used correctly. Her use of pronouns varied in accuracy even after the end of the third year, and possessive pronouns sometimes presented difficulties; for instance, at 33 months, Cynthia climbed over the arm of a chair on to her mother's lap, saying, "You said she wanted to sit on her lap."

"Struggle" is in fact the wrong word to apply to Cynthia's attempts to link speech more closely with meaning, since vocalization gave her great pleasure, and her mother capitalized on this by playing many verbal games with her. But it cannot be said that Cynthia could carry on a simple conversation and verbalize past experience in the way that a sighted child can at this age. On the Maxfield and Buchholz Scale for blind children she passed the three speech items if "talks in short sentences" is interpreted somewhat liberally. She rarely dropped words from imitated sentences. Cynthia tended to drop part of the sentence itself, usually the beginning. Cynthia's two-word phrases were all part of what she had heard. The idiosyncratic phrases which the sighted child invents for his own use, such as "allgone milk, allgone dog," which contain a topic and a comment, did not appear to be present.

This child worked through a great deal of what can be termed echolalia and situational phrases in the process of acquiring excellent speech. While blind children show wide individual differences, the study of a case such as Cynthia's may suggest ways of helping blind children who retain a great deal of echolalia, or who become arrested during other phases which Cynthia passed through so enjoyably.

Cynthia remained at home until she was 5 when she went to a weekly boarding school for blind children. She was there for 6 years and was regarded as an exceptionally able child. She also has considerable musical ability. She is now at a grammar school for blind girls.

In comparison with other blind children, the delays she showed in certain areas of her speech development probably interfered with her drive to independence. There were many wishes she could not express directly and much simple verbal information that she did not understand. However, these delays did not, in the long run, hinder her speech development at all. Indeed, in her play with language she may have been demonstrating strategies useful to some blind children. The great pleasure she derived from playing with words and from vocal interchanges with her mother must have contributed to her later linguistic ability. It underlines the fact that we can usefully keep language a pleasurable area for blind children. Perhaps we should meet them halfway by offering not only nursery rhymes but rhyming games and using similar measures.

CONCLUSION

I have attempted to trace the course of speech development in two blind children in order to throw more light on how they acquire it and on some factors that may be responsible for the arrests often found in such children. Wider individual differences would be revealed in a larger number, but it appears that, as with sighted children, a pleasurable mother-child relationship has to be established in order to motivate speech. Only through such a relationship do blind children learn to use language to act on their objects and on their environment.

Blind children seem to use speech, almost as the sighted use vision, as a tool with which to recognize and build up an image of their world. Apparently they also use it to hark back to earlier experiences for the purpose of mastering the past and the present. These experiences, because of their familiarity, give them a feeling of safety and often pleasure.

If we accept this, we should try to help them work over and organize the past in their own terms; and we should be alert to any indication that they need to do this. It is probable that blind children are often confronted with new experiences by well-meaning parents and others before they have assimilated the previous ones. This may be one of the reasons for the arrests and withdrawals they so often show.

Blind children also appear to use speech as an area of play to a far greater extent than sighted children, since model toys have little appeal for them. This too is an area where we could do much more to promote their development.

The ego of the blind child is faced with damage to its perceptual apparatus. Echolalia and situational phrases appear to be an attempt to master and organize experience in the face of this damage. If this is true for blind children, it would be interesting to investigate how far it may be true for others who show similar anomalies, such as borderline and educationally subnormal children.

BIBLIOGRAPHY

BLOS, J. W. (1974a), Traditional Nursery Rhymes and Games. *New Outlook,* 68:268–275.

———— (1974b), Rhymes, Songs, Records, and Stories. *New Outlook,* 68:300–307.

BROWN, R. (1973), *The First Language.* Cambridge, Mass.: Harvard Univ. Press.

BURLINGHAM, D. (1972), *Psychoanalytic Studies of the Sighted and the Blind.* New York: Int. Univ. Press.

FRAIBERG, S. (1968), Parallel and Divergent Patterns in Blind and Sighted Infants. *This Annual,* 23:264–300.

———— (1971), Intervention in Infancy. *J. Amer. Acad. Child Psychiat.,* 10:381–405.

———— (1977), *Insights from the Blind.* New York: Basic Books.

———— & ADELSON, E. (1973), Self-Representation in Language and Play. *Psychoanal. Quart.,* 42:539–562.

GOUGH, D. (1962), The Visual Behaviour of Infants in the First Few Weeks of Life. *Proc. Roy. Soc. Med.,* 55:308–310.

KATAN, A. (1961), Some Thoughts about the Role of Verbalization in Early Childhood. *This Annual,* 16:184–188.

KEELER, W. R. (1958), Autistic Patterns and Defective Communication in Blind Children with Retrolental Fibroplasia. In: *Psychopathology of Communication,* ed. P. H. Hoch & J. Zubin. New York: Grune & Stratton, pp. 64–83.

LOPEZ, T. (1974), Psychotherapeutic Assistance to a Blind Boy with Limited Intelligence. *This Annual,* 29:277–300.

LURIA, A. R. (1961), *The Role of Speech in the Regulation of Normal and Abnormal Behaviour.* London: Pergamon.

MARCY, T. G. (1975), Sensory and Perceptual Dysfunctioning in Early Childhood. Read at Symposium on Guidance Program to Maximize Sensorimotor Development of Blind Infants, Univ. South. Calif.

MAXFIELD, K. E. & BUCHHOLZ, S. (1957), *A Social Maturity Scale for Blind Pre-School Children.* New York: American Foundation for the Blind.

NAGERA, H. & COLONNA, A. B. (1965), Aspects of the Contribution of Sight to Ego and Drive Development. *This Annual,* 20:267–287.

NORRIS, M., SPAULDING, P., & BRODIE, F. (1957), *Blindness in Children.* Chicago: Univ. Chicago Press.

REYNELL, J. (1978), Developmental Patterns of Visually Handicapped Children. *Child: Care, Hlth & Develpm.* (Oxford), 4:291–303.

SANDLER, A.-M. & WILLS, D. M. (1965), Some Notes on Play and Mastery in the Blind Child. *J. Child Psychother.,* 1:7–19.

SHERIDAN, M. (1960), *The Developmental Progress of Infants and Young Children.* London: H. M. Stationery Office.

SMITH, F. (1971), *Understanding Reading.* New York: Holt, Rinehart & Winston.

TREVARTHEN, C. (1974), Conversations with a Two-Month-Old. *New Scientist,* 62:230.

WARREN, H. C. (1933), *Dictionary of Psychology.* London: Allen & Unwin.

WILLS, D. M. (1965), Some Observations on Blind Nursery School Children's Understanding of Their World. *This Annual,* 20:344–364.

THEORETICAL
CONTRIBUTIONS

Reconstruction and the
Process of Individuation

PHYLLIS GREENACRE, M.D.

I

IT IS MY INTENTION TO DISCUSS CERTAIN VICISSITUDES OF DEVELOP-
ment in the first year of infancy, and to focus especially on the
reciprocal processes of separation and individuation. At this early
time growth and maturation proceed at an extraordinary pace
and can be viewed from many different angles. It is difficult to do
justice to the complex set of forces already at work at a time that
we used to consider simple, protected, and almost nirvanalike. I
hope to indicate some of the ways in which disturbances in separation and individuation affect and may increase later neurotic
problems. What I can contribute is drawn from clinical experience in the course of many years of analytic and psychiatric work.
I am of course dependent for background knowledge on the
psychologists and psychoanalysts as well as the physiologists and
pediatricians who have made and are still making careful observational studies of growth and development both of body and behavior in these first years. Such studies have furnished material
from many different angles and have yielded important findings.
I have been especially stimulated by the work of Winnicott and
of Mahler. Winnicott's understanding of the transitional object,

Dr. Greenacre is a member of the Faculty of the New York Psychoanalytic
Institute, and Professor of Clinical Psychiatry, Emeritus, Cornell Medical
College.
This paper was presented at the Margaret Mahler Symposium in Philadel-
phia, May 19, 1978.

as the bridge between the *me* and the *not me,* has a definite bearing on any consideration of the process of individuation. Mahler's careful studies, carried on over a period of years, within the frame of reference provided by her as an analyst, have given me a particularly good organization of findings helpful in my clinical work with adults. It is probably significant that both Winnicott and Mahler were originally pediatricians.

The first big occasion of separation is, of course, birth itself. This is due not only to the labor of the mother. The pressure of growth together with the forces of maturation in the full-term fetus has a part in initiating the work of changing an intramural environment into an extramural one. The change itself is important as it begins to define a separateness that was not possible in utero. The infant must now depend on a recurring union with the mother in body-to-body contact in the course of nursing and cuddling. At the same time muscle and rhythm responsiveness is stimulated by the handling inherent in the manifold activities of maternal care. There is thus a constantly fluctuating reunion with and separation from the mother (or her surrogate) simultaneous with an increasing forward thrust in the infant's need to satisfy developmental demands. In a "good" infancy these mother-infant enterprises supplement, encourage, and blend with the infant's autonomous activities. With it all, there occurs a change which involves the total body economy and balance. For example, during the first 9 months after birth, the subcutaneous tissue increases rapidly in thickness, while the rate of growth of the body as a whole is decelerating. Thus a good thermal protection through heat conservation in the infant is established at a time when separation from the mother is occurring along with increasing exploration of the external world, as part of the infant's autonomous push. It is an intriguing thought that the infant develops an internal protective blanket of fatty tissue, which is a forerunner of the security blanket that he soon finds for himself and can accept or dispose of according to need.

It is evident that in these early months a subtle and intricate organization takes place in the healthy infant, based on an innate capacity for synthesizing and integrating experiences to make a seemingly new and unique individual. The very complexity and multifaceted quality of the organization increase the range of sensitivity and may add to the vulnerability. But it may also lend safety as the infant's ongoing maturational push is opening up *overlapping, alternate, and sometimes reciprocating ways* of functional response. The ability to absorb discomfort or distress due to untoward conditions may be sufficient, unless distress is extreme, acute, or of such duration that the total homeostatic organismic equilibrium is severely threatened. This fortunately is not very common.

Distress may arise in either partner, mother or infant, and be communicated from one to the other. Thus when the mother is burdened with severe physical or emotional problems, the return to the mother for comfort may be inadequate and unsuccessful. Instead, a reciprocal "borrowed" disturbance in the infant may arise. If the mother is especially anxious about the baby and is on the verge of panic for other reasons, then a peculiar reverberation of tension may mount in both partners, each one increasing the other's disturbance to a bewildering extent.

In this connection I am reminded of a mother-infant state of reciprocal disturbance which I encountered a number of years ago, before problems of separation and individuation had been much recognized. A pediatrician consulted me about a case of a weird mother-infant relationship which had been brought to him by the mother. She was an unmarried woman of 40, a former actress, and the mother of a baby several months old. As she approached the 40s, she had become more aware of her wish to have a child and was determined to accomplish this. The father seemed not to have played much of a role in her life except as the means to this end. She now lived alone, taking exclusive care of the baby. She never left the baby for more than 20 minutes. She would wait until the baby was asleep to make necessary purchases. If she returned before the 20 minutes were up, she usually found the baby asleep. If she overstayed the 20 minutes, the baby would be awake and watchful, seeming to follow with the eyes the mother's every movement. Developing gradually, this state of affairs had reached a point in which neither mother nor baby could sleep much beyond the span of 20 minutes, seemingly out of need to verify the presence of the other. I recall that nocturnal sleep was disturbed, but am not sure to what extent the 20-minute schedule extended into the night with any regularity.

This information came to me from a hospital outpatient service in the early 1930s during the long period of economic depression, when I had barely begun my own work as an analyst. I do not recall what advice I gave: whether I threw up my hands in despair, or gave the enthusiastic but probably impossible advice of the novice, suggesting that the mother be analyzed.

This small clinical vignette is so isolated that it can only provoke speculation about the background that produced it. There was, however, a convincing cohesiveness in the situation which gave it significance. At any rate, it alerted me to a realization of the degree to which one channel of contact (in this case, vision in an eye-to-eye contact) can dominate and substitute for the other channels. There seemed to be a primitive, mutual, compulsive urge to touch each other through vision in order to continue life. Vision here had a prehensile quality, but it also carried an eerie basic communication. One can guess that this pathological but determined mother had herself suffered some deficit or other disturbance in being mothered and had developed a fear of body contact which was felt as dangerous and yet longed for. Her seeking a career as an actress was harmonious with her need to identify with someone else (i.e., to play a role) and in this disguised way show herself on the stage to verify her own desirability through the response from an audience. Whether she determined to have a baby in order to comfort herself in her loneliness, or as proof of being a full woman, or for other powerful unconscious reasons, the end result was that she had produced another version of herself. She now desperately wished to be free of this incubus of a baby.

There are, of course, many gaps in this account. My recollection is that the infant was in the second half of the first year. I cannot recall details as to the stage of communication by sound—either babble or crying, except the infant's crying on missing the mother if she overstayed her leave. Nor do I know what degree of locomotion had been achieved, except that the baby was not walking. Presumably the mother took care of the infant's physical needs, but by the time of the consultation there was little indication of cuddling. My impression was that a visually dominated rhythm had been established early by the mother's strong nonconscious wish to keep the baby as part of herself, with the result that the infant's independent functioning was retarded.

Spitz (1957) saw the early normal union of vision and action in the service of communication at a distance when he observed that the infant generally develops a *yes* or *no* response through nodding the head up and down to keep the desired object in view to mean *yes,* and shaking the head sideways to banish from view the unwanted object, to mean *no.* There is thus acceptance or disposal of an object according to whether or not it is permitted admission to the eye.

Life is full of alternating needs to be alone and to be with others. Perhaps the simplest and most persistent form of this is the alternation of sleep and wakefulness—the need to follow the stimulation of multiple contacts with the external world by withdrawal into the isolation of sleep. With time the urgency of this alternating need of infancy diminishes in frequency as the infant becomes attuned to the rhythm of day and night. In early infancy, the ability to sleep seems to depend largely on the combination of satisfying warmth of the body surface with the internal satiety of being adequately fed, i.e., warmed within. Some infants spontaneously give up night feeding even within their first few months. This may possibly be coordinated with the increasing importance of vision which mediates distance. A growing familiarity with the mother's face is established, supplements and gradually supersedes the need for direct contact with her breast or body. It implies the very dawn of visual memory, which at first may be uncertain and unreliable, but will be reinforced as development continues and permits increased separateness. Night then is not a complete aloneness if the cradle or crib is snug and warm.

Ambivalence gradually emerges from this pervasive rhythm of alternation. The forward movement of (neutral) aggression, i.e., autonomous movement propelled by continuing growth and maturation, at first probably gives rise only to feelings of comfort and discomfort as bodily needs are satisfied or not. As separation proceeds, some capacity for object relations together with incipient aim-directed activity is possible. It seems to be associated with or depend upon the beginning of visual memory. Aggressive forward movement now may become either agreeably satisfying or disagreeably frustrating. It is only at this stage that early versions of love and hostility begin to emerge into potential ambivalence. In the early part of this stage, however, the situation is complicated in that the degree of separateness is so uncertain and fluctuant that the infant seems to attribute to another person or thing the hurts which have originated in his own activities.

Ambivalence has been defined as "the simultaneous existence of opposite feelings, attitudes and tendencies directed toward another person, thing or situation. In the most general sense, ambivalence is universal and not important, because there are few affectionate relations which are uncomplicated by some hostility, and many hostile relations are tempered by affection" (Moore and Fine, 1967, p. 14). I believe, however, that a mild degree of ambivalence is inevitable and healthy in most durable relations, that it permits or demands the awareness of opposites and so promotes forward movement through the need to make choices. *Tolerance of some degree of ambivalence in the self and in others is later associated with the acceptance and even appreciation of the uniqueness of the individual.*

Severe ambivalence, however, produces a wrenchingly painful state of affairs which demands either retreat or combat. Exaggerated states of bodily expressed ambivalence may be manifested and somewhat fixated even within the preverbal period. Even after they subside, vulnerable areas of tension are left and may be revived at later periods of conflict. I think here of early struggles over feeding and toilet training which become battle areas at a somatic level, if the infant is being cared for by a zealous but anxious and compulsively driven mother or nurse. The derivatives of such early conflicts then may reappear later in a stubborn obsessional state as well as contribute to the development of a rigid conscience. This is obviously increased when the struggle has become erotized and offers material for masturbation fantasies. In general, whenever any conflict threatens to become overwhelming, the somatopsychic defenses are aroused, but at some sacrifice of the freedom of spontaneous choice of action. This portends some impairment in the development of early ego functioning with an increase in primary and secondary narcissism that later distorts the developing sense of self. This is apparent in the too strong and persistent need for supportive identifications.

II

The first part of this paper is based on and expanded from a discussion of the theory of the parent-infant relationship (Greenacre, 1960). I was aware then that the progressive separation of infant from mother might involve problems of increased ambivalence and narcissism and might also influence the nature of identifications and the later sense of identity. Hoffer's work (1949, 1950) on the body ego had helped me to understand some aspects of fetishism. I had also come to the idea that the earliest aggression arose from maturational push and might in itself entail bodily pleasure. This was close to Hartmann's concept (1939) of an undifferentiated phase before ego and libido were manifest. It was also forecast in earlier articles by Hendrick (1942, 1943). It seemed clear to me that even a primitive form of love and hate could be felt as such only if there was a sufficient *not me* to be the target for such feelings. Otherwise it would be a matter of comfort or discomfort in the infant himself. In the last 15 years the work of Mahler and her co-workers (1963, 1968, 1975) has continued to give substance for pondering and has offered sustaining help in understanding many complications in adult analyses. I now turn to some clinical findings in adult cases that indicate or illustrate evidences of disturbances in these earliest years.

It is not possible to give an account of a complete analysis, showing all the significant details that led to an understanding of what was important in the creation and the relief of the neurotic symptoms. If one attempts too thoroughly to do this, the reader may lose his way in the forest by seeing too much of the foliage of the underbrush. In addition, time, expediency, and the problems of confidentiality make difficulties. I attempt to solve this situation now by taking clinical illustrations from two case histories already published, the first reported in 1951; the second, in 1970.

CASE 1

In September 1946, an unmarried woman in her mid-30s came to me in a very severe panic. As she had been able by extreme self-control to carry on in a responsible position, I decided to attempt extramural treatment. She promptly quieted down and made a clutching but workable transference relation to me.

During the preceding summer both parents had suffered sudden mishaps. Her mother had a slight cerebral accident with a brief facial palsy and, somewhat later, her father cut his finger severely with an electric revolving saw while working in his basement shop. The patient had helped in both emergencies. These events inevitably brought a hint of the time when she might be parentless. They also reactivated a gamut of repressed memories from early childhood, associated with deeply buried and unacceptable ambivalent feelings toward both parents.

On Labor Day, shortly before she came to me, while walking through the city, she experienced a sudden sense of "frozen unreality" when she happened to look up and see the bridge between two parts of a nearby building. When she later noticed the same sort of bridge at a department store, she was overwhelmed by a full-fledged panic and could scarcely find her way home. Bridges at the ground level did not bother her. Only the sight of a bridge in the air overhead was terrifying, even though she had seen these same bridges many times before without difficulty. She took readily to the analytic situation and reacted with relief as though she had come into a safe harbor.

In the opening days of our work, I learned that she was the middle one of three children: one brother was 5 years older and the other 16 months younger. The older brother, D., was an airplane pilot; he was married and had two children, one of whom, a boy of 5, had recently visited. She was now concerned because she had been irritated and felt she had treated this little nephew "unforgivingly." (She was, in fact, unforgiving toward his father for childhood crimes and disappointments, as I was to learn much later.) In the weeks before the panic, she had already had a number of worries about young children. Her mother's minor stroke had followed her return from visiting the younger brother, B., and his wife who had just had their first baby. She also found herself obsessed with anxious thoughts after hearing talk about an unmarried friend whose baby was born through a breech delivery and how unfortunate this was.

On the fourth day of our work there was a sudden breakthrough of an old memory dating back to the age of 4½. She had been able to put it out of her mind for considerable periods of time, but never could really banish it. Revived feelings of shame, humiliation, and even degradation were such that as she grew up she congratulated herself each year that she was that much farther away from this unholy experience. A lively and investigative child, she had gone on a hot summer day to a neighbor's to play with a little boy about her own age. The two children then went into some bushes to pursue mutual researches. Having stripped first, she was completely nude when the boy's mother suddenly appeared, grabbed her by the hand, and whisked her across the street back to the house where she was hurriedly dressed and sent home. She could not remember the end of the event except that she had felt humiliated by the boy's mother putting "stiff brown stockings" on her instead of allowing her to dress herself. She recalled being hot with excitement and humiliation, and that the coolness of a slight breeze on her nude body had been soothing. I was much later to see that the stiff brown stockings probably represented the fecal penis that she had earlier felt was taken away from her.

This painful experience, so insistently remembered, was obviously a screen memory that definitely hid some sexual experience with her brother D., when she was about 9 years old and he a young adolescent. From related dream associations it seemed that she had taken the initiative in this situation with the fantasy of becoming pregnant. Her persistent inability to recall this later event with the brother may have been due to the fact that by 9 her superego was firmer and her guilt was unbearable. Her way out was to repress the memory of the later experience and remain chronically hostile and envious of this brother.

After dwelling on this memory for two or three hours, she did not mention it again for almost a year. Then on a hot day in late summer, after quietly lying down on the couch as usual, she suddenly broke into extreme sobbing. Pointing at a pedestal electric fan placed near the head of the couch, she said angrily that she did not know why, but she felt I was accusing her in this way and she could not tolerate it. It was again some time before this matter of the fan was spoken of. In the meantime she brought out masturbation fantasies that were clearly related to it. In them she had shifted her position to being an onlooker rather than an active participant, e.g., "a delicate young woman was on a pirate ship when the captain undressed and attacked her," ending nicely, "though of course she was willing." Another fantasy concerned a wicked and licentious woman who was nude outdoors when she was attacked by a mythological creature like a sun god. These two fantasies referred rather clearly to her intense oedipal feelings toward her father. These were displaced and acted out in child-hood with her brother or his representative. Thus envy and jealousy had been almost unbearably strong.

This became clear when she recalled an event that had also occurred at about the same time as the old expedition into the bushes. She was then sleeping in a twin bed in a room with her mother when her father entered. "He gave me the feeling of a strange being, an *It*. He got into bed with mother. I heard heavy breathing and there was an atmosphere of struggle. Then *He* or *It* went away again. I did not brood about this. But it seemed strange, and it all took place without any words." The *It* creature thus reappeared as the exalted mythological sun god, and the two events were brought together, representing the two sides of her envious ambivalence toward her father, as well as her glorification of him. At 13, a few months before the onset of menstruation, she had a kind of love affair with her dog, an airedale. Fantasying about him as human, she tried to entice him into mutual genital play. When he failed to cooperate, she felt humiliated and dis-graced. Later, during a lonely time in her 20s, she spent her last cent for a sheepdog who seemed to be a combination of this aire-dale and her early blanket fetish. In latency the blanket had been succeeded by a lucky stone carried in her pocket.

Many aspects of this young woman's life story have been omitted. The original paper was focused particularly on the phallic phase and its unique qualities as a bridge between the anal and the oedipal periods. Under ordinary "good" conditions, individuation is then relatively secure, and the child can feel responsibility for his toilet and other bodily needs. He no longer must experience or use them as part of the closeness to the care-taking parents. He is now aware of memory, of thought and even of dreams, and also concerns himself increasingly with the outer world. He is able to differentiate tangible objects from their intangible representations in dreams and thoughts. The rise of genital feelings not only ushers in the oedipal demands, but gives a general body invigoration as well. At this age, children are doomed to discover that they cannot fly.

This patient's first years, however, had been disturbed in ways that interfered with the adequate development of separation and individuation. Such ambivalence may become tolerable through a suppression of one side of the ambivalent state with an overemphasis on the other side. This predisposes a child to an all-or-none emotional reaction. Under stress this may break down into adoring dependence and intense aversion. These opposites sometimes appear as a splitting of the object into the "good" and the "bad," at first as different aspects of the same person. Later these tend to be projected onto different individuals. Such tendencies, when pronounced, complicate and intensify the oedipal conflict both in childhood and in adolescence. The love then contains more of a wish to please and of possessiveness than of appreciation of the other's individuality; and inevitably on the opposite side there is a tendency to abnormal jealousy and hateful destructive wishes. Such feelings were still expressed in this patient's dreams and fantasies. She attempted to control all anger out of fear of hostile impulses. At puberty she had developed a temporary but intense phobia of touching her father or anything associated with him, and even became apprehensive when she saw his clothing close to hers in the process of being laundered. Envy of her brother's penis and awe of her father's were reflected in crude castrating wishes vividly expressed in early fantasies and later dreams. These frightened her so much that she had developed a tendency to habitual retreat into passive compliance and shyness, repressing all anger.

Gender identity was wavering and uncertain, later expressed in confused secondary ways. Her sense of everyday reality was good, but vulnerable to the extent of occasional bizarre episodes of reality distortion. These appeared in accounts of past experience and in the transference relation.

In the third year of treatment she again brought up the incident

of the insulting fan. She spoke of it as a table fan placed at the
foot of the couch and clearly in her view. When I corrected this,
she became extremely angry, insisting that if I could not remember
things more accurately, she would leave the analysis. The fan with
its rotating blades had symbolically condensed the idea of the
saw that had injured her father as well as the memory of his penis
which was big and destructive. It probably had been seen as above
her in the primal scene that haunted her so; whereas the smaller
fan at the foot of the couch represented the penis of the brother
with whom she had had the experience at puberty, or perhaps also
that of the younger brother with whom she had been constantly
bathed. Some of her nightmarish dreams had been of herself
slicing raw and bloody meat that she was preparing for dinner.
Spying was also a theme in many dreams. Yet with all this in the
background, she had a sufficiently practical and durable set of
reaction formations so that she could carry on responsible work
steadily and efficiently. She sometimes dreamed of herself as
having a *double*.

Although the emphasis in my original paper was on the phallic
phase, I learned a good deal about the first 2 or 3 years of her life
as these were reflected in associations and fragmentary memories.
There was an unusual opportunity to check their validity when,
toward the end of the analysis, the patient produced a baby book
that had been faithfully kept by her mother. While I recognized
that these early conditions were important in accentuating later
conflicts and symptoms, I did not grasp their full significance in
the developmental process of individuation; and I shall now attempt a reevaluation.

She was a normal baby at birth, breast-fed for 3 months. Lacta-
tion may have been inadequate, for subsequent bottle feeding was
pushed so energetically that at 18 months she was "abnormally
fat." This seems, however, to have been considered a desirable
achievement. Toilet training was completed by 12 months, though
she had not yet begun to walk. It was considered that her overfeeding had interfered with her walking and at 18 months this
was discontinued, and some solid food began to be offered. Up to
this time she had had nothing to chew upon.[1] By 22 months, she

1. Sybille K. Escalona has suggested that this delay in walking may have

was thinner, had grown greatly in height and achieved walking. Nothing was reported about the beginning of talking, but at Christmas, when she was almost 3 years old, she was chanting, "I am going to be born."

If her first year was one of sedentary stuffing, the second was eventful. The mother had become pregnant again when the infant was only 7 months old, and concern about this may have accelerated the toilet training. Recent observations indicate that a baby in the first year often reacts quite early to the mother's pregnancy as the mother tends to be absorbed and withdrawn. Certainly by the first half of this little girl's second year, the pregnancy would also have crowded her out of the mother's lap, for her brother was born when she was 16 months old, before she herself was walking independently or taking solid food. It was a situation to make an anxious mother more anxious, and an older infant develop a primitive envy and ambivalent identification with the new interloper. It may, in fact, have contributed to her later feeling of having a "double."

For several years, from the time the little brother was 6 months old and she 22 months old and just walking, they were bathed in the same tub. She apparently solved her envy by identifying with him in an unusually peaceful, though sometimes rivalrous way. In an association to a dream about water, she reported that the bathing together had made them "one and the same, of the same flesh and blood, through the spray of the bath water." She also developed a bathtub masturbatory play by letting sprayed water stimulate her clitoris. Her penis envy was not so much of this brother, for he was more or less part of her anyway, than of the one 5 years older, who urinated in her presence and later masturbated before her.

New changes in shape and form constantly preoccupied this young woman. These seemed to involve both genital excitation

---

been due largely to the interference of the normal body rhythms by the overfeeding—i.e., that the baby was fed so constantly that no degree of hunger could be experienced. Oral aggression also would seem to have been given little opportunity to express itself through the deprivation of chewing. No details of the systems of training were recorded—only the fact of supposed successes.

and feelings of total body size. Twice later in life she had rather sudden shifts in weight, possibly patterned after these early changes. She also automatized the different parts of her body, saying, "My clitoris wants to be touched," "my foot means to kick you," etc., and from time to time had illusory—almost hallucinatory—distorted perceptions. Seeing me once in a public place, she was insistent that my hat had, as part of its trimming, something which stuck out straight in front.

I never saw the parents, but the impression formed that the family was a rather tight little group and that the parents had been and attempted to remain rigid social and moral guides for their children well into adult life. Duty had invaded and absorbed many of the functions of love. The patient was so deeply identified with her parents that she could not realize how much she rebelled against them. Her father was a teacher. Both parents were college graduates who valued formal education highly. Even when she was in a "very nervous state" for 2 or 3 years at puberty and it was thought necessary to remove her from school, she kept up with her class and lost no time in her school progress. She was obviously a bright, responsive child for whom formal learning offered an acceptable and organizing defensive system. A vivid and active imagination early became erotized and was expressed mostly in compelling masturbatory fantasies in which she might be either sex. These were increasingly repressed until the realistic demands of puberty brought a period of prolonged confusion. This seemed to be a forerunner of the acute disturbance that brought her to me.

The primitive, frightening quality of the fantasies required a massive repression with denial. Not sufficiently converted or transformed into any artistic form, they were partly sublimated by her investment in special educational work with adolescents. These fantasies and the associated primitive impulses were reproduced in an extraordinary series of dreams. She still lived at home, much under the influence of her parents. It is probable that the suggestion of the imminence of their death threatened her whole adult superego organization, which had been her main protection.

This patient can be compared to and contrasted with the first case. Already in her early 40s she had had a period of analysis and several of psychotherapy before she consulted me, asking whether she should continue her current treatment, change analysts, or discontinue treatment altogether. She had held responsible positions, but an extreme underlying ambivalence would break its containing bounds and disrupt both work and personal relations by attacks of rage. Her story emerged during a series of five consultative interviews, which followed a period of several years of analysis. I had also seen her for an initial consultation and had then recommended that she undertake analysis. The information here was a composite of all three sources. As in the case of the first patient, it was necessary to examine the earliest years in order to understand the bases and nature of her ambivalence, with its gross disturbance of body awareness—especially of genital identity. In her adult life, she was to develop a periodic illusion of possessing a large penis with which she might shock others if they knew of it. There also were distorted perceptions of external reality which she sometimes exploited, dramatized, and acted out, accompanied by threats of suicide. Vivid and persistent fantasies led to forays into life which promised well at first, but tended soon to break down.

She was the only child of parents, themselves only children. Her mother had been a flirtatious young woman, drawn into early marriage with a young man who threatened that otherwise he would commit suicide. The baby was born 10 months later in this worsening marriage; and by the time she was $2\frac{1}{2}$ years old a divorce banished the father, whom she did not see again until her young adulthood. She seemed never to have idealized him as his place had always been somewhat absorbed by the maternal grandfather, who was devoted, indulgent, and full of ambitions for her future. He was definitely the dominant and successful one in the family group. Her first $2\frac{1}{2}$ years were ones of tension and overstimulation due to the parents' incessant quarreling. With the father gone, the mother became depressed and sought a total and pathological absorption in the little one, sleeping with her both at night and in the course of daytime naps and offering her breast to be sucked. This was ostensibly to distract the child from frequent masturbation, as the little girl had already developed the habit of rubbing her genitals with a crumpled-up part of the sheet. It was certainly a state of morbid symbiosis in which mother and child regressed together to an early infantile stage.

This period contributed to the later development of character traits that frequently were handicapping but sometimes exploited with seeming usefulness. Throughout it all she showed a remarkable alertness—a willingness to attempt to make great changes in her life with a watchful hold on external reality. She seemed a very practical woman with a capacity to organize work. In specific situations, however, this might break down through temper outbursts. All in all her sense of reality had a peculiar durability even though her perceptions of her own body and of specific things in the world around her might temporarily be grossly distorted and then selectively denied. The too great plasticity of the sense of the body self as well as of the developing ego contributed to bizarre distortions of perception and unusual somatic symptoms. Yet one felt that there was a good but not remarkable core of autonomous developmental pressure.

To return to the life story: by the time the child was 4½, the mother reemerged from her depression and presently left her little daughter in favor of a lover of whom the grandparents disapproved. Between 4½ and 7 she did not see her mother but remained with her grandparents, writing daily "letters" to her mother. Now the grandfather began to put her in her mother's place. He planned for her future and was closely affectionate with her. He demanded that she be a pretty and feminine-appearing child, and daydreamed with her of how she would ultimately succeed to his business. He loved her as long as she fulfilled his wishes. She in turn learned to control situations with feminine tears—with alternate rage, if tears were ineffective. She remembered less of the period from 4½ to 7 than of the one from 2½ to 4. When the mother remarried, the girl felt herself as a surrogate for her mother.

A quiet and studious little girl in school, she had an exciting, secret, romantic fantasy life at home. Masturbation continued throughout. Her interest in the mouth-vagina changed to a concern about the clitoris. This in turn was accompanied by erotic fantasies of watching a man with an enormous penis about which he felt helplessly frustrated. While this fantasy contained both seduction and revenge and the genital elements were stronger than previously, there also were efforts at establishing a sense of body separateness, supplemented by the sight (i.e., thought) of the big penis. As masturbation had given her a sense of importance, she was disappointed when she learned that a girlfriend also had discovered it.

As a teen-ager she was a good student, but drab and not popular. With great determination, at 20 she retrained herself to be like her mother, to appear pretty, chic, and flirtatious, and promptly made a marriage that lasted only 3 months. She was afraid of intercourse, and the penis seemed like a cannon. In response she had severe rages, at herself for being a failure as a woman, and at her husband for being a man. Earlier she had had suicidal fantasies, possibly influenced by knowledge of her father's suicide threats, which had, however, never been repeated after the parents' divorce. The idea of death was clearly associated with going to sleep, probably as the culmination of childhood masturbation with a mixture of alternating oral and phallic components. She imagined a man with a huge penis; and she suffered severe globus hystericus, which subsided only when she slept.

Leaving her husband, she was afraid of being alone and so returned to her mother and stepfather. On the first night, when they went out for the evening, she took a nonlethal dose of sedatives, which precipitated a period of hospitalization. After this, she replaced her mother with a woman friend and moved to a nearby city where with some supportive therapeutic help she undertook self-sustaining work and did rather well. At 26, she came to New York, held a good job successfully while she lived a frantic life with a succession of lovers, at the same time undertaking more therapy with a woman. But still, each time she became seriously interested in a man, she developed the old globus hystericus symptom. In addition, a new difficulty arose: she periodically felt that her eyeballs were being pulled out of her sockets and she could not control their direction—which usually pointed to a woman. These symptoms were relatively, not absolutely, sex assigned. Sometimes the globus appeared with a woman and the eye symptoms with a man.

It seems to have been about this time, after a period of depression, that she developed a compromise symptom, which rather amused her: she now imagined that she herself had huge male genitalia, which would shock others if they knew about her condition. This was an acceptable illusion. Revenge seemed now to have been converted into controlled and triumphant humor. She was nonetheless rather disconcerted by her illusory achievement and so sought consultation, which initiated a period of 5 years of psychoanalytic treatment.

III

I have revived these two case histories as they could be presented in fairly full detail. It was also possible to get some follow-up reports on these patients' later lives. In both cases developmental patterns rooted in disturbances of the preverbal period can be found reappearing—reshaped, augmented, or diminished at critical periods in later years. It has long been recognized that early severe traumatic conditions or events might adversely affect later development. It was thought, however, that such early disturbances, grounded largely in body responses, would be organized as part of the general constitutional equipment and later could not be reached in psychoanalytic treatment. In other words, the assumption was that what occurred in the preverbal period was permanently embedded and could not be brought into words and communicated in speech. The content of these first years was thus considered to be beyond the limits of metapsychology and of psychoanalytic treatment proper.

Recent observational studies have shown—what nearly every mother knows—that a sharp dividing line seldom exists between verbal and preverbal communication. Infancy is a time zone in which speech emerges in irregular stages, from body reactions that have accompanied and focused the infant's attention on particular significant sounds. These may evolve into hybrid words that come both from the *me* and the *not me*. I think here of the various early words for the bowel movement that are sometimes echos of body sounds and sometimes approximations of exclamations of the mother or nurse. It is interesting in this connection that the word *verb* (itself meaning *word*) is a part of speech denoting motion or action. The inception of verbalization may progress coincidentally with the increase in the infant's autonomously directed motion.

As a matter of fact, few analysts limit attention to the patient's words but are aware of the degree of tension expressed in a variety of ways—the movements, gestures, sweating, coughing, twitching, and other evidences of nonverbal responsiveness. Frequently these are understood as part of a transference reaction or of some concurrent problem and conflict. This is true, but from experience I have found that patients who have had undue disturbances early show such reactions more plentifully and more sharply than others and often have rather florid physical complaints, formerly often referred to as "hypochondriac." The body participates in the analytic situation to an unusual degree, essentially with a primordial cry to get back to an illusory comforting mother.

These body responses may appear as symptoms that are part of a long-standing somatized anxiety; or they may erupt in episodic physical distress, activated in the transference during the analytic hour. Commonly they appear in seemingly inexplicable affecto-motor moods of dreariness, irritability, and fear of loss of basic transference contact. If the original infantile distress has been acute and unrelieved, rage rather than irritability may occur. In any case, such elements derived from early infancy may be incorporated in dreams, as part of a time-layered collage of extraordinarily rich and varied symbolization, and often contain primitive body representations.

The range of empathic responsiveness in the analyst depends largely on his awareness of the degree of his own sensitivity to such changes not only in the analytic situation but in himself in other life situations. The major critical problems of emotional development—the oedipal conflicts, castration fears, and states of blatant penis envy—are severe and unusually openly expressed, sometimes giving a misleading impression of insight. They are, however, oriented toward narcissistic aims with a weakness in object relatedness.[2]

Returning to consider the role of memory in the work of reconstruction, I would emphasize that screen memories can rarely be understood and interpreted through immediate free association, as may sometimes be done with dreams. As screen memories have evolved through years, they commonly have considerable stability as part of their defensive function, thus lacking the rich fluidity in symbolism so characteristic of dreams. The analyst must carry in mind the many events and landmarks of development in the analysand's life, somewhat as one follows the development of a character in literature. Then the full significance of the events of later childhood and adulthood becomes more readily apparent, while the patient's awareness of the analyst's presence and participation adds depth and naturalness to interpretations.

Further, I think that memory does not begin just with the development of language and the ability to put the impression of new happenings into words. Rather it would appear that rudimentary reactions, in great variety, pleasant and unpleasant, may be related to, but not identical with, the phenomenon of imprinting in some animals.[3] Some impression may be made on young

2. For an excellent discussion of the stage of organization with the period of rapprochement (Mahler) see Blum (1977).

3. A recent report of a psycholinguistic study (Curtiss, 1977) is of interest here. It deals with a "modern-day Wild Child" who was discovered at 13 years, 7 months, after suffering extreme deprivation and abuse since the age of 20 months. She had been shut up by her paranoid schizophrenic father, put in a small room, harnessed to a potty chair, allowed minimal food, movement, and almost no verbal contact. The account is of the first 5 years after her discovery. During this time she had gained a limited ability to use words, although she was well past the age when this was thought possible. She was able to indicate with words that her father had beaten her with a stick at some time during her speechless period. This seems to suggest that experience may be "encoded" before spoken language is developed, and possibly be reproduced in one way or another later.

Evidently the urge for communication is very great. I recall the deprivation experiments begun by Dr. and Mrs. Wayne Dennis in 1940–41. The subjects were a pair of twins who, from 2 to 10 months of age, were handled with only the minimal stimulation necessary to provide food, cleanliness, and warmth. (In other words, they were not abused.) At 10 months, however, when

infants as they meet a new situation which requires or allows an appreciable change in the general organismic equilibrium. The memory reaction is strengthened if the new experience is repeated and becomes part of the infant's accepted milieu; or, if it is definitely unpleasant, it must be protested against in some appropriate way. These first impressions are body bound and expressed through whatever channels of discharge are available. Speech and language emerge later as enormously economizing functions in the service of directed communication, implying and furthering an increase in object relatedness. They tend to cover and to absorb the nonverbal memory impressions from the earlier months.

IV

The clinical and observational findings discussed here bring up certain questions as to how this material may become useful. Certainly, it is of value in understanding the intensity and stubbornness of some neurotic states and perversions. These are not psychoses, although they have often been regarded as such, and therefore usually considered to be not accessible to classical analysis. Does this portend some possible modification of theory or technique?

In any case, the better understanding of the patient's problems may be reflected in the therapeutic attitude and interpretive responses of the analyst due to the widening of *his* or *her* empathy. In addition, it may lead to further study of the nature of some defense reactions (especially those of denial) and of disturbances of incorporation and primitive projection. These, in turn, hinder early object relatedness and may disrupt integrative processes generally. The roots of these untoward developments seem to go back to early infancy. There is the alternative question, whether it may provide substance for new conceptions of mental hygiene for infancy.

The group of so-called "borderline" patients who in recent

---

they were held with forcible body restraint and marked pressure was applied to the nose (provocative stimulation intended to test rage responsiveness), the babies smiled, seemingly out of attachment to the experimenters, and the experiment broke down.

years have come to seek analyses with only a modicum of success has contributed a practical stimulus to a progressive interest in ego psychology. It is tempting to discuss why this group of patients has emerged so strongly during the last two or three decades.

Is this phenomenon due largely to the greater spread of knowledge of and demand for psychoanalytic treatment, together with the limitation of classical psychoanalysis in treating such cases? Or is it a change occurring in the fundamental structure of current neuroses, due to conditions in the outer world during the massive upheavals of the last 50 or 60 years—upheavals that certainly had an impact on the organization and expectations of family life and especially on parent-infant relationships?

We are just now seeing patients in their early or mid-30s who, having been conceived either just before or during World War II, did not know their fathers until they were 2 to 5 years old, and often then in unnatural emotional situations and in strange new surroundings. Working with such patients, one is impressed with the difficulties ensuing from father deprivation in infancy. This is not the only or most important evidence of special disturbances in disorganized family relationships, and is given only as a current illustration.

As adolescents in the 1960s, many of these war-born children became members of massive group demonstrations, and some subsequently went on into activist organizations, as well as adopting the pseudo-family commune way of life. The regression which inevitably took place under these conditions had paradoxical results in that the demands for individuality became reduced and reversed with a final loss of the sense of individual realization and responsibility. The "sexual revolution," together with the emergence of new contraceptive techniques, and the feminist movement may have brought changes in ideals and expectations in marriage and in child care in ways that might affect the structure of neuroses when today's infants become young adults in the future.

All this is against a background of momentous changes in world conditions. Freud (1916–17) spoke of how much the discovery that the earth is round jolted man's narcissism by depriving him of the illusion of his position as being the center of the universe. In our time the atom bomb has made real the fantasy of the possibility of world destruction; the flight to the moon has also turned fantasy into reality in a mind-boggling way, complicating our sense of reality, including that of time and space. Man seems, generally, to have adjusted rather readily to these portentous events in that he no longer disbelieves them. Two concepts of reality are being established, and man also suffers both an attack on his narcissism and a compensatory narcissistic inflation in expanding fantasies and expectations.

This paper, however, is focused with the telescope turned in the opposite direction—to decipher the significant developmental processes in infancy having to do with the realization of individual autonomy. As the interest in early ego development has increased, different theories have emerged, stressing various elements in the ego as of leading importance—the backbone, as it were, of the early ego structure. Narcissism, the self, identity, object relatedness, splitting, and even the progressive formation and use of the transitional object have each been described as the pivotal determining element in the development of healthy or disturbed ego functioning. These represent developmental trends in individuation that may have varying degrees of importance, depending on the timing and the intensity with which they are evoked, together with incipient defense reactions, which may appear first as somatic responses (Greenacre, 1958). The somatic elements may contribute significantly to the production of somatized anxiety symptoms which, under some circumstances, reappear in psychotic delusions regarding the body. They may also increase the intensity of the developing superego, or play a part in strong enclosing character defenses. The situation is always one in which there is an interplay between developing ego tendencies and manifestations of libidinal phase progression. We are not yet, in my estimation, ready to explain the variety of borderline conditions. A great deal more work is to be done.

BIBLIOGRAPHY

BLUM, H. P. (1977), The Prototype of Preoedipal Reconstruction. *J. Amer. Psychoanal. Assn.*, 25:757–786.

CURTISS, S. (1977), *Gene*. New York: Academic Press.

DENNIS, W. (1941), Infant Development under Conditions of Restricted Practice and Minimum Social Stimulation. *Genet. Psychol. Monogr.*, 23:143–189.

FREUD, S. (1916–17), Introductory Lectures on Psycho-Analysis. *S.E.*, 15 & 16.

GREENACRE, P. (1951), Respiratory Incorporation and the Phallic Phase. *This Annual*, 6:180–205.

———— (1958), Toward an Understanding of the Physical Nucleus of Some Defense Reactions. In: *Emotional Growth*. New York: Int. Univ. Press, 1:128–144.

———— (1960), Considerations Regarding the Parent-Infant Relationship. *Ibid.*, 1:199–224.

———— (1970), Notes on the Influence and Contribution of Ego Psychology to the Practice of Psychoanalysis. *Ibid.*, 2:776–806.

HARTMANN, H. (1939), *Ego Psychology and the Problem of Adaptation*. New York: Int. Univ. Press, 1958.

HENDRICK, I. (1942), Instinct and Ego during Infancy. *Psychoanal. Quart.*, 11:33–58.

———— (1943), The Instinct to Master. *Psychoanal. Quart.*, 12:561–565.

HOFFER, W. (1949), Mouth, Hand and Ego-Integration. *This Annual, 3/4:49–56.

———— (1950), Development of the Body Ego. *This Annual*, 5:18–24.

MAHLER, M. S. (1963), Thoughts about Development and Individuation. *This Annual*, 18:307–324.

———— & FURER, M. (1968), *On Human Symbiosis and the Vicissitudes of Individuation*. New York: Int. Univ. Press.

———— PINE, F., & BERGMAN, A. (1975), *The Psychological Birth of the Human Infant*. New York: Basic Books.

MOORE, B. E. & FINE, B. D. (1967), *A Glossary of Psychoanalytic Terms and Concepts*. New York: Amer. Psychoanal. Assn.

SPITZ, R. A. (1957), *No and Yes*. New York: Int. Univ. Press.

WINNICOTT, D. W. (1953), Transitional Objects and Transitional Phenomena. *Int. J. Psycho-Anal.*, 34:89–97.

———— (1960), The Theory of the Parent-Infant Relationship. *Int. J. Psycho-Anal.*, 41:585–595.

Persistence of Denial in Fantasy

ANTON O. KRIS, M.D.

> An ego which attempts to save itself anxiety and re-
> nunciation of instinct and to avoid neurosis by deny-
> ing reality is overstraining this mechanism. If this
> happens during the latency period, some abnormal
> character trait will develop.
>
> ANNA FREUD (1936, p. 81f.)

> One of Freud's favourite sayings was: "Man muss ein
> Stück Unsicherheit ertragen können" (One must learn
> to bear some portion of uncertainty).
>
> HANNS SACHS (1944, p. 145)

AS PART OF A LARGER STUDY OF THE FORMS AND FUNCTIONS OF FREE
association, my attention was drawn to a particular pattern in the
analysis of several "narcissistic" adult patients that seems to me
to resemble the latency child's use of denial in fantasy. Typically,
in this pattern, the patients speak freely and fluently, are involved
in what they are saying, earnestly endeavoring to express all
thoughts as they come; and regularly the result is a rebuttal of
their own sense of inadequacy, sometimes complacent, often self-
justifying and self-aggrandizing. The psychoanalyst easily recognizes that the unconscious aim of these associations has all along
been to reach such a gratifying conclusion, to disarm guilt and
counter fears of weakness.

Just when one expected to hear of failure, shame, and doubt,
for example, one young man regularly asserted superiority, satisfaction, and certainty. In another instance, a woman's fears of sex-

---

Dr. Kris is a member of the Faculty of the Boston Psychoanalytic Institute.

ual inadequacy and of never getting married and having children were replaced by overemphasis upon her satisfaction with interminable sexual fantasies about her male analyst. And a man who was virtually paralyzed by ambivalences and who was overwhelmed by fears of bodily injury never tired of reporting his wishes to return to the sunny South of his earliest years and to embark on adventure trips that were filled with courageous action and physical prowess.

Attempts by the analyst to approach the unconscious aim of avoidance directly in such instances lead rapidly to more denial, to devaluation of the analyst, and to withdrawal. An intervention pointing to the patients' emphasis on self-gratification rather than on free expression and understanding is heard as criticism—unfair criticism, at that. For patients regularly believe that such a characterization refers to their conscious intentions instead of to unconscious ones. They feel that the analyst does not acknowledge their conscious dedication to the basic rule. The evident increase in the patients' anxiety and the need for renewed vigor of their defenses only derail the process of association. Insight does not lie that way.

In these circumstances the analyst may suppose that he faces the Charybdis of an endlessly self-gratifying avoidance and the Scylla of destructive confrontation. The analyst's impression, I believe, closely parallels the patients' experience. In such either-or dilemmas, which appear to be insoluble because either alternative seems to lead to intolerable loss, intrasystemic conflicts in all three systems, id, ego, and superego, are always present (Kris, 1977). Their analytic resolution requires a very different management than is needed for intersystemic conflicts. When the analyst attempts to demonstrate the defensive aim of avoidance in the associative pattern I am describing, his approach is the one that regularly succeeds in the interpretation of intersystemic conflict, where analysis of the defenses can be counted upon to reveal the instinctual forces against which they have been deployed. The analysis of intrasystemic conflicts, however, requires a different approach. In their case it is necessary to demonstrate to the patients the mutually frustrating nature of their paired instinctual wishes and the contradictory nature of paired ego and superego attitudes. The analyst must foster the expression first of one side and then of the other of these multiple pairs in successive alternations. In the pattern of free association under discussion here, such a demonstration becomes even more difficult than usual, owing to the extreme sensitivity of these patients to feelings of humiliation and rejection in the transference situation. Even to be shown that they are frustrated is for them a danger calling for defense. Denial as a defense is employed against the perception of projected unconscious guilt.

All "narcissistic" patients whom I have seen, no matter what earlier developmental injuries they may have sustained, perpetuate the additional injuries of the oedipal period in an intensely self-critical attitude (Kris, 1976). Therefore, the gratification obtained in the denial-oriented pattern of association cannot initiate the pendulumlike process of expression of one side and then the other of the frustrated instinctual pairs. While the analysis can make substantial progress in the expression and gratification of the passive libidinal wishes, especially those of preoedipal origin, it is as though the pendulum, blocked by unconscious guilt operating in tandem with castration fears and fears of rejection in loving, cannot swing across the midline to facilitate expression of the active libidinal wishes, especially those of the oedipal phase.

Such conditions determine the choice of an approach that I have found helpful in a number of analyses. Though I present it here schematically, every analyst will recognize that I am only stating a theme, not scoring the full orchestration of the analytic tone poem. This approach starts with the observation of the associative pattern described and then, because of the threatened impasse, turns outside the analysis to study a pattern of behavior in the patients' present life, as they report it in analysis, that can be summarized as a failure to tolerate frustration. This failure may or may not be accompanied by an attitude of narcissistic entitlement (Murray, 1964). It is always accompanied by unconscious guilt. In situations of tension these patients will invariably show some tendency to impulsive avoidance. Of great importance is the intolerance of uncertainty and the consequent difficulty in resolving all forms of ambivalence [1] (intrasystemic conflicts).

1. The concept of ambivalence was, originally, used in psychoanalysis to refer to conflicting feelings of love and hate toward one person. I find it more useful to designate all intrasystemic conflicts, whether in id, ego, or superego,

The process of helping such patients develop greater frustration tolerance is a laborious one for both patient and analyst. It has led, in the patients I have in mind, to a reconstruction of the latency years. Current problems with self-control can be traced to that time of life. This observation fits well with the recognition of a resemblance between the pattern of associations described and the child's use of denial in fantasy. In the latency period, as in their present lives, these patients made use of varying proportions of denial in fantasy and denial in action for defensive purposes. In analysis the pattern of denial in fantasy may appear more prominent because of the demand for putting thoughts, sensations, images, feelings, and wishes to take action into words.

The finding that disorders of development may occur at any age needs no special introduction here. Difficulties in understanding "narcissistic" patients, however, have led some clinicians to attribute all such disorders to a very early phase of self development and object relations. Perhaps the tendency to view denial mechanisms as invariably "primitive" defenses contributes to this tendency (Geleerd, 1965). Patients with very early disorders in development have an especially difficult time in the latency period when they face the task of developing mastery over their own impulses and achieving tolerance of frustration and uncertainty. There are other disorders in the first years of life more narrowly among the precursors of frustration tolerance that may also compromise further development of this capacity in the latency period. Some of these disorders appeared to play a part in the lives of the patients I refer to here. Those earlier contributions, however, were not uniform among my patients, while those of the latency period appeared to be so.

The failure to develop the basis for adequate self-control in the latency period and the reciprocal need to rely excessively on denial mechanisms have their effects in the immediately subsequent problems of adolescence. For in adolescence, with the intensification of impulse, a host of intrasystemic conflicts needs to be resolved—between primary attachments and later ones, and between genital and pregenital, homosexual and heterosexual, and active and pas-

---

as ambivalent. I would not find it useful to extend the meaning of ambivalence to include intersystemic conflict, though there, too, one holds two opposing positions.

sive wishes—no easy task under the best of circumstances. The analysis of the patients under discussion must help them complete this task.

Adolescents must also gain a new sense of independence in their evaluation of the world around them and a corresponding sense of their own integrity. The need to rely upon denial mechanisms to ward off unwelcome perceptions, both from inside and from outside, interferes with attaining these capacities. In the sphere of self-regulation, which must move to new levels in adolescence, the need for denial, especially of unconscious guilt, may utterly invalidate the orienting signal function of affects, with devastating results.

One frequent complaint of these patients—all but one of whom, it happens, were living with both parents during the latency period—is that their parents did not respond sufficiently to their distress, especially to anxieties connected with separating from home in the latency years. (The one patient whose parents were divorced at the beginning of his latency years was especially sensitive to separation and loss, although both parents maintained relationships with him.) On further study one recognizes that the parents of these children may get few clues to the anxiety. Denial mechanisms supervene. Denial in fantasy and the minor impulse-control problems of these patients in the latency years are very easy to miss and very painful to interrupt. The ordinary latency experience for parents and for children is full enough of anguished confrontations; much more so for the child strained by excessive anxiety. Parents who may have their own unconscious reasons for avoiding the children's anxieties can hardly be blamed for failing to turn their quietly well-behaved neurotic child into an anxious, irritating one. Somehow the analyst must permit such a development to occur.[2]

2. "Somehow" covers a good deal of technical ground. I take it for granted that there are differences among analysts and among the several analyses of any one analyst in such a matter. My emphasis, therefore, is on describing patients' experiences, developmental deficiencies, and mechanisms. Even the one specific suggestion I have made already, to move the focus of attention away from the transference, to study behavior outside the analysis as it is reported in the analysis, is a matter of degree and variation and, in any case, only a partial and temporary measure that is not intended to minimize events within the analysis (Gray, 1973).

While these patients complain of their parents' failures to respond to anxieties, they do not complain of their parents' failures to help them develop self-control. They are aware enough of their own lack of self-control, but they blame only themselves, though denial will be used to obliterate perception of the self-criticism much of the time. This situation can be described in a number of ways that may be of use in understanding the patients' situation. Conditions must be established to permit mutual awareness of the problem of self-control. This requires repeated clarification of who is critical of the patient, the patient (unconsciously) or the analyst. These patients also need some clarification of their potential for developing self-control, the basis of hope, for they are utterly pessimistic about mastering this part of their problems. Reconstruction of the events of the latency period regularly shows too little parental support for the child's own efforts and, in some cases, unequivocal seduction by the parents into loss of self-control. Often the child is treated as more grown up than is possible for a child, and is expected to maintain self-control and other aspects of self-sufficiency, too much, too early. In this soil of relative neglect, denial mechanisms flower. In half my cases, however, there was an additional component: misbehavior was ignored or even encouraged; and sexual excitement and aggressive outbursts were stimulated by the parents, without their being aware of it. These latter experiences regularly reappeared in the transference.

The development of frustration tolerance and self-control requires an alliance between children and their parents that these patients did not have sufficiently in the latency years. Such an alliance to foster the development of the child's taking on more and more of the responsibility for self-regulation is part of ordinary growing up. The shift of responsibility from parents to child, at any phase of development, is dependent on a variety of influences, but in the long run they must not exceed the child's tolerance, or unwelcome defensive measures will ensue. In the latency period, the alliance for the development of the child's frustration tolerance and self-control may be strained in many ways. I have already mentioned excessive anxiety as the child emerges from the oedipal phase, insufficient parental support for the child's own efforts, excessive expectations for early self-control, and parental seduction, as typical factors. Others include illness and injury to the child, maturational failures (especially in the sphere of learning disabilities), physical and emotional withdrawal by parents, loss of supporting figures (such as the death of grandparents or the departure from home of older siblings), and parental illness that creates a threat of impending death (which tends to produce a special strain in the tolerance of uncertainty). In the analysis of these adult patients, where the therapeutic goals would seem to imply a natural revival of such an alliance for the development of self-control and frustration tolerance, obstacles arise that demonstrate another source of their self-critical pessimism—a sense of the impenetrable circularity of their deficiencies.

This source of their pessimism derives from a belief that takes shape in adolescence, though it has its precursors in earlier phases of development—that they must choose between parental support and bodily satisfaction. This belief, which the patients apply to all situations in which they ask for assistance, including psychoanalysis, represents an either-or dilemma, a conflict that seems insoluble because either alternative appears to lead to intolerable loss. Revision of the belief requires the resolution of the component intrasystemic conflicts of the dilemma. These include instinctual conflicts between primary and secondary objects and between active and passive aims of libidinal wishes. In the ego and superego there are conflicts between such pairs as gratification and frustration, immediacy and postponement, dependence and autonomy, potentiality and actuality, and between reality and fantasy. To resolve these conflicts the patients must develop self-control and tolerance for frustration and uncertainty, which, in turn, requires the establishment in the analysis of an alliance for the patient's development of these capacities. Unfortunately, the difficulties of forming such an alliance are compounded by fears of too great dependence, by fears of having to give up *all* expression and satisfaction of bodily desires, by a feeling of being insignificant, by a wish for a speedier approach to pressing problems, and so on—in short, a vicious cycle. In my experience, these patients have all too correct an intuitive grasp of the problem posed by these conditions. Analytic resolution of this problem and its components makes up a significant part of their analyses.

The problem of deficient self-control and tolerance of frustration always links up with conflicts over masturbation. In my experience, these patients generally engage in an intense masturbatory sexual life alongside a variably satisfying heterosexuality. (None of the patients I am referring to engaged in homosexuality in the adult years, as it happens.) In the analysis, derivatives of early childhood masturbation conflicts are reviewed at the same time as they are remobilized in present conflicts over masturbation. The multiple meanings and functions of the masturbation must be identified repeatedly. It is necessary, I find, to distinguish between function, such as the avoidance of a partner, and meaning, such as the gratification of wishes that may be forbidden in the presence of the partner. Adult masturbation, though it reflects immaturity and failure to resolve conflict, may also represent a means of partial self-control. For example, masturbation may be an outlet for sadistic components of loving that cannot otherwise be held in check. Or masturbation may gratify homosexual components of loving and thereby preserve the heterosexual relationship. As the analysis gradually contributes to a resolution of the corresponding intrasystemic instinctual conflicts, it permits more satisfying solutions than obligatory masturbation.

When new hope has developed from the process of analytic insight, and when the capacity to tolerate frustration has been strengthened, the focus of the analysis can return to the point of departure, the pattern of denial in fantasy. The analyst does not relinquish the extra role assigned to him in the transference—for only the patient can decide on that—but he can now exert his influence within the analysis in his usual way, studying the associations and clarifying their multiple meanings. Slowly the fears that determine the associative pattern can be identified. Gradually the frightening oedipal transference, the major stimulus for denial, can be approached in the analysis, but no matter how many years have gone into preparing the way, its intensity makes it seem to have come too soon. One can well understand why patients and analysts alike might choose to pass it by. It would be less than candid, in that regard, not to acknowledge that one of my patients still could not tolerate the full intensity of the castration fears after many years of otherwise successful analysis and major gains in the conduct of his life. He has persisted, however, in efforts toward mastery of the remaining problems since we agreed to interrupt his analysis.

Among the half dozen patients I have treated in this way, preoedipal pathology has been variable, though all had suffered significant strain in the preoedipal phases of separation from their mothers. Such strain and other preoedipal difficulties did not, however, provide a basis for differentiating between these patients and others who do not make use of an associative pattern of denial in fantasy to the same extent.

To summarize, I have described a pattern of free association which appears in the analyses of "narcissistic" patients and which seems to be the counterpart of the child's use of denial in fantasy to ward off feelings of weakness and insecurity of oedipal and preoedipal origin. This pattern serves a self-gratifying function as well as a defensive function; it poses a significant problem in analysis, because the patients who employ this pattern have failed to master the latency task of developing tolerance for tension, frustration, and uncertainty. They have, I believe, persisted too long in the use of denial in fantasy and denial in action. They are therefore ill-equipped to master through analysis the intrasystemic conflicts which were not adequately resolved in adolescence and which continue to plague them, since the analysis of these conflicts requires more tolerance for uncertainty than they can muster.

An approach to the therapeutic problem is outlined, which begins with a focus on present-day problems of impulse control and failures of frustration tolerance. It gradually reawakens the hope for an alliance for the development of self-control, abandoned in the postoedipal period. In the course of this aspect of the treatment, the patients develop new strengths to apply to the still unresolved ambivalences, especially those between oedipal and preoedipal wishes. The oedipal transferences in the analyses of these patients, even when the way has been prepared in this manner, remain unusually difficult to analyze, especially because of the intensity of the patients' fears.

BIBLIOGRAPHY

FREUD, A. (1936), The Ego and the Mechanisms of Defense. *W.*, 2.

GELEERD, E. R. (1965), Two Kinds of Denial. In: *Drives, Affects, Behavior,* ed. M. Schur. New York: Int. Univ. Press, 2:118–127.

GRAY, P. (1973), Psychoanalytic Technique and the Ego's Capacity for Viewing Intrapsychic Activity. *J. Amer. Psychoanal. Assn.*, 21:474–494.

KRIS, A. O. (1976), On Wanting Too Much. *Int. J. Psycho-Anal.*, 57:85–95.

────── (1977), Either-Or Dilemmas. *This Annual*, 32:91–117.

MURRAY, J. M. (1964), Narcissism and the Ego Ideal. *J. Amer. Psychoanal. Assn.*, 12:477–511.

SACHS, H. (1944), *Freud: Master and Friend.* Freeport: Books for Libraries Press, 1970.

Reflections on the Psychoanalytic Process and Its Therapeutic Potential

HANS W. LOEWALD, M.D.

AS A SPECIAL FORM OF PSYCHOTHERAPY, PSYCHOANALYSIS CONSTI-
tutes a unique mode of personal relationship. It shares certain
aspects with other kinds of psychotherapy and personal relationships, for instance, with those between child and parent, patient
and physician, student and teacher, between friends and between
lovers. But the relationship between analysand and analyst is quite
different from all of them. There appears to be something inher-
ently unnatural and contradictory about it. In an important sense
it is engaged in for the purpose of a deeper understanding of
human relationships and of their impact on the organization of
the individual's inner life in time—although this purpose often
is but vaguely, if at all, grasped by the analysand when he enters
treatment. While there is this engagement, there is at the same
time, and from the beginning, a countermovement of disengagement. I am not speaking here of resistance, at least not in the
usual sense, but of the fact that the dissolution and abnegation of
whatever factual reality the relationship tends to assume are part
and parcel of the analytic method from the start. The reason is
that individuation and what we consider mature object relations,
while originating and culminating in intimacy, involve and are

Faculty, Western New England Psychoanalytic Institute, New Haven, Conn.
Contribution to Panel on "Conceptualizing the Nature of the Therapeutic
Action of Psychoanalysis," held at the Fall Meeting of the American Psycho-
analytic Association, New York, December 16, 1977.

dependent on separation, alienation, and renunciations along the way from infancy to adulthood. Without these there cannot be effective internalization, that is, the building of a stable self that can maintain viable object relations.

The analytic relationship, then, comes into being as a sort of self-played dramatic play in and by which the history of the individual is reexperienced, restructured, acquires new meanings, and regains old meanings that were lost. But this relationship is never allowed to materialize fully as an actual relationship. It has the substantiality and the evanescence of a play, as well as that quality of a child's play: it seems to exist for its own sake and at the same time to be a rehearsal for real life.

The analytic method of treatment requires simultaneously unusual restraints and endurance of frustration together with an uncommon quality and degree of intimacy, spontaneity, and freedom—and this, although in different ways, from both partners.

Except in child analysis, both participants are adults, with the age difference often insignificant or nonexistent, yet the relationship is asymmetrical, much of the time experienced by the analysand as unjustly unequal. If the analysis progresses well, this asymmetry and sense of inequality gradually recede, not unlike what happens between parents and children as the children grow into adolescence and beyond, if things go well there.

The relationship between analysand and analyst is comparable to adolescent and oedipal relationships and their derivatives, but also to the infant-mother "dual unit." Much of the analytic work centers around oedipal conflicts, but more and more, in many cases, also around developmental defects and distortions related to those early phases of the individuation process described by child analysts. In this connection, the self-object differentiation, until recently considered an essential condition of what we have believed to be scientific objectivity and analytic objectivity—this dichotomy can, to say the least, no longer be taken for granted as the single or basic mode of cognition and mental interactions. Is it the relevant mode and basis for all mental transactions between analysand and analyst, or is there a deep unconscious level on which this dichotomy is not valid? If the latter, for the sake of a more encompassing objectivity vis-à-vis the psychoanalytic process and its therapeutic potential this needs to be further elucidated. We are far from understanding much about it.

There are other problems I want to mention, some of them related to the above. What are the preconditions for analysis? Is its scope becoming too wide, or is it, as traditionally understood, too narrow? Is the psychoanalytic process one of objective investigation of "psychological facts," or is it "interpretation of meanings?" If the latter, are the meanings there, to be uncovered by us as analysts, or are we, although not arbitrarily, providing meanings? Are the patients providing the meanings, or the psychological facts, as a function of our active receptivity as analysts? Are "meanings" something that arises in the interactions between analysand and analyst?

It is questioned, in view of rapid, sometimes radical, changes in and dissolutions of cultural norms and child-rearing methods, whether we still can speak of an average expectable environment and in conjunction with it of an "average expectable physical and mental equipment" of the child (the latter expression used by Anna Freud, 1976, p. 259).

These and many other questions, doubts, novel conceptual approaches, often are disconcerting and troublesome; they are at times formulated too naïvely or too stridently, or do not give due weight to important aspects and factors involved in very complex problems. But I believe that they are raised where psychoanalysis is most alive, endangered, and troubled—yes, but not in danger of ossification. At the International Congress in London in 1975 much was heard of the malaise of psychoanalysts (Green, 1975; Anna Freud, 1976), as though it were a new phenomenon. But is malaise, *Unbehagen,* discontent, not a condition of life for psychoanalysis, one of the reasons for as well as a result of the rise of psychoanalysis? Does this go for a therapeutic analysis too? If a result of psychoanalysis is malaise, suffering, is it therapeutic? Does its therapeutic potential reside, as Freud (1916–17) suggested, in a subtle but crucial shift in the quality of suffering? Is malaise, as Anna Freud seemed to imply in her discussion at that Congress, incompatible with excitement and satisfaction?

Most important questions are—as is true in our clinical work— not raised in order to be answered with a yes or no or a clear-cut reply, but in order to address oneself to and reflect on issues that are brought to the fore by the question or that arise within its context.

Let me turn briefly to some pragmatic considerations. A therapeutic analysis, as a treatment process extending over a long period of time, is a blend consisting, even in the hands of the most purist analyst, not only of verbal interpretation of free associations, fantasies, dreams, and other verbal and nonverbal material, in terms of transference and resistance. Aside from their content, the timing of interpretations, the context in which they are made, the way they are phrased, the tone of voice, are important elements of therapeutic action. Clarifications and confrontations are used, historical discrepancies are pointed out, comments and interpretations are made that are not or only indirectly related to the analytic transference itself. Tact, basic rapport and its fluctuations, the analyst's breadth of life experience and imagination, the manner in which intercurrent events in the patient's life, incidents before, during, and after the analytic hour, are handled—all these and other factors are significant ingredients of the therapeutic action. They constitute the actual medium without which the most correct interpretations are likely to remain unconvincing and ineffective. So-called educational measures, at times encouragement and reassurance, are used. If used judiciously, they often make possible and enhance the more strictly psychoanalytic interventions, and this not only in the initial phases of an analysis. Psychoanalysis, a distinct and unique therapeutic method, in actual practice makes use, if sparingly, of therapeutic measures that are in themselves not analytic, while inspired and guided constantly by the model of the psychoanalytic method. A clinical analysis and the nature of its therapeutic action are more complex, more lifelike than any theory or model. Attempts at conceptualizing the therapeutic action always will stress certain aspects at the expense of others.

The conceptualization of therapeutic action at any given historical moment also is a function of particular predilections, biases, and innovations of that moment, of preoccupations with specific clinical problems, theoretical issues, and research interests.

To this must be added the impact of fashions whose origins are not always apparent and which are often determined or strongly influenced by extra-analytic cultural currents. And we often encounter reactions and overreactions to preceding slants and fashions.

I return now to more strictly psychoanalytic considerations of the psychoanalytic process. The complexities and intricacies of relationship between analysand and analyst have come under more careful scrutiny in recent years. It is no longer only a question of investigating the patient's transference and resistance, of considering the analyst's stance as objective-empathic observer and interpreter or of his possible countertransference and counterresistance as interfering factors. The origins of the psychoanalytic exploration of the nature of the patient-analyst relationship, as a relationship, can be traced back to the teens of the century when Freud, Ferenczi, Federn, Tausk, and others began to concern themselves with the problems of narcissistic identification, introjection, projection, the ego ideal, ego boundaries. What we term object cathexis was recognized as developing out of less differentiated "emotional ties" called identifications. The differentiation of, and the establishment of boundaries between, self and objects came into focus as developmental processes. Thus, that distinction itself could no longer be taken for granted as the unquestioned single basis for psychoanalytic investigations. There are kinds of relatedness between what conventionally we refer to as self and object, which call into question the universal validity of these very terms. We have come to see that there are levels of mental functioning and experience where these distinctions are not made, or made only fleetingly and in rudimentary form. These are deep unconscious layers showing modes of interpsychic relatedness, of emotional ties that are active under the surface in both analysand and analyst, and thus in *their* relatedness, forming ingredients of the therapeutic potential. The psychic reality or validity of these more deeply hidden unconscious levels is no more dubious than the psychic reality of unconscious oedipal currents and conflicts and their manifestations in the transference—that is, seen from a perspective which goes beyond conscious mentation (the original meaning of the word "metapsychological"), but their strangeness and uncanniness are more pronounced. These layers of experience, too, coexist with the more advanced levels of mental functioning and organization of mental content, and continue to exert their influence throughout life.

Schematically speaking, I would say that in the classical transference neuroses unmastered oedipal conflicts and their derivatives are revived and reworked in the psychoanalytic situation of controlled and limited regression, which enables the analyst to interpret those unconscious contents and their forms of mentation in terms of conscious content and form of organization. The analyst has to have a flexible and firm hold on his conscious, objective, frame of reference, a frame of reference the analysand tends to lose or to maintain too rigidly. The analyst, as empathizer, in order to be able to interpret has to experience with the analysand on the analysand's primitive level of functioning. Unless the analyst's own oedipal attachments and their inherent conflicts, while having been and repeatedly being "mastered" by him, remain for him alive and available, true empathy does not take place. His interpretations, although correct as to abstract content, are not likely to touch the patient so that he can make them his own. This is a side that Freud did not dwell on, although undoubtedly he was aware of it. Freud emphasized the patient's autonomous defenses against assimilating interpretations. The validity and pertinence of such autonomy, however, recede as we penetrate to deeper unconscious levels, where there are communication and interdependence between the unconscious of the patient and that of the analyst.

What is true for the classical transference neuroses (with their main basis in the oedipus complex) also goes for those disturbances that are included in the widening scope of analysis. If I again speak schematically and omit a great many complex clinical problems, these disturbances (narcissistic disorders, borderline cases, etc.) can best be understood as rooted in those deeper unconscious levels where the distinction between self and object is at a vanishing point, blurred, uncertain, unstable, or even nonexistent. As we became more aware of and better acquainted with these forms of mental functioning, we also have come to recognize that problems in the classical neuroses, which had been seen mainly in the light of psychosexual conflicts rooted in the oedipal phase, are often importantly codetermined by disruptive, distorting, and inhibiting influences occurring during earlier phases. Such recognition and the ability to work with these problems analytically are dependent on the analyst's awareness and mastery of his own problems in this area—an extension of the principle that an analyst can understand and help his patient only as far as he understands himself and is ahead of the patient in the degree of mastery of his unconscious. Problems of self-object differentiation, with its inherent issues of the polarity between individuation and merging union, probably are not less but more universal and deep-seated than psychosexual conflicts of the oedipal nucleus of neurosis. They are what some have called the psychotic core of our mental life, an expression that should be understood in the same sense in which we speak of the oedipus complex as the nucleus of neurosis. Such expressions refer to pathogenicity, not to pathology itself. All of us are heirs to this psychotic core. That is the nugget of truth in Melanie Klein's work, as much as many of us disagree with her emphasis, her metapsychological elaborations and speculations, and her technical procedures.

Many patients coming to analysis have, sustained by a sufficiently favorable early environment, mastered this psychotic core enough so that no or little explicit analytic work need be devoted to it. But with many patients in analysis nowadays a good deal of work has to be devoted to the analytic revival and working through of such problems. "Nowadays" means the present world in which patients and analysts alike have grown up and live. Many patients and many analysts are different from those half a century and more ago, and so is analysis. How could it be otherwise? It is not that human nature has changed since then, but shifts in inner and outer reality and their interaction have brought to the fore differently centered conflicts and disruptive influences, revealing to the psychoanalyst levels and phenomena of unconscious processes and their derivations that earlier could hardly have come into clear focus.

In my analytic experience, oedipal conflicts—to use that shorthand expression—are no less important today than they have always been. And their neglect, when it occurs, is an overreaction to exclusive preoccupation with them. But it is not surprising that the analytic situation so frequently today is compared with that developmental stage in which the phenomena and pathogenic issues of self-object differentiation, of the initial stages of individuation, of the formation of a cohesive self and of object relations, first come into view, namely, the infant-mother dyad. The mental functioning and the derivatives of that developmental phase today are a focus of analytic exploration and interpretation. These archaic levels and their sublimated equivalents in the adult are revived and become available in the analytic situation—as is true of the oedipal level—through the medium or vehicle of transference and resistance, i.e., through the analysis of the patient's relatedness with the analyst. The patient-analyst relationship in its totality is highly complex, has many facets, levels, and stages. I shall come back to this briefly later on. On the archaic level now under discussion, the patient-analyst relatedness is not an object relationship in the usual sense. On that level of his mental life— and I oversimplify here for purposes of exposition—the patient is not, does not experience himself as, a self clearly distinguishable from the analyst as an object; by the same token, the analyst is not experienced as clearly distinguishable from the patient as self. Kohut (1971) speaks of narcissistic or self-object transference— transference insofar as there is not a lack of relatedness, not a "withdrawal of libido into the ego," but a lack of differentiation between two relatable entities that could be called self and object.

Unless the analyst grasps that he is, on the now pertinent level of the patient's mental functioning, drawn into this undifferentiated forcefield, he will not be able to interpret adequately the transference meanings of the patient's communications. To do so, he has to be in touch with that mental level in himself, a level on which for him, too, the distance and separateness between himself and the patient are reduced or suspended. Ego boundaries, the whole complex individuating organization of self-object differentiation, tend to dissolve. The difference between the patient and the analyst is that the former is at the mercy of that primitive level (inundated by it or disavowing it), whereas the analyst is aware of but not given over to it. The undifferentiatedness of that level also involves a dedifferentiation of the secondary process difference between words and their referents ("things"), between words as sound entities and their "meanings" or what they symbolize. Such dedifferentiation entails special qualities of intimacy, intensity, and poignancy of communication, both verbal and nonverbal, or, in the absence of empathy, of total, though temporary, alienation (depersonalization and derealization).[1]

The analyst—as is true, though on a relatively more advanced level, in the case of the more familiar transference manifestations—for a stretch joins the patient on a potentially common level of experience. On that basis the analyst can translate, as it were, that form of experience, by means of articulate and specifying language, onto a level that is further differentiated, thereby enabling the patient to join the analyst, for a stretch, on the path to higher differentiation and articulation of experience.

Having spoken of the archaic pole of analysis, I now turn briefly to its overall conditions and intentions which make feasible and justify the whole undertaking. I come back here to the complexity and the apparent contradictions of the analytic relationship. I wish now to stress the risks of misunderstanding and distortion when the analytic situation is compared with the early parent-child dyadic relationship, as illuminating as this comparison is in many respects. When all is said and done, the widening scope of analysis notwithstanding, the analytic situation, in contradistinction to other, often related psychotherapeutic settings, presupposes or is encompassed in an adult overall setting—at least as far as work with adults is concerned. I am not competent to speak of the necessary modifications and qualifications in regard to child analysis.[2] The analysis of adults, no matter how much given to regression or immature they are in significant areas of their functioning, is a venture in which the analysand not only is in fact, chronologically, a grownup, but which makes sense only if his or

1. For a discussion of primary process and secondary process mentation in their relations to language, see Loewald (1978).
2. It is to be considered whether, in the case of child analysis, the "adult overall setting" is provided by the understanding "cooperation" of the parents or parent. If such cooperation is not available, child analysis apparently tends to become difficult or impossible.

her adult potential, as manifested in certain significant areas of life, is in evidence. The predominantly verbal channeling of expression and communication, the restraints on action, the high degree of tolerance for frustration, the required capacity for reflection, as well as the unique spontaneity and freedom of responsiveness as elements of the analytic situation—even if some or all of them are available in anything but their optimal form—these characteristics make psychoanalysis an adult undertaking.

Thus there is a grid of rational adult mentation through which the analytic experience, and specifically the transference in all its primitive and more advanced variations, is sifted or screened. Analysis as a relatively continuous process, sustained over a protracted period of time, not constantly disrupted by irrational *manifest* behavior, requires the patient's capacity for this kind of rational mediation as a fairly reliable compass and overall guide. The engagement and development of this capacity frequently need the overt or silent support of the analyst, but the analyst cannot create it. This does not mean that analytic methods, including transference interpretations, and analytic knowledge and insights cannot be used at given times in cases where analysis as a sustained clinical process is not feasible. And it is to be emphasized that analysts can and do learn a great deal about the unconscious and about transference from patients who for practical purposes are unsuitable for sustained therapeutic analysis—often learning things about unconscious processes and transference phenomena that they then can use in their strictly analytic work. This actually has been the case ever since Freud and the early pioneers began to concern themselves with problems of psychosis.

Anna Freud (1976) spoke of the difference between understanding a mental aberration and the possibility to cure it, suggesting that there is no obvious reason to assume "that any mental affliction which is open to analytic understanding is open also to analytic cure" (p. 260). This issue has interested me for years. I think that any answer to the problem has to wait for further insights concerning the structure and function of psychoanalytic understanding. At present our insight is insufficient. But I suspect that there is no psychoanalytic understanding worthy of the name that leaves that which is to be understood altogether untouched and unchanged, if one is to judge from the act of understanding that takes place in a piece of analytic work during an hour. It is true that our understanding has to be communicated to the patient in an interpretation. Yet, it seems to me that an interpretation is not so much the *result* of understanding as it is the means by which understanding proceeds; this has to do with the intimate inter-relations between thought and language. Understanding as an act—as distinguished from a storehouse of knowledge that we make use of for understanding—is impossible unless the patient lends himself and is open to our understanding, although he may not know that and may fight against it; and it is to *his* powers of understanding that we speak when we interpret. In this sense, while understanding does not spell "cure," it is a therapeutic step. Perhaps it could simply be said that a therapeutic step occurs when the patient feels understood. It is a curious fact, however, that unless the patient feels understood, we do not feel that we have understood him. Understanding would seem to be an act that involves some sort of mutual engagement, a particular form of the meeting of minds. As applied to self-understanding, it would in-volve the mutual engagement of different mental levels.

Psychoanalytic interpretations are based on the analyst's self-understanding, and self-understanding is reactivated in the act of interpretation to the patient. Self-understanding originates in the early interactions between child and caring parent. For the ana-lyst, his self-understanding is resumed, vastly increased, enriched, and deepened in his own training analysis. On that basis—firmed up and articulated by the rest of his training—he is enabled to understand the patient if the latter is open to it. Interpretation is an activity in which the analyst mediates or conveys self-understanding or its possibility to the patient, something the patient then is enabled to make his own or internalize as an intrapsychic activity.

Psychoanalytic interpretations establish, or make explicit, bridges between two minds, and within the patient bridges be-tween different areas and layers of the mind that lack or have lost connections with each other, that are not encompassed within an overall contextual organization of the personality. Interpretations establish or reestablish links between islands of unconscious mentation and between the unconscious and consciousness. They are translations that do not simply make the unconscious conscious or cause ego to be where id was: they link these different forms and contents of mental life, going back and forth between them. There are interpretations upward and interpretations downward. What is therapeutic, I believe, is the mutual linking itself by which each of the linked elements gains or regains meaning or becomes richer in meaning—meaning being our word for the resultant of that reciprocal activity. In the reinitiation and promotion of this process the interpretative activity of the analyst and the specific contents of interpretations are the enabling factors; he envisages and holds for the patient that context which makes linking possible.

One last comment, having to do with pleasure. Interpretations may gratify the patient. All of us know how patients may exploit or try to exploit the giving of interpretations for the sake of direct instinctual gratification. We also know that there are interpretations that are, at least at first, anything but gratifying to the patient. On a different level, however, the interpretations that the patient assimilates and makes his own are and should be gratifying the patient's desire for responsive understanding and articulation of his deepest needs and highest wishes. These are gratifications that reverberate, together with the frustrations inherent in analysis, throughout the whole spectrum of mental life. On that foundation, shaky as it still is likely to be at the termination of analysis, separation from and renunciation of the analyst become possible and in the end an inner requirement.

BIBLIOGRAPHY

FREUD, A. (1976), Changes in Psychoanalytic Practice and Experience. *Int. J. Psycho-Anal.*, 57:257–260.
FREUD, S. (1916–17), Introductory Lectures on Psycho-Analysis. *S.E.*, 15 & 16.
GREEN, A. (1975), The Analyst, Symbolization and Absence in the Analytic Setting. *Int. J. Psycho-Anal.*, 56:1–22.
KOHUT, H. (1971), *The Analysis of the Self.* New York: Int. Univ. Press.
LOEWALD, H. W. (1978), Primary Process, Secondary Process, and Language. In: *Psychiatry and the Humanities,* ed. J. H. Smith. New Haven & London: Yale Univ. Press, 3:235–270.

MAHLER, M. S. (1968), *On Human Symbiosis and the Vicissitudes of Individuation*. New York: Int. Univ. Press.

SYMPOSIUM (1954), The Widening Scope of Indications for Psychoanalysis. *J. Amer. Psychoanal. Assn.*, 4:567–620.

The Psychoanalytic Theory of Cognitive Development

PINCHAS NOY, M.D.

FREUD'S MAJOR CONTRIBUTION TO THE PSYCHOLOGY OF COGNITION lies in his formulation of a dual theory, one which conceptualizes the cognitive processes as being composed of two sets of processes, each operating according to its own organizational rules. In his biography of Freud, Jones (1953) states, "Freud's revolutionary contribution to psychology was not so much his demonstrating the existence of an unconscious, and perhaps not even his exploration of its content, as his proposition that there are two fundamentally different kinds of mental processes, which he termed primary and secondary" (p. 397).

The studies of Freud as well as those of psychoanalytically oriented clinical and experimental researchers since Freud have proved repeatedly that the distinction between the primary and secondary processes involves practically all areas of cognitive functioning—thinking, perception, communication, and others.

This study represents an attempt to show that:

1. Every cognitive function operates according to two different organizational modes: one mode submitted to the organizational rules of the primary process, and the other to those of the secondary process.

2. The normal development of the cognitive apparatus as a whole as well as that of any of its separate functions requires that

---

Dr. Noy is a member of the Israel Psychoanalytic Society, and a part-time teacher (as a Visiting Professor) in the Hebrew University in Jerusalem.

both the primary and the secondary processes reach optimal levels of development and maturation.

3. Normal, mature cognitive functioning in any area depends upon there being a sound balance between primary and secondary process operations.

4. The organizational modes of primary and secondary processes reflect the two main forms of adaptation that characterize humans—the autoplastic and the alloplastic forms.

On the basis of these four assumptions, I will use autonomy as a criterion for distinguishing between the primary and secondary processes, proposing a new developmental theory of cognition and discussing its implication for psychoanalysis.

THE DEVELOPMENT OF THE TWO MODES OF ORGANIZATION

Almost all of the contemporary theories of cognitive development approach cognition as a one-track system, and its development as a linear process proceeding along a single developmental line. The fact is that although psychoanalysis has repeatedly attempted to assimilate part of several of these theories, such as those of Piaget or Werner, it has never been able to adopt any of them *in toto*. The dual concept of primary and secondary processes is so deeply rooted in psychoanalytic conceptualization, that any developmental theory which does not view cognition as being composed of two systems, forms, modes, levels—or, at least, as a continuum stretched between two organizational centers—can never be integrated into psychoanalytic metapsychology.

The question, then, is: if psychoanalysis could not adopt any of the prevailing theories of cognitive development, why has it never developed its own theory? The reason seems to lie in the still current inability to formulate one common theory regarding the structure and function of the primary process. Without such a formulation, a developmental theory can never be formed.

In classical psychoanalysis, the primary process was regarded as a primitive, infantile, chaotic, unstructured, and pleasure-oriented mode of ideation, which, as Cameron (1963) states, "includes throughout life the primitive rock-bottom activities, the raw strivings and strange unconscious maneuvers of the human being. It includes prelogical archaic symbolism, a peculiar interchange of expressive vehicles, a tendency to condense the cathexes of several drives into one, and an absence of such logical necessities as negation, resolution of contradiction, and the recognition of time and spatial relations" (p. 155).

Many psychoanalysts still adhere to this assumption, e.g., Kligerman (1972), who "criticized some recent attempts to elevate the role of primary process in creativity," and stated that the "Primary process is a primitive discharge mode, and as soon as it undergoes modification into higher levels of organization it is no longer primary process. The tendency to apply the term to highly sophisticated non-verbal operations leads only to theoretical confusion" (p. 28). The relation between the primary and secondary process was conceptualized, in line with the Jacksonian model, with the latter regarded as "overriding" and controlling the primary processes, "secondarily revising" the products, and inhibiting the free activity, of the primary (Klein, 1970). Conveniently, neurophysiological research managed to prove that the substrate of the secondary processes is found in the higher cortical centers, while that of primary processes is found in subcortical centers, especially in the limbic system and the hypocampus (for a comprehensive survey of the pertinent neurophysiological studies, see Meissner, 1968).

The view of the primary processes as primitive, chaotic, and unstructured gradually began to change in the 1950s. One of the first to influence this change was Ehrenzweig (1953) who, basing himself on studies of artistic activity, claimed that the primary processes include organizational and ordering abilities to an extent that may sometimes exceed even those of the secondary processes. In 1967, Ehrenzweig contended that while the secondary process organizes perceptual data into gestalts and tends to focus mainly on details, the primary process scans the entire perceptual field in an undifferentiated manner, taking in entire structures. This undifferentiated mode of scanning, which may be a disadvantage in logical reasoning, may prove to be an advantage for creative achievements in art and science.

Holt (1967) tried to analyze the concept of the primary process from the structural point of view. He writes, "the central point of my argument is the proposition that primary process is not synonymous with chaos, with random error" (p. 367), and concludes, "we can conceptualize the primary process as a special system of processing information in the service of synthetic necessity" (p. 383). Moses (1968), referring to the formal rules governing unconscious id material, writes about the primary processes: "These are organizational forms that differ from those of secondary process functioning, but they are organizational forms nonetheless" (p. 211).

I have suggested (1969) that the primary process be conceptualized as neither inferior nor superior to the secondary process with regard to organizational properties, but only as *different*. Both groups of processes are to be regarded as equally developed, structured, refined, and efficient; their only difference lies in their processing mental data according to different organizational criteria. In 1973, I compared the two processes to two programs processing the same information in one computer, and suggested the term "horizontal processing" for the secondary process mode and "vertical processing" for the primary process mode. I argued that the difference between the primary and secondary processes is mainly functional, and that the differences in their organizational modes merely reflect the function assigned to each process. The function of the secondary process is to handle everything related to reality orientation, i.e., perception and inner representation of reality, control of reality-oriented behavior, and information exchange through communication. The function of the primary process is to handle everything related to the regulation, maintenance, and development of the self, i.e., assimilation of new experience into the self; accommodation of the self to changing experience and growing reality demands; and integration of the self to safeguard its cohesion, unity, and continuity. For this reason, I define the secondary process as *reality-oriented* and the primary process as *self-centered.*

The mental apparatus needs two different sets of organizational process because the functional requirements of reality orientation are so different from those of self-regulation that each demands its own specific instruments, mechanisms, and modes of processing mental material. Ordinary cognition always combines primary and secondary process operations, constantly fluctuating between the two organizational poles in order to cater to the changing functional requirements. If the mental task is more reality-oriented, cognition shifts in the direction of the secondary process pole (as in reality-oriented problem solving, verbal communication); and if the task is more self-centered, cognition shifts in the direction of the primary process pole (as in dreaming, fantasizing, contemplation). In some rare but blessed instances, cognition succeeds in embracing the whole range of its primary and secondary process operations and in synthesizing the organizational modes of each. This is what happens at the heights of spurts of creativity in art and science, and in moments of insight in psychoanalysis, those rare moments when reality and self blend into one experience (Noy, 1978).

It is interesting to note that those parts of this theory which regard the primary and secondary processes as differing only in their organizational modes have recently been supported by neurophysiological research. Modern studies on the lateralization of the brain cortex proved that the dominant left hemisphere operates dominantly according to secondary process modes. Galin (1974) assumed that while the left hemisphere is specialized for verbalization and linear, analytic logic, "the right hemisphere uses a nonverbal mode of representation . . . a nonlinear mode of association . . . its solutions to problems are based on multiple converging determinants rather than a single causal chain . . . grasping the concept of the whole from just a part" (p. 574). Hoppe (1977) states, "The right hemisphere senses the forest, so to speak, while the left one cannot see the woods for the trees" (p. 220).

Those who uphold the experimental approach to psychoanalysis will find sustenance in the fact that a theory such as that of Ehrenzweig (1953, 1967), who knew nothing about the studies of brain lateralization, can be supported by objective research. On the other hand, the cynic will exploit this to claim that it provides a good "lesson" for anyone who takes scientific objectivity too seriously. Instead of experimental research being the basis for formulating psychological theories, it has somehow managed "objectively" to support the fashionable theory. When everyone re-

garded the secondary as overriding the primary process, neurophysiology proved that the secondary process is located in the
cortex and the primary process in the lower subcortical nuclei;
but when the view changed so that both processes were regarded
as equal but only organizationally different, neurophysiology
proved that they are located at exactly the same height in both
hemispheres.

The lack of consensus concerning the structure and function of
the primary process has prevented psychoanalysis from coming to
any agreement about its course of development. In fact, classical
psychoanalysis did not attribute any development at all to the
primary processes. Freud (1900) wrote, "But this much is a fact:
the primary processes are present in the mental apparatus from
the first, while it is only during the course of life that the secondary processes unfold, and come to inhibit and overlay the
primary ones; it may even be that their complete domination is
not attained until the prime of life" (p. 603).

In line with this statement, the primary process was regarded
by most psychoanalysts as inherent, already present in infancy.
With the evolution of the secondary processes the former are
thrust into the unconscious to remain there, according to the law
of the unconscious, without change forever. As formulated by
Freud (1915), "The processes of the system *Ucs.* are *timeless;* i.e.
they are not ordered temporally, are not altered by the passage
of time; they have no reference to time at all" (p. 187). This
means that the primary process is to be regarded as something that
springs from nowhere, and develops toward nowhere, a strange
group of functions for which there is nothing similar to be found
among all other biological functions!

Rapaport (1960), who surveyed Freud's theory of the primary
and secondary processes, admitted that "Freud did much to clarify
the relationship between these two types of thought process, . . .
but many aspects of their relationship, and in particular their
maturational and developmental relationship, remained ambiguous" (p. 836). Holt (1967) tried to define the reasons for the confusion concerning the eventual developmental course of the primary process: "One circumstance that makes this position seem a
perverse or paradoxical one is the ambiguity of the term primary

process, for it is used by psychoanalysts to refer to modes of acting and experiencing affect ("process of discharge") as well as to a kind of cognition" (p. 364). As a mode of action it is conceptualized as one of immediate discharge, in the service of the pleasure principle which does not tolerate any constraints or delay. Therefore, "it would be surprising indeed if an inability to tolerate delay had to be attained by a process of growth" (p. 365). However, Holt regards the primary process as "the product of development" only if it is approached as a system of cognition (p. 365).

Both Rapaport and Holt tried, each in his own way, to suggest a theory for the development of the primary process. In Rapaport's view, "the secondary process does not simply arise from the primary process under the pressure of environmental necessity, but, like the primary process, arises from an undifferentiated matrix in which its intrinsic maturational restraining and integrating factors are already present" (p. 842f.). The course of development of both processes is determined by "intrinsic maturational factors, which can be modified by experience" (p. 846), but there is a difference in regard to the factors determining the development of each process: "The intrinsic maturational factors involved in the primary processes are related to the instinctual drives, and those involved in the secondary processes are related to instinctual-drive restraints and synthetic functions" (p. 844).

Holt (1967) takes a slightly different stance, stating that "The position I wish to develop is that primary-process thinking (or ideation) is not present at birth, and does not arise from the undifferentiated phase by a simple process of bifurcation, but that it presupposes many of the stages of what Piaget . . . has called the development of sensorimotor intelligence. . . . The basic facts of cognitive development, therefore, lay the groundwork for the primary and secondary processes alike" (p. 364).

The problem with both of these approaches—and I identify with their essentials—is that they outline the development of the primary process only until the maturational phase when the secondary process "takes over" and dominates conscious cognition, but say nothing about what happens to the primary process later on. To the best of my knowledge, this issue has never been tackled explicitly. The question of the further development of the primary process therefore remains unsettled. Everything said in the psychoanalytic literature about later cognitive development, the development of reality representation, of language, and even of representation of the self, relates only to the development of the secondary process. It would seem as self-evident that, at a particular point, the developmental course shifts from the primary to the secondary process, and that only the latter continues to mature and develop, leaving the primary process in its infantile-primitive form forever.

I have previously (1969) suggested a new approach to the development of the primary process based on the "self-centered" vs. "reality-oriented" theory. I believe that the primary processes never cease their development, but continue to evolve and mature hand in hand with the secondary processes and all other cognitive functions. The developmental course of both processes is determined by the function each is assigned: the secondary processes continue to develop as a part of all the reality-oriented functions of the cognitive apparatus and the primary processes as a part of the self-regulating functions. As time passes, the secondary processes become more and more specialized in order to deal efficiently with reality. This development is expressed in the evergrowing ability to perceive, represent, and understand reality, the capacity to solve problems, and the ability to use language. The primary processes, at the same time, become more and more specialized to deal efficiently with the expanding self. The development is reflected in the child's growing ability to assimilate complex emotional experience and master the phase-appropriate traumas, to accommodate the self to an evermore demanding environment, and to maintain the integrity and cohesion of a self which is gradually beginning to differentiate into its dimensions (the "actual self," the "ideal self," the "social self").

While the rate of development of the secondary processes can be measured by using ordinary intelligence-testing techniques (such as the enrichment of the semantic vocabulary, the ability to articulate ideas, the power of abstraction), the developmental rate of the primary processes is more difficult to measure. The products of primary process operations are hardly ever expressed in any measurable overt behavior, but can only be inferred through measures such as the progressive enrichment of the individual's symbolic life, the increasing complexity and "sophistication" of his dreams, and the expansion of his artistic interests. (An interesting task for the future would be to devise a simple and standardized "IQ test" to gauge the performance level of the primary processes.)

The cognitive apparatus with all its functions develops according to an inborn maturational program that determines which skills and abilities will appear at each developmental phase, what course of development each of these will follow, and the final state of specification that each will attain at maturity. This program, of course, determines only the framework of the individual's potentialities, while the specific developmental course and outcome of each skill and ability always depend on the interaction of constitutional and environmental factors.

My thesis is that the primary and secondary processes form two developmental lines whose courses of development are determined by the same intrinsic maturational factors. Each new cognitive skill that appears in its appropriate phase influences both processes to the same degree, and each new stage of refinement of any of these skills is reflected equally in the operations of both. This means that each process displays, at every developmental phase, the same ability to categorize, make mental representations, and operate in all other areas of cognitive functioning. The difference between the two processes, in the realm of any of the cognitive functions, remains always in the mode of organization only, a mode which reflects the specific functional requirement assigned to each process: self-centeredness for the primary process and reality orientation for the secondary process.

I shall now try to demonstrate this thesis by focusing on five typical cognitive functions—categorization, mental representation, representation of the self, representation of reality, and causal reasoning—and describe the developmental course of each function in order to show (1) how the emergence of self-centeredness and reality orientation as two different organizing principles brings about the differentiation into primary and secondary process modes; and (2) that normal functioning in any area must be based on the balanced participation of both modes of operation.

Categorization [1] is the mental function that sorts out, arranges, and organizes into discrete entities the data which flow into the apparatus from the sense organs, the interior receptors of the body, and the archive of memory. This inner ordering activity begins at birth and continues to develop and improve throughout life. At first, perceptual data are presumably organized around innate sensorimotor schemata, basic drives, and physical needs (what Rapaport [1951] called "drive organization"). With the growing ability of the infant to distinguish between the various qualities of his sensations, wishes, needs, and responses, each new quality is used as a new criterion for further categorization. Objects become categorized according to the specific need that they satisfy or sense that they stimulate; events, according to the wish they are related to, and so on. With the accumulation of more and more categories, the growing repertoire becomes arranged into a hierarchically ordered system in which each group of similar categories becomes united under a more generalized category, so that a multilevel pyramid is gradually formed. As more and more attributes of any of the objects, events, and phenomena are used to form new categories, each item becomes cross-categorized several times. For example, a duck, which belongs to the category of birds by its form, belongs to food by its substance, and to toys by its function for the child. This gradually formed pyramidlike network of categories expands in three directions: its base broadens by progressive *differentiation* (the developmental principle of Werner, 1948), its apex becomes elevated by higher *generalization,* and its center becomes denser by continued *cross-categorization.*

All these types of categories are formed by the process which I would call "the primary mode of categorization." They are always organized around self-centered criteria, i.e., organizing criteria derived from sensual qualities, wish fulfillment, need satis-

1. Logicians distinguish between "categorization" and "classification." For the sake of brevity, I shall use the term "categorization" to denote both processes.

faction, and other experiential states. Images are formed, events are organized, and inner object representations are reconstructed only in relation to the drives and needs they satisfy or frustrate, the particular sense they impinge upon, and the significance they have for the experience of the self (e.g., the "self-objects" described by Kohut, 1977).

When reality orientation emerges as a new organizing principle, new possibilities for categorization open up to the mental apparatus. No longer are only those criteria that are related in some way to the self used for categorization, but any item derived from reality, even if it lacks any personal significance, can from now on be used as a criterion for organizing new categories. This new organizing principle gives rise to what I would call "the secondary mode of categorization." In this mode, objects are related according to what they *are*, and not merely to what they *do;* events are perceived on their own, and not only as affected by or affecting the self; and the interrelation between the various objects and events is understood as an objective occurrence, without the self necessarily being involved. For example, milk, which until now has been grasped only as a white substance that satisfies the need to be nourished, as a liquid that supplies a good feeling of warmth in the mouth, can now be perceived as a special category of food, and understood in connection with the cow that produced it or the milkman who sells it.

Being / Doing

The secondary categories also become organized into a hier-archically ordered, pyramidlike network, which, like the primary network, continuously expands in three directions: by the addi-tion of more differentiated subcategories along the base, of more generalized supercategories at the apex, and by cross-categorization in the center. The gradual dissolution of categories organized in reference to the self and the ascent in the hierarchical level of gen-eralization enable the mental apparatus to form new kinds of categories, units that include all qualitatively different attributes related to a given object, event, or phenomenon. The categories that serve secondary process thought as its main operational units are what we call *concepts*. Concepts always tend to attain the high-est level of generalization and, once on this level, to embrace all the attributes which may have any relation to the organizing cri-terion of that particular category. For example, a concept like *productive/introspective*

"mother" embraces all females in the world, whether human or animal, who bear offspring, and also includes all the attributes (behavior, feelings, wishes) that characterize the relation of mothers to their offspring; or the concept of "work" that denotes any act in the world in which an animal, human, or even a machine invests energy in some productive task.

With the emergence of the ability to form concepts, the former primary categories gradually undergo secondary transformation. The self-centered categories formed around a need, sense, wish, or emotional experience become disconnected from their relation to the self, assume an objective existence of their own, and turn into generalized notions that denote any instance where the particular object, event, or phenomenon may exist. This process of transformation does not cause the primary categories to disappear, but from now on both kinds of categories continue to exist and grow side by side, and both are used concomitantly as means for organizing mental data. For example, the color red, on its secondary level is a concept that denotes all phenomena in the cosmos where an object radiates light waves located on the lower end of the spectrum. On the primary level, however, it connotes a particular sensual experience, which, according to the specific history of the individual, is related to such self-experiences as warmth, emotional upheaval, or lust.

My thesis is that the secondary categories are never formed to *replace* the primary ones, but are always added as another level. In the years of childhood development, therefore, two qualitatively different networks of categories are formed, which reflect the two modes of organizing information that are characteristic of the mental apparatus. According to the primary process mode, objects, events, and phenomena are organized as *experience,* which always involves some self elements, and according to the secondary process mode, as *knowledge,* an inner representation of some hypothetical outer reality which is composed of things, beings, and events that act, change, appear, or disappear without any relation to the self. With the consolidation of the two networks, any single item of information is *categorized twice,* first as a subjective experience and then as a piece of objective knowledge.

We have to assume that there are some inner processes that constantly transform data perceived and organized by one of the modes of categorization into the other mode. Inner needs and wishes which are first processed according to the primary mode undergo "secondary revision" into secondary-process-organized categories; and perceptual input originating in reality which is first processed according to the secondary mode undergoes "primary revision" into primary-process-organized categories. The process of secondary revision can be demonstrated in the attempt to verbalize dreams or to articulate an emotional experience, and the process of primary revision in the attempt to transform occurrences into personal experiences.

The two modes of categorization and the continuous transformation from one mode to the other also determine the organization of *memory*. Any information stored in memory is always organized twice: once in the network of primary categories, as self-related personal experience, and again in the network of secondary categories, as objective categorized knowledge.

In normal cognitive development the two networks of categories continually grow and expand, as both primary and secondary modes of categorization are indispensable for normal cognitive functioning and for adaptation. Each mode reflects one of the two main forms of adaptation that characterize humans: self-centeredness and reality orientation. The permanent cooperation of both modes and the continuous transformation of information from one organizing mode to another make for the special flexibility and high adaptability of human thought, which succeeds in mediating between the demands of the self and the requirements of reality by integrating self-interests and reality considerations. Any disturbance in the course of development in one mode may endanger the normal balance between the two, thereby causing varying degrees of psychopathology. This is what happens in schizophrenia, where, owing to a disturbance of the secondary mode, the primary mode dominates cognition; in contrast, in obsessive-compulsive neurosis, disturbance in the primary mode causes cognition to be dominated by the secondary mode.

MENTAL REPRESENTATION

This term refers to the special ability of the mental apparatus to retrieve perceptual input in the absence of the sensory stimulus that originally provided this input. Visions are seen, voices heard, people felt as present, even when immediate sensory stimuli are not present to impinge on any of the sense organs. This ability to retrieve information from memory is almost never complete, and it is very rare that any sensory experience can be reproduced exactly as it occurred originally. In most cases, the original experience can only be *represented,* whether by a part, by one or by several of its sensory aspects, or by an agreed-upon sign. The process of *mental representation* may be viewed as a screen at the entrance to the archive of memory, on which the archivist can project, at the request of the user, any of the contents stored inside. This is a very unusual screen, which has not yet been duplicated in any man-made instrument. It is possible to project upon it not only visual images, but all kinds of sensory images, such as voices, smells, touch, and even the accompanying emotional atmosphere. This screen is the sole available access to memory, and no one is permitted to enter the archive itself to examine the contents stored there. Therefore, everything that can be known about the contents themselves will forever depend on what the archivist is ready to project on the screen and on the specific way he chooses to *represent* it.

We do not know in which developmental phase the processes of mental representation begin to operate. Freud assumed that in the first months of life the infant already can hallucinate the presence of the missing nourishing breast. Piaget (1963) claimed that there is no proof that a child is capable of forming the image of a missing object or event before the second year of life. It is clear, however, that the ability for mental representation is very crude in the beginning and that the child can only roughly represent a missing object or event on his inner mental screen.

This ability for mental representation develops in the course of maturation from its initially imperfect performances in two opposite directions:

1. With time, representations become richer and fuller, including more and more elements of the various aspects of the originally represented content, thereby succeeding in copying it more faithfully. This line of development, called *imagery*, almost never attains its possible perfect form. With regard to some of the senses, *percept identity* it may proceed relatively far, e.g., a visual or vocal image which represents the original visual or vocal percept fairly well; but with regard to other senses, such as smell or taste, the development is minimal, and only very few individuals are able to recall such a percept from memory in anything more than a sketchy manner.

Individual differences of imagery development are enormous, perhaps more so than in any line of cognitive development. People differ in their dominant sensual modality of imagery, in the degree of vividness with which they are able to reconstruct an image, in the extent to which their image resembles the original content, and so on. Most never attain the ability to form an image, via any of their sensory modalities, which will be a faithful copy of the original content. The few who possess this ability (which Jaensch [1930] called "eidetic imagery") in one or several of their sensory modalities are regarded as being endowed with a "special talent," e.g., the musician who can reproduce the sound of a whole orchestra in his imagination, or the painter who can faithfully visualize an entire landscape in all its details.

2. With time, the representation becomes more economic in its use of elements of the original, so that with each subsequent phase fewer elements are required for the representation of the whole. This line of development, called the development of *sign representation*, aims at attaining the state in which any rich and full *word / thought identity* content, such as all the aspects of an emotional experience, or all the components of a concept, will finally be represented by only one tiny cue, such as a word or a written sign. The capacity to represent mental contents via minimal signs makes possible the development of all the systems used in human communication, whether verbal or nonverbal.

Of course, the two diametrically opposite forms of representation reflect only the two extremes of the continuum of means available for mental representation, while a multitude of possible intermediate forms exists. In addition, the two opposites are not mutu-

ally exclusive, as any content can be represented alternately by
both imagery and sign representation or by both simultaneously
on different levels of consciousness.)

The choice of the form of representation depends mainly on the
functional requirements of the apparatus at any given moment. If
the mental task to be fulfilled is the assimilation of an emotional
experience, mastery of a trauma, or finding a new pattern of adaptation, the "holistic" method of imagery is preferred, where as
many elements as possible of the original experience to be worked
through are represented. But if the task is to embrace as much in-
formational data as possible in order to solve a rational problem
or to communicate a complex idea to others, the economic method
of sign representation is preferred because it permits the maximum amount of information to be evoked in a minimal amount
of time.

According to my thesis, there is no inherent difference between
the primary and secondary processes insofar as their ability to use
any of the available methods of representation is concerned. But,
naturally, owing to their different functional requirements, the
primary process tends to rely more on imagery, and the secondary
process on sign representation. This is because the self-centered
primary processes are involved mainly in the tasks of assimilation
and inner mastery, while the reality-oriented secondary processes
are involved mainly in realistic problem solving and communication. This does not mean, however, that when a particular task of
self-assimilation requires economic sign representation, or a task
of realistic problem solving requires vivid imagery, either of the
two processes is not able to put the best-suited method of representation to use. In fact, the difference between the representational capabilities of the primary and the secondary process lies not
in their varying ability for imagery vs. sign representation, but in
the basic criteria used for the organization of both imagery and
sign representation. In the case of imagery, the difference lies in
the fact that the primary process mode is confined to self-related
images, i.e., imaginary visions and sounds, which are in some way
related to needs, wishes, or past emotional experiences; while the
secondary process mode is free to reconstruct any type of image,
even one that is not connected with a need or wish or that bears

no personal significance whatsoever, e.g., the historian who may vividly imagine the daily life in ancient Rome, the architect who can "see" how a building will look before he draws up his plan, or the psychoanalyst who attempts to reconstruct in his mind the emotional atmosphere of his patient's childhood. The same is true for sign representation. According to the primary process mode, cues used to signify a mental content can be derived only from the repertoire of personal memory traces that bear some relation to present or past self-experiences; but in the secondary process mode, any arbitrary mental item can be used to signify a given content.

The limitation of the primary process mode to self-centered means of representation is well demonstrated in the dreamwork. Freud (1900) states, "All the material making up the content of a dream is in some way derived from experience, that is to say, has been reproduced or remembered in the dream" (p. 11). He says repeatedly that "the dream-work cannot actually create speeches" (p. 418), and where "spoken sentences occur in dreams and are expressly distinguished as such from thoughts, it is an invariable rule that the words spoken in the dream are derived from spoken words remembered in the dream-material" (p. 304). Fisher (1954) goes even further: "it is entirely possible that *the dream work cannot compose a new visual structure any more than it can a new speech*" (p. 422). This, however, does not mean that the dreamwork, by its processes of condensation, displacement, and reversal, cannot project a seemingly new creation of the inner screen; what it means is that if we examine the components of these new images carefully, we will see that *all* of them always derive from personal experiences.

The difference between the primary and secondary process modes of sign representation is highly significant for an understanding of the development of human systems of communication in particular, and of civilization in general. The primary process mode of representation enables the mental apparatus to use signs to denote a given content, but owing to the fact that its repertoire of signs is restricted to self-related elements, any "language" based on these signs must always be a personal one, which varies from one individual to another according to his own experience (what Piaget [1963, p. 125] calls "the system of individual significants").

The secondary process mode, which is free from this restriction and can use any item as a sign to represent its contents, can use collective, socially shared, and agreed-upon signs, whose usage is the precondition for the formation of language.

A necessary condition for the acquisition of language and secondary process thought is the ability to isolate verbal signs from their signified meaning. In order to facilitate this isolation, the verbal sign in itself must remain as neutral as possible and arouse a minimal emotional response to its very appearance, sound, and shade.[2]

Because the signs used by the primary process mode of representation are always, by their very self-centered nature, related to emotional or other experiential significant meaning, they can never attain the degree of neutrality requisite for their usage in a socially shared language. We can see that even if primary process thought uses words or other collective arbitrary signs, such as those which occur in dreams, art, or schizophrenic thinking, it can never disengage itself from the primary meaning of the words. Thus, the primary process deals more with the sound, color, shape, or rhythm of the words than with their designated meanings. Only the secondary process mode of representation can supply a repertoire of signs disconnected enough from self-related meaning to enable them to be used as socially shared, agreed-upon signs, and neutral enough to enable the necessary isolation between the sign and its meaning, which is required for the formation of any system of language.

The two modes of mental representation continue to develop hand in hand and, as will be further illustrated in the two special cases of mental representation—the representation of the self and the representation of reality—normal, mature mental activity is

2. It is interesting to note how rarely onomatopoeic words appear in any of the developed languages, in spite of the fact that they are regarded as being the first verbal signs to have appeared. It almost seems that language tries as much as possible to reject any word which, by its too close association to its signified meaning, makes it difficult to isolate the sign from the signified. This also happens with what are called "obscene words," which are regarded as "emotionally contaminated" because of their close association with drives and wishes and therefore have to be continually deleted from ordinary language.

always based on the balanced operation of both modes. The two modes are also reflected in the organization of human communication, which is based on a mixture of two kinds of signs: "secondary signs" produced according to the secondary process mode of representation and "primary signs" produced according to the primary mode. Both modes are present in ordinary conversation where objective, factual information is transmitted by the meanings of the words and sentences and the subjective experiential information through the rhythm, clang, modulation, and the "music" of the voice.

Most students of communication approach language as a system consisting of two levels of communication. Carnap (1955) distinguishes between the "expressive function" and the "representation function" of language. Wittgenstein (1921) describes two kinds of communication—that which transmits factual and theoretical information and that which transmits values and states of experience. Parry (1967) distinguishes between information with a cognitive content and information with an affective content. Langer (1942), who describes language as a system of symbols, distinguishes between "discursive" and "non-discursive" symbols. Aranguren (1967) writes, "It is necessary to distinguish between the descriptive or cognitive and the emotive aspects of language" (p. 27). Russell (1940) distinguishes between the ability of language to indicate facts and its ability to express the state of the speaker. Although each of these writers uses a different vocabulary, in practice all of them refer to the same two modes, called here primary and secondary process modes of communication, and all of them regard these two modes as the essential components of any system of human communication.

THE REPRESENTATION OF THE SELF

When I suggested (1969) that the primary process be defined as self-centered, I in no way meant that the self as an organization, structure, or image should be regarded as a pure primary process product. By the same token, the representation of reality is not determined by the secondary process alone. In fact, the representation of the self as well as the representation of reality depend on a combination of primary and secondary process operations. A mature, normal self image is thus based on a combination of primary and secondary modes. According to the primary process mode, a person perceives himself as from *within,* as a collage of sensations, wishes, needs, and experiences. According to the secondary process mode, a person perceives himself as from *without,* as a group of objective phenomena, an object among other objects, a collection of physical substances and forces. For example, I perceive my leg in two ways, once as something belonging to me, which I can feel through my senses of touch, temperature, and weight as well as through other proprioceptive senses, and again as a part of my body, something I can look at, touch, and know the functions of. On the primary level my leg is an experience, and on the secondary level it is a concept, while its total image is normally a combination of the experience and the concept. When one of the two aspects does not exist, as is the case in a "phantom limb," where the leg is felt but is known to be missing, or in paraplegia, where the leg cannot be felt but is known to exist, a normal image of the leg as a part of the "body self" cannot be maintained.

This double perception and representation pertain to any part of the body, to the body self as an overall image and to the subordinate self in all its dimensions. The all-inclusive self image is an inner representation made up of the two aspects, which I would call the "experiential self" and the "conceptual self." A healthy sense of selfness results from a sound balance and optimal fit between these aspects, in which every self experience is supported by the appropriate conceptual self knowledge, and all self knowledge goes hand in hand with suitable experiences. Any imbalance or mismatch between the two aspects is expressed in the feeling of depersonalization, a disorder which, while it may be the result of many possible disturbances in any of the parts of the experiential or conceptual self, always indicates an inability to fit the two aspects together in an optimal manner (for a similar approach, one that connects depersonalization with disturbances in the self and outlines the various possible disturbances, see Frances et al., 1977).

I relate the experiential self to the primary process and the conceptual self to the secondary process because each of these two aspects reflects one of the two major forms of human adaptation and survival. The primary mode of processing sensations, feelings, and emotions enables the organism to react effectively to dangerous situations and to assure its physical existence. For example, the sensation of pain will force a person to remove his hand from a fire; hunger pangs will drive him to seek food; fright will motivate him to flee from danger. The secondary mode, in which he perceives himself as a physical entity in time and space and as an object among other objects, enables the organism to adapt to the conditions of its natural environment and to adjust to society. These two modes of adaptation and survival, the self-centered and the reality-oriented ones, normally supplement one another. For example, man's ability to satisfy a need such as hunger or sex is enhanced by his capacity to evaluate objectively his social environment and to plan his actions accordingly. On the other hand, his attempt to adjust to a new social environment is influenced by his specific emotional responses to the members of his society.

From the standpoint of development, the experiential aspect of the self always precedes the development of the conceptual aspect. Lichtenberg (1975) says that "the sense of self can be seen as arising during the infantile stage as islands of experience that then, bit by bit, are formed into more ordered groupings of images" (p. 482). I suggested (1969) that these early experiences be called "self-nuclei," in analogy with the old term "ego-nuclei" (p. 169). Gedo and Goldberg (1973), who also use the term "nuclei of the self," say, "It is from such antecedent nuclei that the cohesive, whole self is gradually built, in parallel with the realistic sorting out of the variety of part objects, into cohesive wholes" (p. 65).

I think that it is not only "in parallel with the realistic sorting out," but that the emergence of reality-oriented thought itself causes the consolidation of the disparate self experiences into a cohesive whole. In other words, under the influence of the emerging conceptual self the various "islands" of the experiential self are blended into the all-inclusive self image. The maintenance of the unity and continuity of the self can be assured only by the double representation of the self as an experience and as a concept.

THE REPRESENTATION OF REALITY

The inner representation of reality, like the representation of the self, is normally a combination of two modes of perception and representation. According to the primary process mode, reality is represented as a collection of places, events, objects, and situations that satisfy (or fail to satisfy) needs, fulfill wishes, arouse expectations, stir emotions, and impinge upon various past experiences. According to the secondary process mode, reality is represented as an assemblage of objects and phenomena that have an independent existence, subordinated to some objective physical rules which determine their creation, evolution, and interrelationship. For example, the town I live in is represented in my imagery as a collection of places, each of which is connected to a particular past experience: here is the corner on which I met my first girlfriend; here is the street where my aunt lived. From another aspect, it is an assemblage of streets, places, buildings, whose pattern is known to me and whose plan I can reproduce in my mind. On the primary level, the town is a collection of experiences; and on the secondary level, a concept I carry with me. The complete image is normally a combination of both the experience and the concept. This combined image provides me with a sense of familiarity, with the sound feeling of being and acting in a real environment to which I am connected by personal memories and experiences and in which I feel "at home." Should one of the two aspects be missing—for example, being conducted blindfolded around a new town, having many meaningful experiences, but never knowing exactly where I have been; or were I to visit a new city and tour its streets while referring to a map, but having no connection with it through personal experiences—I would feel estranged and alienated from the reality surrounding me.

The inner image of reality, or any part of it, always comprises two aspects, which I would call the "experiential representation of reality" and the "conceptual representation of reality." A healthy sense that something is "real" results from a sound balance and optimal fit between the two aspects. Any imbalance or mismatch between them is expressed in the feeling of derealization, a symptom in which the individual complains about feelings of unreality and unfamiliarity of the familiar.

Feelings of depersonalization and derealization generally appear together, because any imbalance between the experiential and conceptual modes of representation usually affects both the creation of the self image and the inner representation of reality. We see these two symptoms in such a broad spectrum of psychopathological states—from cases of severe schizophrenia, through borderline or narcissistic personality disorders, to transient neurotic disturbances—that the symptoms in themselves have no prognostic value, until the exact disturbance that prevents the normal fit is located.

As in the case of the self image, in reality representation, too, each mode reflects one of the two major forms of human adaptation and survival. According to the primary mode, the reality represented on the inner screen seems to serve only the self; to gratify its needs, fulfill its wishes, and assist in its functions of assimilation, accommodation, and integration. In contrast, the reality represented according to the secondary mode serves reality orientation: it assists in the accurate perception of the environment and the significant objects, the understanding of what is going on, and the adjusting of behavior to meet the requirements of reality.

The primary process mode is responsible for the images of reality that are reconstructed by fantasy, dream, and the arts, a reality image which almost always deviates from the objective in the direction of the pressing needs of the self. This mode is best demonstrated in the dream, which never attempts to reconstruct a faithful copy of reality; and if such a reality picture or occurrence appears, it is always tailored solely with the aim of aiding wish fulfillment or any other need of the self which instigated the dream.

When Freud stated that dreams are concealed wish fulfillments, he did not claim that the dreamer simply imagines his wish as being fulfilled (which often happens in daydreams). Because Freud (1900) knew that *"a wish which is represented in a dream must be an infantile one"* (p. 553), he realized that in most cases such a wish not only cannot be fulfilled in adult life, but even cannot be imagined. Therefore, in order to fulfill such a wish to some degree, the dream must first create an imaginary reality situation in which the fulfillment of the forbidden wish will be possible without violating the standards of the superego. Once it succeeds in doing so, the dream usually does not even continue to imagine the fulfillment of the original wish itself, like a good movie, which ends at the point where the central idea has just become clear.

For example, a patient dreamed that he and his best friend were lost in the desert. They wandered endlessly, starving and thirsty, and he felt that he had no chance of being rescued. When he reported the dream, he asked the classical question, asked certainly by generations of analysands: "Freud claimed that every dream is a concealed wish fulfillment. How is it possible that I wish to die in the desert in such a terrible manner?" He was right. It did not seem that that was really his wish. His unconscious wish, however, was to have homosexual relations with his friend, a wish which he could never realize, and could not allow himself even to dream about. But if they were to be lost in the desert together and had no hope of ever returning to civilization, perhaps it would be possible then?

To build such "in-the-service-of-the-self" imaginary reality is also one of the major functions of art. The most naïve fairy tales and the most elaborate forms of literature and drama, all try to create an imaginary reality in which the reader can freely identify with the hero through whose deeds he can gratify his own wishes (see also Waelder, 1965).

The secondary process mode of reality representation is quite different in that here the major concern of the mental apparatus is how to succeed in reconstructing on the inner screen an image of reality that will be the most accurate copy of a presumably existing objective reality. In contrast to the primary mode, the aim here is to prevent wishes and needs from interfering and to maintain the "purity" of the actual reality from the "contaminating" effect of the self's needs.

From the standpoint of development, the experiential aspect of reality representation always precedes the conceptual aspect. The child at first selects only those memory traces of reality for projection on his inner screen that may in some way help him cope (satisfy or enable to bear frustration) with his basic needs. Only later, with the development of the secondary processes, does he gradually begin to reconstruct an inner representation of reality as it really was or is. As the child grows older, this secondary process representation is used more and more to check the tendency of the primary process to distort reality in the service of the self. In the transition years, while the optimal fit between the two aspects is not yet achieved, we can see how the child often tends to distort even conceptual reality to serve his needs, wishes, or conflicts. For example, a boy of 6, when asked to draw the plan of his apartment, extended the corridor between his room and his parents' room to twice the length it was in reality. Since the boy felt that his parents were always trying to keep him far away from their "privacy," he perceived their room as being far away from his own. Such distortions of reality, which may be regarded as normal in childhood, gradually become "corrected" with the passage of time by the growing influence of the developing secondary process mode of reality representation, until the optimal fit between the two is achieved, and each aspect acts to maintain the other, to establish "reality constancy."

CAUSAL REASONING

One of the earliest central functions of the mental apparatus is the tendency to relate things, events, and phenomena to each other. Thus the child generally succeeds in bringing order to his universe. The creaking of the door becomes related to the appearance of his mother, the sight of the boiling pot on the stove becomes associated with the experience of eating, and so on. As Koestler (1964) said, "Goethe's 'connect, always connect' seems to be the motto of the child as, out of the fluid raw material of its experience, it selects and shapes patterns and relations" (p. 620).

In time, the child gradually learns that A and B are not arbitrarily connected, but that A causes B, or that B is the result of A. Once this learning occurs, the child begins his attempts to master his universe by making hypotheses about a chain of events, by assuming that B appeared or occurred *because* A caused it (causal thinking) or that A occurred *in order* that B will be affected by it (teleological thinking). The establishment of this tendency to perceive and order things, events, and phenomena into a chain of causes and effects is called *causal reasoning*.

This tendency is also reflected in the structure of language. A sentence is never built as an arbitrary chain of words, but consists within a structure where each word explains and modifies the meaning of all the others. The use of language requires, therefore, the development of what is called "propositional logic," i.e., the ability to relate meaningfully one word to another.

It seems clear to most psychoanalytically oriented students of cognition that causal reasoning and propositional logic abilities are exclusively characteristic of the secondary process, as the primary process is unable to make any meaningful connections. Bogen (1969), in studying the differences between the two hemispheres of the brain, assumed that while the dominant left hemisphere (the secondary process) has a propositional capacity, the right one (the primary process) has an "appositional capacity." I believe that there is no difference between the primary and secondary processes with regard to their ability for causal reasoning and propositional logic; they differ only in regard to how the causal connections are made. The primary process always connects things in a self-centered mode. In other words, two elements can be connected only on the condition that at least one of them in some way represents the self and its needs. This means that a reality occurrence can be perceived only as caused by or affecting the self in some way. The secondary process, being able to connect things according to a reality-oriented mode, is free to relate objective things, events, and phenomena to each other, without having to assume any relation to the self. For example, if the individual, by his primary process mode, can explain the appearance of a thunderstorm only as a means to punish him, or the rain as a response to his prayers, by his secondary process mode, he can understand that the storm and the rain have an intrinsic causal connection that has no relation to his sins or his prayers.

As was the case with all the other criteria of cognition, it is clear that the two modes represent the two major forms of human adaptation and survival. Those who tend to ignore the ability of the primary process to make causal connections are biased by the fact that these connections often are wrong in terms of reality, and overlook the immense significance that such connections have from the point of view of the self and its striving for survival. By his ability to differentiate "good" from "bad" food, to perceive others in terms of their intentions toward him, to understand events to be the results of his own actions, the human being suc-

ceeds in adapting himself fairly well to his environment and ensuring his survival by escaping from dangers.

The development of the secondary process mode of causality
makes possible the emergence of a new kind of adaptation. By being able to connect things causally among themselves, without the
involvement of the self, the growing child learns the rules which
determine the occurrence of events around him, understands that
there are objective reasons for what happens, knows what to expect, and in time learns how to intervene actively in the objective
chain of events in order to change them according to his will.

The two modes of causality determine the lifetime development
of human thinking. The primary process mode is represented in
magical thinking and is involved in the development of myths,
religions, and arts. The secondary process mode is represented in
purely logical reasoning and is responsible for the development
of science. Like any other kind of normal cognitive activity, daily
ordinary thinking is a combination of the two modes, with each
contributing to the performance of the other—the primary process
mode of causality supplies the self-centered motivation for seeking causal connections between events in the objective world,
while the secondary process mode is used to check the intuitive
primary one and confirm objectively the understandings arrived at.

THE DEVELOPMENT OF THE TWO FORMS OF ADAPTATION

The various contemporary theories of cognitive development and
the development of intelligence can be roughly divided into two
major groups—those that perceive it as a linear process commenc-
ing in lower animals and proceeding to the intelligent animals
such as apes, until it reaches its highest developmental levels in
man; and those that conceive human intelligence to be the result
of a new beginning, the product of a unique evolutionary leap
which produced a totally new line of development. The first
group, regarding human intelligence to be only *quantitatively* different from lower animal forms, naturally tends to focus its studies
on animals, in the hope of isolating the basic features of cognition
in their "pure culture." The second group, believing that human

intelligence is *qualitatively* different from that of animals, believes that the characteristics of human intelligence can be learned only by studying human beings.

The debate between the proponents of these two approaches seems to reflect the difference between primary and secondary processes. I contend that the primary process of humans represents the linear development of cognition and the secondary process represents a new beginning, which is unique to man. In other words, a "clever" animal, such as a dolphin or chimpanzee, even if it someday reaches its highest potential intelligence, will always remain confined to a primary process, self-centered intelligence, because by linear development alone it will never attain any of the qualities characteristic of the secondary process, reality-oriented intelligence. Indeed, attempts to improve intellectual achievements in animals, like that of teaching apes to use language (Premack, 1976), proved that although they may learn to categorize, represent images, use signs and symbols, and even make causal connections, they can never disengage their cognition from the immediate needs of the self. Consider the following example:

A dog living on our street, generally quite a goodhearted animal, barks angrily at any person carrying a basket. The reason is certainly that the supermarket delivery boy always kicks him. This dog learned to place people into two categories—friendly ones without baskets and dangerous ones with baskets—a categorization which certainly helps him to evade troubles. If he were a more intelligent dog, he would perhaps also learn to differentiate between various groups of men carrying baskets and not attack an innocent old lady. But no matter how clever he might be, he would never go beyond recognizing people solely according to how they behave toward him. The cat in our street, whom my daughter feeds, is much cleverer. She seizes any opportunity to get into our home, and she can read the mood of every member of our family. She ignores our attempts to draw her out when we are feeling playful and scurries off when we are really angry. She knows that my daughter likes her, and that I can hardly bear her, so that she is clever enough to direct her pathetic wailings only to my daughter and does not try to arouse my pity. But she also will never be able to understand the interchange between my daughter and me, and therefore will never entertain the idea that she might be able to manipulate my daughter against me, for example, by trying to have my daughter stop me from kicking her out of the house. This cat has reached the limits of her "cleverness"—although she can accurately read feelings and attitudes of people, it can only be to the degree that she herself is involved. She will never be able to know anything about our feelings, attitudes, responsibilities, or any interchanges between us in which she herself is not involved.

The secondary process in humans, as we know today, is the only biologically central information-processing system that succeeds in disconnecting its functioning from the immediate needs and compelling forces of the self. It can develop programs to sort out information, to categorize it, to connect it into causal chains, and to represent it on its own, according to the contiguities, similarities, and interrelations between the various items of information. Since the secondary process does not develop to replace the primary one, man becomes the only living being equipped with a doubly structured cognitive system that operates according to two different organizing principles. One part operates according to the old approved principle of self-centrism, common to all "intelligent" living beings; and the second part operates according to the principle of reality orientation, a new creation unique to the evolution of man. This double arrangement makes for the specific flexibility of the system, as the organizational center can shift freely from one mode to the other according to changing functional requirements.

The two basic modes represent two different forms of *adaptation* characteristic of human cognition, each of which is efficient and would suffice by itself to ensure man's basic survival and propagation. In the attempt to comprehend the special advantage of man's ability to utilize two different forms of adaptation, I now will focus on their essential difference.

According to the primary process mode, everything perceived and recalled from memory is sorted out, categorized, and understood in terms of the self and its needs. The object is represented in terms of whether it satisfies, frustrates, or threatens; the event, in terms of how it influences or can be influenced by the self. This

enables the individual to distinguish between what is good or bad
for him and what is comforting or dangerous; to understand how
the changing conditions around him may influence him; to find
the best method of satisfying his needs and to learn how to avoid
dangers. By the use of the secondary process mode, an individual
can categorize and understand the events and phenomena in terms
of reality; he can comprehend the inner relations between the
various objects on their own; he is able to discern regularities,
detect repetitive and similar patterns of order, and derive rules
that determine the occurrence of the events. Thus, the essential
difference is that while according to the primary form an individual can successfully adjust to his environment by modifying
himself in accordance with changing reality requirements, only
by the secondary form is he able to modify reality and adapt it to
his own needs. The primary process form of adaptation is an *auto-*
plastic one, while the secondary process form of adaptation is an
alloplastic one,[3] a higher form of adaptation that is achieved when
a person has the capacity to apply his knowledge of the rules determining the occurrence of events in reality, for the purpose of
actively manipulating reality and modifying it in the service of
the self.

The two forms of adaptation determine man's attitudes and behavior for his entire life. The primary form is reflected in his emotional and "intuitive" responses, and the secondary in his logical
reasoning. The permanent cooperation of the two ensures the synthesis of self-interests and reality considerations that is necessary
for optimal adaptation.

The Development of Autonomous Thought

I have so far focused on the fact that the development of the secondary process, including its application to cognition and adaptation, is dependent on the emergence of reality orientation as a
new organizing principle. Now I shall examine the characteristics
of reality-oriented cognition, in order to show how a section of
cognitive processes succeeded in becoming disengaged from the
traditional subordination to the self and its needs.

3. These two terms were introduced by Ferenczi (1919).

Freud (1900) contends that the secondary process develops out of the primary one in response to the requirements of reality to restrain and control the free discharge of the drives: "The bitter experience of life must have changed this primitive thought-activity into a more expedient secondary one" (p. 566). For Freud, thinking is a central organizing activity *compelled* to deal with and solve problems created by the intrinsic opposition between the drives striving for gratification and reality requirements. For Freud, then, the development of the secondary process is nothing more than an exchange of one master for another, owing to "the bitter experience of life." Instead of serving the drive in its search for gratification, a part of the thought processes exchanges its master to serve reality in its attempts to impose constraints on drive discharge. Rapaport, who in his numerous studies on thinking maintained Freud's basic approach, took a somewhat different stance in his last paper devoted to this topic (1960): "Since the synthetic function emerges here [*Totem and Taboo*] as a new function unique to the secondary process, independent of the demands of instinctual drives as well as those of reality, it is no longer a mere superimposition upon the primary processes by the dire necessities of reality. In the terminology of present-day psychoanalytic ego psychology, we would formulate this state of affairs as follows: the secondary process and its synthetic function are *autonomous ego functions* in relation to both instinctual drives and external stimulation" (p. 841f.; my italics). Thus, secondary process thought differs from primary process cognition not only in the organizing principle to which each is submitted, but, in contrast to the primary process which is always subjected to the self and its needs, the secondary process is autonomous, not subjected to any master. Its capacity to orient itself toward reality, to categorize, to represent, and to discern causal connections, regularities, and the rules determining reality events stems from the fact that it is *not* subjected to reality, so that reality cannot dictate the forms and strategies which the secondary process will use.

The special ability of secondary process thought to deal with reality is determined by the fact that it is *free* to choose those models for organizing experience, categories for conceptualizing knowledge, and strategies for analyzing and solving problems which are the ones best suited to deal with reality. The problem is never if they *fit* or do not fit a given objective reality, but only if they have proved to be the most effective means of dealing with such reality.

Indeed, the concept of the autonomy of thought already is inherent in the philosophy of Kant, then called "the Copernical revolution of philosophy." Kant (1787) went against the accepted view of his time which regarded consciousness as a mere mirror that only passively reflects outer reality. He looked upon it as an active instrument that perceives, organizes, and gives meaning to reality. Thought concepts and organizational categories do not reflect nature's phenomena and rules, but they are a priori given instruments by which the human mind projects *its* order and lawfulness on the phenomena of nature: "Namely, that we can know a priori of things only what we ourselves put into them" (p. 23).

The concept of autonomy is prevalent in psychoanalysis today, used mainly to describe the status of the ego vis-à-vis the id and environment. My concept of autonomy, when I speak of the secondary process, is much wider than that used by Hartmann and Rapaport in reference to the autonomy of the ego. For them, autonomy means a relative independence and distance of ego functioning from the id and environment. I conceive of the secondary process not only as independent from the demands of the self and the requirements of reality, and not even as just free to decide *how* to cope with a given problem, but as free to decide whether or not to deal with the problem at all.[4]

4. The relation between the tripartite model (id. ego, superego) and the thought processes (primary and secondary processes) is still an unsettled problem. Freud (1940) said, "We have found that processes in the unconscious or in the id obey different laws from those in the preconscious ego. We name these laws in their totality the *primary process,* in contrast to the *secondary process* which governs the course of events in the preconscious, in the ego" (p. 164), but he did not say which processes the unconscious part of the ego obeys (a part that includes the defense mechanisms). Rangell summarized the panel on "The Psychoanalytic Theory of Thinking" (see Arlow, 1958): "the functioning of the primary process must be regarded, according to the discussion, as an aspect of all three systems of the psychic apparatus, ego, id and superego" (p. 151), which really means that the secondary process too is an aspect of all the three systems, and the two groups of concepts are over-

The primary process as manifested, for example, in dreamwork, may deal with wish fulfillment, problem solving, assimilation of experiences, etc. But in all cases, a person is never free to select the contents of his dream, to choose the time for dreaming, to decide about the strategies to be used, or even if he wants to dream at all. When secondary process thought is employed, however, he is not only free to decide about all these parameters, but may, if he wants to, deal only with a part of the problems, make all kinds of mistakes, and solve the problems in the most maladaptive or self-destructive way, bearing all the consequences implied. The main difference between the autonomy of the ego and the autonomy of thought is, therefore, that while the ego is obliged to cope with the problems aroused (as demonstrated especially in post-traumatic neurosis, where the ego may try for decades to cope in vain with the original trauma) and is never free to abstain from its attempts at mastery, assimilation, and integration, autonomous thought always has its freedom of choice—if, when, where, and how to act.

How was autonomous thought established? What were the conditions that made this unprecedented turn in phylo- and onto-genetic development possible; a turn which enables a portion of cognitive processes to separate their natural attachment from the needs of the self and become autonomous? There is no reliable experimentally supported answer to this question, and it seems that there will never be one, so that all we can do is to speculate. To my mind, the emergence of autonomous thought is dependent on one single factor—the development of *the ability of thought to think about itself.* It is what Dewey (1933) called "reflective thinking" and defined as "Thought is, as it were, conduct turned in

---

lapping. In line with my views on the models in psychoanalytic meta-psychology (1977), I would simply approach the two groups of concepts (ego, id, superego, on the one hand, and primary and secondary processes, on the other) as two different models, describing the mental apparatus from two different points of view, and therefore stop bothering about the possible relation between them. I will also describe primary and secondary thought as systems and take the liberty to use, in regard to autonomous thought, the same metaphorical terms as are used in ego psychology—terms that imply that autonomous thought possesses its own regulatory mechanisms and controls.

upon itself and examining its purpose and its conditions, its resources, aids, and difficulties and obstacles" (p. 108).

To understand the meaning of a system of thought which is able to think about itself, I return to the contrast between the dream and logical thinking. We may be able to recall the contents of a dream, and often even be aware of the latent meaning expressed by the manifest dream. But we can never explore the "laboratory" of the dreamwork (without the aid of the psychoanalytic process) and be aware of the processes by which the material of the latent dream is worked into the manifest dream. This applies also to parapraxes, neurotic symptoms, moments of inspirational insight, and all other primary process operations—in all of which we may be fully aware of the products, but never of the underlying processes that produce them. However, in the case of logical problem solving, for example, in finding a mathematical solution, the process can be stopped at any point; we can "wind the tape back" and reconstruct exactly all the steps of logical operation used for working on the problem—the ways of data selection, criteria used for sorting out and categorization, how these categories are represented on the inner screen, the strategies used for working with the material, etc. This awareness of all the phases of inner processing enables us to establish complete *control* over the operations of secondary process thought and over their expression in behavior and communication. The ability to evaluate the various operations of thought in the light of their results (what in psychology is called K.R., i.e., control by Knowledge of Results) and to compare different strategies makes it possible for us to select and refine the most efficient ones and to discard the rest.

We may assume that for thousands or even millions of years there existed many species of higher animals equipped with cognitive systems in various stages of evolution; these operated as biological central information-processing systems preprogrammed by nature to deal with the information vital for the adaptation, survival, and propagation of the species. At one particular point of evolution an unprecedented capacity appeared in one of the higher primates—the ability of a system to control and direct its own actions. The emergence of this new capacity is presumably the one single turn that started the entire chain of events that

brought about the development of human autonomous thought—
and thereby the growth of human language, civilization, technol-
ogy, science and art.

The development of the reflective capacity of one section of
human cognitive processes (the secondary process) made it the first
biological information-processing system that could liberate itself
from the dependence on fixed preset programs (instincts). It allowed for the modification of these programs according to changing requirements, for the discarding of those that proved useless,
and for the composition of new programs if needed. This development created an entirely novel condition—a biological system
which was no longer dependent upon the programs provided by
nature, but which could *program itself by itself.*

The description of autonomous thought as a system that controls its own course suggests its definition as a "feedback-monitored
system." Indeed, in an earlier paper (1969), I suggested the following formulation for the differential definition of the secondary
and primary processes: "secondary processes are all mental processes dependent on feedback for their maintenance; primary processes are all mental processes not dependent on feedback for their
maintenance" (p. 166). Today I no longer find this definition to
be relevant; first, because we really have no proof that the primary
processes are not dependent on feedback perception, at least on
some mechanistic or unconscious level; and second, because I have
become hesitant about the adequacy of such a concept as feedback
for the understanding of the function of the mind. Ten years ago
this concept was highly fashionable, together with all other concepts of cybernetics and information theory which then seemed
to be capable of clarifying all the perplexities of living systems.
Since then we have learned the limitations of all these concepts.
The term "feedback" was formulated in order to describe the self-
regulating functions of servomechanisms, and as such it is a rather
mechanistic concept implying preestablished arrangements regulating the activity of a system in an automatic manner (see also the
critique of Bertalanffy, 1973, p. 169). Certainly, all the "programs"
activating human autonomous thought include inbuilt feedback
loops, but what characterizes autonomous thought is not its dependence on this feedback, but its *freedom* from the necessity to

respond automatically to any feedback information. Autonomous thought continues to perceive all the required information about how it operates and the results achieved, and it certainly uses this information for steering its own activity and for planning its future moves, but it is not compelled to take this information into consideration. A person may do something while receiving all the information required to warn him that he is on the wrong track, but if for some reason he does not want to be adaptive or reasonable, he may go on pursuing it and ignore all inner and social feedback warning signals (for example, in purposely suicidal behavior).

It is plausible to assume that all biological systems are feedback monitored. What characterizes autonomous thought and distinguishes it from all other systems (and perhaps also from what is regarded as "autonomy" of the ego) is its ability to liberate itself not only from the dependence on the needs of the self and the dependence on reality requirements, but also from the dependence on its own feedback; autonomous thought *may* use itself for self-monitoring, but it does not *have* to do so.

The emergence of the reflective capacity and the establishment of autonomous thought as a system disengaged from the compelling needs of the self and from the pressing demands of reality, and free to manipulate feedback information according to its own purposes, have had a widespread influence on the phylogenetic evolution of the human race. This process is repeated in a condensed form in the ontogenetic development of the individual. I shall summarize the influences it has on uniquely human abilities.

1. Reflective capacity is used as an inner controlling factor which enables the system to check its methods of categorization and modify the schemata used so that categorization may fit the same schemata employed by significant others. Thus, a body of categories and concepts shared by all members of a given society is gradually formed. These categories and concepts serve as the basis for the development of *language,* which is (in its semantic aspect) a system for signifying the socially shared concepts by agreed-upon signs.

2. The development of language as a socially shared communi-

cation system has a reciprocal influence on the development of secondary process thought, whose operational patterns and rules of organization must be adapted to those which govern language (grammar and syntax). Because a part of the system (the primary processes) continues to process its data along the self-centered mode, without any consideration of the reality requirements of language (as represented by the rules of logic), reflective thought must be able to differentiate clearly between the two modes of thought. In other words, reflective thought must develop the ability to differentiate fantasy from reality. Once this ability is established, there is no longer any danger that the growing child will confuse primary-process-dominated imagination with secondary-process-dominated logic, and the way is open to share imagery with others. This is the phase when the child begins to communicate the products of his imagination and to enjoy that of other people's imagination (such as fairy tales). With time, a second socially shared "language" is created, a medium of communication which, in contrast to verbal language that is based on reality-oriented logic, is based on self-centered imagery and the growing ability to share such imagery socially. This is the "language" of *art*.

3. The linguistic ability of man to conceptualize his experience and knowledge so that they may be comprehensible to others allowed for their externalization so that these can become a socially shared body of knowledge available for anyone's use. Language and the invention of writing as a method whereby this knowledge may be stored enabled mankind to transmit accumulated knowledge from generation to generation. With this, a situation, hitherto unknown in the biological world, was created. In the world of living things below man on the evolutionary scale, an individual's experience and knowledge always vanish with the death of their possessor, and each issue must be tackled anew from the starting point determined by its genetically given, inborn programs. Man, on the other hand, is the only living being who can benefit from the knowledge acquired by his ancestors, and each generation can continue its development exactly from the stage reached by the previous generations.

With the passage of time, accumulated knowledge becomes organized into the various systems of *science*, and each one of them develops its specific criteria for the controlled selection, ordering, validation, and usage of the knowledge accumulated.

It took mankind many centuries of scientific development until it discovered the fact that the capacity of secondary thought for reflection can also be used on a higher level—to examine reflectively its own reflective capacity. On this basis the highest disciplines of philosophy and science were developed—epistemology, for inquiring into the ability of the human mind to accumulate knowledge; and psychoanalysis, for studying the abilities of the mind to examine, control, and modify its own activities.

4. The capacity of reflective thought to compare the various strategies of thought, means of communication, and patterns of behavior enables it to select, reinforce, and cultivate the most effective ones while suppressing the rest. This ability is used for continually improving the achievements of autonomous thought and to form a system that will operate on the highest possible level of performance.

In order to enable any child to use the experience gathered by man on how to improve his thought's performances, and to enable him to benefit from all other relevant knowledge accumulated over the generations, *education* was developed as a process for shaping his mind and for supplying it with all the necessary information.

5. The capacity of reflective thought to acknowledge itself enables man to get a fairly reliable image about the structure and functioning of his own mind. By projecting this image onto others, the growing child learns to understand how they respond to him and what motivates their behavior. He simply assumes that other people's minds are similar to his own in structure and functioning. Thus, the ability for *empathy* is established, which not only aids a man in predicting the behavior of others (something every "intelligent" animal can also do), but also allows him to understand the feelings and emotions the other is experiencing.

With the growing ability to differentiate clearly between "fantasy and reality," the process of empathy becomes more advanced, and the growing child succeeds in perceiving that the other also possesses a multilevel mind, composed of images, reality considerations, contrasting emotions, and conflicting motives. This advanced empathy is employed by the higher sciences, such as psychoanalysis, as their basic methodological instrument. Unlike the "exact" sciences, which use only objective, reality-oriented logic as their instrument, psychoanalysis uses all the levels of thought, including reflective introspection and multilevel empathy to study its subject matter.

6. The nature of reflective thought to separate itself into observing and observed parts gives the individual the experience of possessing a divisible self. This is expressed in the various experiences such as the cleavage between emotions and reason, fantasy and reality, wishes and constraints. The ability to pit the observing part against the observed one in order to control it gives the experience (or illusion, depending on one's philosophical attitude) of possessing a "free will" and of being responsible for one's own actions.

The experience of self-control and responsibility serves as the basis for the development of human *ethics,* a socially shared system of moral rules, partly internalized and partly imposed by society, which guides the individual in his thoughts, feelings, and behavior.

These six abilities—to use language, to create art, to develop science, to improve methods for education, to feel empathy, and to submit to ethical rules—are all unique to human beings and are all an outcome of the human development of the reflective capacity and the establishment of the secondary process as an autonomous thought system.

THE STRUGGLE FOR AUTONOMY

The autonomy of the secondary process is not a quality that, once achieved, is warranted forever; it requires the investment of a permanent effort to guarantee its boundaries. Drives, basic needs, and various demands of the self all strive continually to gnaw into the boundaries of autonomy and to reenslave parts of the autonomous section of thought to their service.

These efforts of the inner forces to enslave the autonomous thought are expressed in the various psychopathological states. All neuroses are characterized by varying degrees of loss of autonomy, as in the obsessive-compulsive, where more and more portions of thought activity lose their autonomy and become enslaved by the drives and the demands of the self. The extreme state is seen in the schizophrenic psychosis, where all remnants of autonomy are lost and the entire secondary process thought becomes self-centered; for example, the paranoid patient who may display the highest intellectual ability, but whose excellent logic is totally enslaved in the service of the self, so that he is no longer able to pay attention to any objective reality considerations.

In this never-ending struggle between autonomous thought and inner enslaving forces, autonomous thought does not concentrate its efforts only on passively protecting its boundaries, but actively hits back and tries to expand its boundaries into the territory of the obligatory primary process, self-centered thought. This expansion is expressed particularly in the phenomenon of *creativity,* an achievement which is always carried out by a combination of secondary process thought enriched by primary process elements (Noy, 1978). The primary processes participating in the creative process typically bear all the qualities of autonomous thought processes, a fact which supports the theory that they are stirred into activity not by a process of "regression in the service of the ego" (as Kris [1952] assumed), but by a temporary (or permanent) expansion of the autonomous section of thought to include a part of the territory originally belonging to the obligatory primary processes.

The unending struggle between autonomous and obligatory thought creates a dynamic state in which the boundaries between the two systems may shift back and forth according to the relative strength of the various forces involved. The exact placement of the boundaries varies from one individual to another, and in the same individual in different periods of his life. There are situations in which the primary process boundaries are expanded far into the territory of the secondary process, so that considerable parts of it lose their autonomy to become enslaved by the demands of the self (this happens in almost all mental diseases), and other situations in which the boundaries are thrust in the inverse direction, so that considerable parts of the primary process become autonomous. In cases in which such a situation becomes a permanent state, involving one particular section of the primary process, a special artistic talent may emerge. Such a talent is typically based on one or several primary processes which originally belonged to the group of obligatory primary processes; but in the gifted individual, it became detached for some reason from its original group, attained autonomy and therefore continued its development together with all other autonomous secondary processes to become a part of the individual's regular cognitive processes (for possible reasons for such a development, see Noy, 1968, 1972). For example, for the gifted musician, his particular talent to hear and distinguish ten different voices at the same time is a regular cognitive activity, like someone else's ability to distinguish the voice of his son out of the voices of other children.

The permanent danger that autonomous thought will be flooded by the obligatory self-centered processes requires it to be constantly on the alert and to employ various controls. The main guarantee for the maintenance of autonomy is, of course, the capacity of reflection. The same capacity which allows autonomous thought to examine and control its own functioning also helps it to discern any self-centered motives which succeeded in infiltrating the network of autonomous reality-oriented thought. This reflective "defense" activity may be preconscious or conscious, and occupies our minds as a constant part of regular thought activity. For example, a college teacher is a member of a committee to select new students for training. He is a conscientious man, and tries to evaluate the applicants as objectively as possible, without allowing his biases to distort his judgment. He may sympathize with one of the students interviewed, he may be attracted to a second or repelled by a third, but he forces himself to suppress self-interest and to adhere to the objective data. Every day practically all of us face similar problems with which we should deal objectively. We must then make every effort to "isolate emotions from reason," "not let our biases influence our judgment"—all are efforts to prevent self-centered interests from interfering with autonomous thought.

The continuous efforts to safeguard the autonomy of thought are directed not only against the enslaving influence of the demands of the self, but also against the pressure of reality. The maintenance of the optimal autonomy necessary for efficient reality orientation requires that the operating thought processes be isolated from the urgent pressure of immediate reality demands. The pilot who enters into a critical aerial combat knows that his chances of winning are dependent upon his ability to keep his cool and to forget for the moment that his very existence is dependent on his ability to solve the reality problem with which he is confronted.

We know, of course, from psychoanalytic practice, that any autonomy is at best only a relative autonomy. Even in those cases where an individual is absolutely sure that he has succeeded in eliminating all self-interests or reality pressures from his objective reasoning, analysis will certainly prove that many self-interests are still involved in all the phases of his process of thinking. Reflective thought can never attain a complete elimination of the various self-interests and reality pressures. It can only hold them at an optimal distance which may be sufficient for autonomous thought to function without too many disturbances. Because this conscious controlling activity is insufficient to maintain required autonomy on its own, the reflective efforts have to be supported by the employment of various defense mechanisms, mostly unconscious. The most important of these is the defense of *isolation* between the secondary and the primary processes. This defense pertains to one of the most amazing phenomena of human mental life—our inability to understand the "language" of the primary process. All of us have an average of five dreams a night, make meaningful errors in speaking and writing, create or enjoy complicated artistic creations, produce neurotic symptoms—without being able to recognize their meaning. It is a paradox that although we all speak this common, ancient, native "language" very well, we are mostly unable to understand it. And it took several thousand years of human civilization to develop, until one genius, Freud, succeeded by simply listening to his own dreams, and learning the basic rules of this language's syntax and grammar.

Freud (1900) explained the phenomenon of isolation by introducing the metaphorical concept of the "censor," a hypothetical unconscious mechanism whose function is to prevent any contents dangerous to our inner mental equilibrium from entering into consciousness. Yet, this explanation of Freud's really referred only to the fact that we cannot allow ourselves to acknowledge the existence of many of our mental *contents,* but not to the more general phenomenon of our inability to acknowledge the *processes* by which these contents are formed. This fact—that the very "language" of the dream, parapraxes, and other primary process products remain incomprehensible to conscious scrutiny, even if they do not deal with any forbidden material—remains unexplained.

I believe that this phenomenon is a part of the general defense mechanism that autonomous thought enacts in order to defend itself against the danger of being flooded by the obligatory self-centered processes. It succeeds in protecting itself from the engulfing demands of the self only by pretending that it does not recognize the "language" of the self-centered processes at all. It treats them as something which originates outside, is encoded in a foreign language, like the belief in the "Sandman" who brings the dreams, the "Muse" who inspires creativity. When some of these primary processes become accessible, it is mostly not because autonomous thought dared to look beyond its boundaries, but because the expansion of these boundaries has caused parts of the original territory of the primary process to be included (as in creativity or special artistic talents).

The inability of autonomous thought to acknowledge the processes which are beyond its boundaries seems to be the *negative* manifestation of its reflective capacity to acknowledge itself. The activity of the mind can be compared to a long staff-room divided by a big mirror. The very fact that this mirror enables the clerks in one half of the room continuously to examine themselves while working prevents them from seeing the clerks working in the other half of the room. Thus, the function of reflecting and concealing are the two sides, the positive and the negative, of the same mechanism.

One cannot consider the defense of isolation or "the negative reflection" to be only a pathological manifestation. Education almost always establishes and reinforces this defense. Children are taught to think "reasonably," to articulate their ideas and emotions in a clearly conceptual manner, and not to let their emotions distort their judgment. The degree of social pressure to reject all the primary process modes of organization from adult discourse and manifest behavior varies from one culture to another, and is today at a maximum in the Western industrial societies. The primary process mode of categorization is typically regarded as "self-ish" or "primitive"; the primary mode of imaginative mental representation, as "childish" or "autistic"; the primary mode of self and reality representation, as "emotional" or "sentimental"; the primary mode of causality, as "mystical" or simply as "nonsense"; and all, if expressed openly in communication, as "infantile" and indicating a failure of education or a lack of maturity.

The processes of education and social pressure force the growing child to isolate his primary process operations from logical reasoning. A part of these operations is repressed to become the "language" of the unconscious, and another part (which varies from one individual to another) remains conscious and is expressed in daydreams, fantasies, contemplation, and artistic creation. As far as possible, the child learns to eliminate this conscious part from his manifest communication and behavior (to talk sense and to behave rationally) and to treat it as a "private language," which may be indulged only on condition that others have no access to it.

My thesis is that the state of isolation between the secondary and the primary processes, which is forced on the child's mind by his own defensive needs and reinforced by the demands of education and society, is somehow alien to human nature. The price that modern man has to pay for maintaining his logical reasoning, objective judgment, and competence while dealing with the complicated social, economic, and business world around him is in his progressive alienation from his emotional life and his inner resources of motivation. Because man can never pay the full price of this sacrifice, he is forced to look for some compensatory activity which will allow him to undo the unnatural isolation and to synthesize his primary and secondary operations into one act in a legitimate and socially acceptable way. This is the essence of all *artistic activity*—in creating, performing, or enjoying art. The "language" of art, by its very nature, is based on an integration of primary and secondary modes of communication; its structure is based on a combination of primary and secondary process rules of organization, and its perception requires a synthesis of primary and secondary process modes of experiencing and reasoning.

One additional question has to be asked: what is the relevance of the theory of the autonomy of thought to psychoanalytic practice? Most of the psychopathological states with which psychoanalytic therapy deals are the result of the failure of autonomous thought to protect its territory from the enslaving dominance of the obligatory self-centered processes. The weak apparatus defends the shrinking autonomy of its secondary processes by reinforcing the defense mechanism of isolation. But the strong apparatus has the power to hit back and, through the process of creativity, to expand the boundaries of autonomous thought and once more to dominate parts of the lost territories. In this struggle, psychoanalytic therapy joins forces with the ego to hit back; and, like creativity, it endeavors to enable autonomy to prevail over more and more areas dominated by the obligatory self-centered processes (for the similarities between insight in psychoanalysis and creativity in art and science, and the polarity between neurosis and creativity, see Noy, 1978, 1979).

By facilitating the development of the transference neurosis, psychoanalysis attempts to evoke the various past and present self-interests to come to light; by following the threads of free association, it penetrates into the depths of the self-centered processes; and by utilizing the instrument of interpretation, it exposes previously inaccessible levels of the mind to the scrutiny of reflective thought.

The process by which psychoanalytic therapy attempts to get control over the blind compelling forces of the drives, needs, and other demands of the self is essentially the same as the one which autonomous thought employs in its struggle to disengage itself from the obligatory demands of the self and the immediate pressures of reality—that is, both rely on reflective capacity and strive, by continuous examination and modification of their own processes and operations, to get control over autonomous thought functioning. A person's ability to push back the forces of the self, which in the various psychopathological states succeeded in gaining control over parts of the autonomous thought, is dependent mainly on the strength of the ego, enforced by the analyst's interpretations, to expand the scrutiny of reflective thought into the "dark" areas, thereby increasing the scope of autonomy.

In addition to the important effect of gaining control over parts of the drives, needs, and other demands of the self, the expansion of the boundaries of autonomy has another effect hitherto unrecognized by psychoanalytic theory—the effect of *restoring cognitive balance*. Normal cognitive development and functioning are dependent, as I have attempted to show, on the optimal fit between the two modes of organization. The defense mechanism of isolation, by creating an asymmetrical situation in which the secondary process modes of categorization, mental representation, etc., are conscious and open to reflective scrutiny, and the primary process modes are repressed beyond the boundaries of reflective scrutiny, violates the sound balance between the two modes. This imbalance is expressed clinically, especially in various disturbances of the self image, as well as in several other difficulties in cognitive functioning.

By focusing the scrutiny of reflective thought on the primary process modes, and by the expansion of the boundaries of autonomy to include at least a part of these processes in the territory of autonomous thought, psychoanalytic therapy succeeds in restoring the sound balance between the two modes. To the degree that *both* modes of categorization, representation of the self, etc., can be brought under the light of reflective thought, the discrepancies between them can be acknowledged, analyzed, and modified, and the optimal fit between the primary and secondary process modes, in any of the cognitive areas, can be achieved.

Freud, in 1933, formulated the aim of psychoanalytic therapy: "Where id was, there ego shall be" (p. 80). In line with the view presented here, we could formulate an additional aim for therapy: "Where obligatory ideation was, there autonomous thought shall be."

BIBLIOGRAPHY

ARANGUREN, J. L. (1967), *Human Communication*. New York: McGraw-Hill.
ARLOW, J. A. (1958), Report of Panel: The Psychoanalytic Theory of Thinking. *J. Amer. Psychoanal. Assn.*, 6:143–153.
BERTALANFFY, L. (1973), *General System Theory*. Middlesex: Penguin Books.
BOGEN, J. E. (1969), The Other Side of the Brain: II. *Bull. Los Angeles Neurol. Soc.*, 34:135–162.

CAMERON, N. (1963), *Personality Development and Psychopathology.* Boston: Houghton Mifflin.

CARNAP, R. (1955), Philosophy and Logical Syntax. In: *The Age of Analysis,* ed. M. White. New York: New American Library.

DEWEY, J. (1933), *How We Think.* Lexington, Mass.: D. C. Heath.

EHRENZWEIG, A. (1953), *The Psycho-Analysis of Artistic Vision and Hearing.* London: Routledge & Kegan Paul.

———— (1967), *The Hidden Order of Art.* Berkeley: Univ. Calif. Press.

FERENCZI, S. (1919), The Phenomena of Hysterical Materialization. In: *Further Contributions to the Theory and Technique of Psycho-Analysis.* London: Hogarth Press, 1950, pp. 89–103.

FISHER, C. (1954), Dreams and Perception. *J. Amer. Psychoanal. Assn.,* 2:389–445.

FRANCES, A., SACKS, M., & ARONOFF, M. S. (1977), Depersonalization. *Int. J. Psycho-Anal.,* 58:325–331.

FREUD, S. (1900), The Interpretation of Dreams. *S.E.,* 4 & 5.

———— (1915), The Unconscious. *S.E.,* 14:159–215.

———— (1933), *New Introductory Lectures on Psycho-Analysis. S.E.,* 22:5–182.

———— (1940), An Outline of Psycho-Analysis. *S.E.,* 23:141–207.

GALIN, D. (1974), Implications for Psychiatry of Left and Right Cerebral Specilization. *Arch. Gen. Psychiat.,* 31:572–583.

GEDO, J. E. & GOLDBERG, A. (1973), *Models of the Mind.* Chicago: Univ. Chicago Press.

HARTMANN, H. (1939), *Ego Psychology and the Problem of Adaptation.* New York: Int. Univ. Press, 1958.

HOLT, R. R. (1967), The Development of the Primary Process. In: *Motives and Thought,* ed. R. R. Holt [*Psychol. Issues,* 18/19:344–383]. New York: Int. Univ. Press.

HOPPE, K. D. (1977), Split Brains and Psychoanalysis. *Psychoanal. Quart.,* 46:220–244.

JAENSCH, E. R. (1930), *Eidetic Imagery and Typological Methods of Investigation.* London: K. Paul, Trench, Trubner.

JONES, E. (1953), *The Life and Works of Sigmund Freud,* vol. I. New York: Basic Books.

KANT, I. (1787), *Critique of Pure Reason* [Introduction to the Second Edition]. London: Macmillan, 1953.

KLEIN, G. S. (1970), On Inhibition, Disinhibition and "Primary Process" in Thinking. In: *Perception, Motives, and Personality.* New York: Alfred A. Knopf, pp. 281–296.

KLIGERMAN, C. (1972), Report of Panel on 'Creativity.' *Int. J. Psycho-Anal.,* 53:21–30.

KOESTLER, A. (1964), *The Act of Creation.* London: Pan Books.

KOHUT, H. (1977), *The Restoration of the Self.* New York: Int. Univ. Press.

KRIS, E. (1952), *Psychoanalytic Explorations in Art.* New York: Int. Univ. Press.

LANGER, S. K. (1942), *Philosophy in a New Key*. Cambridge, Mass: Harvard Univ. Press.

LICHTENBERG, J. D. (1975), The Development of the Sense of Self. *J. Amer. Psychoanal. Assn.*, 23:453–484.

MEISSNER, W. W. (1968), Dreaming as Process. *Int. J. Psycho-Anal.*, 49:63–79.

MOSES, R. (1968), Form and Content. *This Annual*, 23:204–223.

NOY, P. (1968), The Development of Musical Ability. *This Annual*, 23:332–347.

―――― (1969), A Revision of the Psychoanalytic Theory of the Primary Process. *Int. J. Psycho-Anal.*, 50:155–178.

―――― (1972), About Art and Artistic Talent. *Int. J. Psycho-Anal.*, 53:243–249.

―――― (1973), Symbolism and Mental Representation. *The Annual of Psychoanalysis*, 1:125–158. New York: Int. Univ. Press.

―――― (1977), Metapsychology as a Multimodel System. *Int. Rev. Psychoanal.*, 4:1–12.

―――― (1978), Insight and Creativity. *J. Amer. Psychoanal. Assn.*, 26:717–748.

―――― (1979), Form-Creation in Art. *Psychoanal. Quart.* (in press)

PARRY, J. (1967), *The Psychology of Human Communication*. London: Univ. London Press.

PIAGET, J. (1963), *The Psychology of Intelligence*. Paterson, N. J.: Littlefield, Adams.

PREMACK, A. J. (1976), *Why Chimps Can Read*. New York: Harper & Row.

RAPAPORT, D., tr. & ed. (1951), *Organization and Pathology of Thought*. New York: Columbia Univ. Press.

―――― (1960), Psychoanalysis as a Developmental Psychology. In: *The Collected Papers of David Rapaport*, ed. M. M. Gill. New York: Basic Books, pp. 820–852.

RUSSELL, B. (1940), *An Inquiry into Meaning and Truth*. London: Allen & Unwin.

WAELDER, R. (1965), *Psychoanalytic Avenues to Art*. New York: Int. Univ. Press.

WERNER, H. (1948), *Comparative Psychology of Mental Development*. New York: Int. Univ. Press, 1957.

WITTGENSTEIN, I. (1921), *Tractatus Logico-Philosophicus*. London: Kegan Paul.

Play and Adaptation

ERIC A. PLAUT, M.D.

PLAY HAS NOT HAD A PROMINENT ROLE IN PSYCHOANALYTIC THEORY, except for childhood play. This stems from Freud's view that play is normally restricted to childhood and, in the course of development, is replaced by fantasy, transformed into creative activity, or subordinated to the reality principle. Play, however, is an activity of central importance throughout life. It is universal, not only in man, but also in many higher animals. It exists in all known cultures. In this paper I propose to develop an ontogeny of play extending throughout life and to consider some implications that such a revised role of play has for the psychoanalytic view of conflict and adaptation.

Freud saw play as helping the child master anxiety through action. The child experiences play as unreal, yet "linked to reality."

> It would be wrong to think he does not take that world seriously; on the contrary, he takes his play very seriously and he expends large amounts of emotion on it. *The opposite of play is not what is serious but what is real. In spite of all the emotion with which he cathects his world of play, the child distinguishes it quite well from reality; and he likes to link his imagined objects and situations to the tangible and visible things of the real world. This linking is all that differentiates the child's play from 'phantasying'* [Freud, 1908, p. 144; my italics].

Commissioner, Connecticut Department of Mental Health, Hartford, Connecticut.

I am indebted to Professor Donald McIntosh, whose knowledge and insight contributed so much to the substance of this paper, and to Susannah Rubenstein, whose editorial skills contributed so much to its presentation.

217

Creative artists preserve and renew the pleasures (or fore-pleasure) of play by the use of "forbidden" wishes through alteration, displacement, and disguise. Freud (1908) wrote that "the essential *ars poetica* lies in the technique of overcoming the feeling of repulsion in us which is undoubtedly connected with the barriers that rise between each single ego and the others" (p. 153). The adult daydreamer "carefully conceals his phantasies . . . because he feels he has reasons for being ashamed of them. . . . Such phantasies, when we learn them, *repel us or at least leave us cold*" (p. 152f.; my italics). This repulsion may be understood dynamically as the result of the subordination of the pleasure principle to the reality principle and the subsequent repression and displacement of pleasure-bound activity through the activity of the ego and the superego.

Freud's personal assessment of pure fantasy undistilled into art can clearly be seen in these passages. For all his fascination with artistic creativity, Freud could not free himself from his conviction that adaptation to external reality was the hallmark of maturity, health, and happiness. He stated, "the growing child, when he stops playing, gives up nothing but the link with real objects; instead of *playing*, he now *phantasies*. He builds castles in the air and creates what are called *day-dreams*" (1908, p. 145).

Several further distinctions between child's play and adult fantasy emerge in Freud's writings. The child's play is characterized by the compulsion to repeat (in unaltered form and content) the activities and rules, patterns and circumstances, inherent in games. This in turn is related to the child's intellectual immaturity. The repetitiveness of childhood play is necessary because the child lacks both the ability to link thoughts together by cognitive work and the capacity for verbalization. Play helps children to renounce instinctual satisfactions by creating substitutes that permit partial discharge and to master anxiety by active rather than passive means. Adult play may be aimed at an audience; a child's play usually is not.

In Freud's view (1920), the compulsion to repeat, characteristically observable in children's play, is also the hallmark of dreams occurring in traumatic neuroses; here again the association between normative childhood play and pathological symptomatology of adulthood could be inferred:

> If we take into account observations such as these, based upon behaviour in the transference and upon life histories of men and women, we shall find courage to assume that there really does exist in the mind a compulsion to repeat which overrides the pleasure principle. Now too we shall be inclined to relate to this compulsion the dreams which occur in traumatic neuroses and the impulse which leads children to play [p. 22f].

Freud concluded his remarks on play in *Beyond the Pleasure Principle* by again linking it to the creative artist's role and suggesting that a system of aesthetics with an economic approach might be devised to account for the amount of pleasure and value inherent in artistic works.

Freud's assessment of the role of play must also be understood in the emotional and intellectual context of nineteenth-century European culture, which, among other things, was characterized by a highly ambivalent attitude toward pleasure and an elevation of work to a dominant position in its value system. This view of play as inappropriate to adulthood had not characterized earlier eras. As Aries (1966) put it, "In Western civilization, down to the eighteenth century at least, the words 'games' and 'play' did not signify anything childish" (p. 101). The subordination of the pleasure principle to the reality principle and the linkage of repression to the emergence of higher levels of civilization are evidences of this nineteenth-century trend in Freudian theory. Freud's definition of health is an additional expression of this value system: health is defined as the freedom to love and work (but *not* to play).

Following Weber (1925), I regard play as an ideal type of action. From a psychological point of view, *love, work, and play are the three ideal types of action.* They are the three primary types of motivated behavior, "ideal" in that they are pure types, non-existent in reality in unalloyed form. Such a formulation allows us to integrate the concept "action" into psychoanalytic theory, and to tie together the adaptive and the conflict-based aspects of this theory. Freud's definition of health was clearly an attempt at this. Perhaps because his definition omitted the crucial role of play and because he did not have a workable definition of action, Freud never further pursued his definition of health. As a step in that direction I shall first define play and then explore it from the genetic perspective by developing an ontogeny of play.

DEFINITION OF PLAY

There is no generally accepted definition of play. Many have attempted to define play activity: it has been variously described as motorically diffuse, i.e., nondirected, exaggerated, repetitive, and even wasteful of motion (Millar, 1973), and psychologically syncretic, involving autonomous, synthetic, integrative, and defensive ego functions (Corbin, 1974). In terms of social relations, play has been shown to permit temporary destruction and reconstruction of social hierarchies and value systems (Bateson, 1955). It has been defined as "free motion within limits" (Forrest, 1978, p. 2). It seems likely that imaginative play activity aids in the development of empathy, while simultaneously sharpening identifications and fostering reality testing (Rosen, 1960). Finally, play has been described developmentally in terms of its aims and structures (Millar, 1973; Erikson, 1977).

I define play as a form of action that is *pleasurable, freely chosen, intrinsically complete, and noninstrumental.* In describing play as a form of *action,* I follow sociologists, e.g., Talcott Parsons (1949) and Max Weber (1925), who define action as behavior which has subjective meaning to the actor. My use of the word "action" here is related to, but different from, Schafer's in that Schafer (1973) rejected the use of metapsychological constructs, while I retain them.

Play is action that is pleasurable. A wide variety of pleasurable activities are found in play. Control, manipulation, ritual, and mastery are common. A kinesthetic component is often present. Although many preconscious and unconscious gratifications will be present in play (as in all human activity), characteristic of play alone is that there is always a conscious sense of pleasure.

Play is freely chosen activity. It is free from both internal and external compulsions. It is free from internal compulsion in that it occurs in a temporary state of relaxation of superego control, although conscience continues to operate. It is free from external compulsion in that it is neither socially nor economically required. These are characteristics of play as an ideal type of action. Real play often, if not always, contains elements of both internal and external compulsion. Sports, for example, often have both a "driven" quality and a strong component of peer expectation and competition.

Play is intrinsically complete action. It does not require another person, as does love, although much play and most games involve other people. It exists entirely within its own boundaries and has no importance beyond the duration of the activity, in contrast to work and love, which always have future implications or immediate practical consequences.

Play activity is a carefully regulated function of the ego with clearly demarcated temporal and psychological boundaries. Play activity in adulthood reveals the masterful mature function of the ego, which, temporarily dominating id and superego, integrates their components into ritualized expression within a structured, articulated framework.

While all activity is bounded by structure, it is uniquely characteristic of play that the bounds are freely chosen and are an integral part of the activity, rather than a limitation to it.

Play is noninstrumental. It has no reality consequences. For example, in competitive play, regardless of who wins and loses, there are no implications for the relationship between the competitors. Play involves primarily symbolic objects, not real objects. In that sense it is narcissistic. I view this as a healthy narcissism, in the adult as well as in the child. Moreover, pure play does not produce goods or services, in contrast to work, which always does. Indeed, when play does produce goods or services, as in professional sports, it is alloyed with an element of work.

While it would be useful to attempt similarly detailed definitions of love and work, these are beyond the scope of this paper. Here I will define work as *an activity producing something useful or valuable* (goods or services) and love as *the active expression of valuing another being purely in his own right.* Freud (1930) considered work as the activity most suited to rooting man in reality. His theory of object relations, however, was based primarily on love relationships. The question of the role of play from the point of view of object relations needs further examination, which cannot be attempted here.

THE LITERATURE ON PLAY

Having defined play, I turn to a brief overview of the current literature representative of the widespread scientific interest in the subject. Ethologists, anthropologists, child therapists, and sociologists have written extensively about play (Altmann, 1962; Bateson, 1955; Groos, 1898; Lorenz, 1952; Millar, 1973).

Ethologists have long recognized that play is an inherent aspect of animal behavior in a wide variety of species, including most of the higher mammals, and that it is found both in the mature and the young. Animal play fulfills the four criteria of my definition. Ethologists' studies suggest that animal behavior, like human behavior, lends itself to organization in categories broadly defined as sexual, playful, and work-oriented (in animals, the latter is signified by food-gathering and habitat-building activity).

Anthropologists stress that play is present in all known cultures and, as far as we know, has always been a feature of human activity.

The psychoanalytic literature on childhood play is extensive (Erikson, 1937, 1950, 1977; Peller, 1954; Waelder, 1932; Winnicott, 1971). There is wide agreement about the central role of play in the development of the child and about the severe pathological implications of its inhibition in childhood. Play has also been extensively explored and used in the construction of Piaget's developmental psychology.

The sociological literature has a long-standing interest in the subject of play. Riesman (1954) pointed out that Freud's neglect of play was deeply influenced by nineteenth-century attitudes toward work and play, as a result of which Freud associated work with the reality principle and play with wish fulfillment.

The extensive literature by Marxists (Marcuse, 1969; Marx, 1939; Schroger, 1970; Shapiro, 1970) discusses only work and play as important activities, omitting love. Marxist theory views work as onerous and play as the relief from that burden, at least under capitalism. Under communism, play becomes unnecessary because work is rewarding. The Marxist focus on group behavior as well as its puritanical disregard of sexuality stand in interesting contrast to Freudian thinking, which views work as rewarding, focuses on individual behavior, and gives sexuality a central role.

There is a large body of psychoanalytic literature on play and creativity (Freud, 1908, 1910a, 1910b; Greenacre, 1957, 1959; Kris, 1952; Winnicott, 1971). I shall limit myself to two contributions which are most pertinent to the subject.

For Winnicott (1971), the realm of play is the area of experience between subjectivity and objectivity. The origins of this area of experience are found in the transitional object relationship, which stands halfway between the infant's purely subjective relationship with his mother and later object relationships. He states: "On the basis of play is built the whole of man's experiential existence" (p. 64). While Winnicott did not develop a detailed ontogeny of play, he postulated a development from transitional phenomena to play, then to shared play, and from that to cultural experiences. Winnicott's formulation that play stands halfway between the subjective and the objective is very similar to Bateson's (1955) formulation that play stands halfway between primary and secondary process. Closely related is Kris's (1950) concept of regression in the service of the ego. All three formulations address the dual aspect of play activity. It involves simultaneous access to unconscious id elements and highly structured ego elements. The player faces both inward to his unconscious and outward to reality (Rothenberg, 1976a; Waelder, 1932).

Like Winnicott, Erikson (1977) sees the origins of adult creativity and cultural experience in childhood play. He uses this as a point of departure to develop a detailed ontogeny of the ritualization of experience. For Erikson, play is a quality of behavior and not an ideal type of action. Along the same lines, the bounds and rules of games are (in Erikson's view) to control hostile agrression (in contrast to my view that they are intrinsic to play as an activity). Erikson's description of the role and development of ritual brilliantly combines biological, developmental, social, and historical factors. His epigenetic sequence for ritualization is especially pertinent. He follows the ontogeny he developed earlier, assigning the characteristics of ritual as follows: for infancy, mutuality of recognition; for early childhood, discrimination of good and bad; for the preschool years, dramatic elaboration; for the school age, rules of performance; and for adolescence, solidarity of conviction.

Winnicott and Erikson have documented the long-neglected role of play in creativity and ritualization. However, neither creativity nor ritualization has its origins in play alone. They both require elements of love and work. Indeed, as the highest forms of human activity, creativity and ritualization probably involve the greatest mixture of the three primary types of action.

I close my overview of the psychoanalytic literature with a few comments about the energies involved in play. Their source remains a subject of dispute. The traditional view follows Freud (1915) and was succinctly stated by Waelder (1932, p. 98): "From the standpoint of the theory of instincts, the mastery instinct, like all others, is a blending of love and destruction." Hartmann et al. (1949) expanded on this formulation, using the concept of fusion of neutralized sexual and aggressive energies. Numerous authors (Bühler, 1925; Fenichel, 1945; French, 1952; Groos, 1898; Hartmann, 1964; Hendrick, 1943; Kardiner and Spiegel, 1947; Mittelmann, 1954; Murray and Kluckhohn, 1953; White, 1959), however, have held that a separate instinct is needed to understand play, as well as for other reasons. White's (1963) viewpoint is the opposite of Waelder's: "The playful, exploratory, manipulative behavior of animals and young children . . . provides us . . . with the clearest body of facts upon which to build a conception of independent ego energies" (p. 33).

It is the thesis of this paper that play has equal status with love and work as one of the three primary types of action. Just as the libidinal instincts are the primary (but not the sole) source of energy for love, just as the aggressive instincts are the primary (but not the sole) source of energy for work, so independent ego instincts may well prove to be the primary source of energy for play. This approach lends support to White's position. An extensive exploration of this issue is beyond the scope of this paper.

Ontogenies of Childhood Play

The best-known psychoanalytic ontogenies of childhood play are those of Peller (1954), A. Freud (1965), and Erikson (1950). The work of Piaget (1951), from the point of view of developmental psychology, also has influenced psychoanalytic thinking on the subject. Erikson lists four stages of early childhood play: autocosmic play, centering on the child's own body; play with nearby things, like mother's body; play in the microsphere, the small world of manageable toys; play in the macrosphere, the world shared with others. A. Freud postulates a six-stage transition from body play to toys and from play to work. Her early stages closely parallel Erikson's; her later stages deal with play as a precursor for work. Peller's ontogeny of childhood play is the most detailed. She elaborates the defensive, expressive, formal, social, material, and secondary gain aspects of childhood play. Her four stages are based on the child's developing capacity for object relations: from the body, to the preoedipal mother, to the oedipal relations, to sibling relations. Piaget lists three stages of play: practice play, symbolic play, and games with rules. His second and third stages parallel Peller's third and fourth stages. Erikson's (1977) ontogeny of ritualization parallels Peller's first two stages (he uses almost identical language) and Piaget's stages three and four. These various ontogenies of childhood play are in basic agreement about the major characteristics of play at each stage of the child's development, although they use varying terminology.

An Ontogeny of Play Throughout Life

For my ontogeny of play (see table 1), I have drawn upon Erikson's eight stages of life. I have characterized the play stages as follows: for infancy, recognition play; for early childhood, discrimination play; for the preschool years, symbolic play; for the school age, games with rules; for adolescence, playfulness with boundaries; for young adulthood, integrated play; for adulthood, generation play; and for mature age, creative play. The first four of these stages come directly from Erikson and Piaget, whereas the last four represent an attempt to identify the most important forms of play in the postchildhood years.

The pressure of the resurgence of sexual and aggressive instincts in adolescence leads to attempts to discharge these via play. Play-

Table 1
Play Throughout Life

Life Stages (Erikson, 1950)	Stages of Ritualization (Erikson, 1977)	Stages of Play (Peller, 1954)	Stages of Play (Piaget, 1952)	Ontogeny of Play
Infancy	Mutuality of Recognition	Body	Practice Play	Recognition Play
Early Childhood	Discrimination of Good and Bad	Preoedipal	Practice Play	Discrimination Play
Preschool Age	Dramatic Elaboration	Oedipal	Symbolic Play	Symbolic Play
School Age	Rules of Performance	Sibling	Games with Rules	Games with Rules
Adolescence	Solidarity of Conviction			Playfulness with Boundaries
Young Adulthood				Integrated Play
Adulthood				Generation Play
Maturity				Creative Play

fulness characterizes many adolescent interactions. However, this playfulness often lacks the boundaries that are required to prevent it from degenerating into maladaptive behavior. Adolescent "horseplay" can become overtly hostile or inappropriately sexual. "Playing with ideas" in adolescence is a necessary precursor of adult creativity, yet it can become a vehicle for self-absorption. Masturbation, "playing with oneself," is a normal adolescent behavior unless it renders object finding dispensable (Blos, 1962). In play the boundaries are explicit. In playfulness they are implicit. Containing playfulness within boundaries is an important task of adolescence.

Genitality is the characteristic mode of relating in young adulthood (Erikson, 1950), with marital intimacy as the primary arena for its expression. Mutual participatory play needs to be an integral part of that intimacy. If young adult play is narcissistic or imitative, rather than participatory, it will undermine the relationship. If there is no play involved, the intensity of the intimacy, with all the inevitable unrealistic mutual expectations, can threaten the only recently established independent adult identities. Similarly, play must be an integral aspect of the sexual relationship. Otherwise, intercourse without foreplay depersonalizes the partner and foreplay without intercourse becomes teasing.

For adulthood, I have chosen generation play as the most characteristic, because of the critical role that the parents' ability to enjoy playing with their children has in successful child rearing. Child psychoanalysis has long recognized that meaningful interaction between an adult therapist and a child patient requires that the adult participate in the child's play. Curiously, child-rearing theory and practice have not given comparable weight to parent-child play. Spock (1976) devotes only 2 of 600 pages to the subject. My ontogeny of play, like other psychoanalytic ontogenies, posits that successful adaptation at later stages is predicated on successful integrations at earlier stages. The parent who was not able to play, freely and pleasurably, in earlier stages of his own life will have difficulty enjoying play with his or her children. Because play is such a central aspect of a child's world, the parent who does not enjoy playing with the child excludes himself from full participation in the child's life. The child, in turn, will feel that he is valued only insofar as he is learning to become an adult, not as a member of the family in his own right. In my clinical experience, the parents' ability to enjoy playing with their children is a significant indicator of the quality of functioning of the family as a unit.

For maturity, "creative play" is most characteristic. Here I have in mind not only the social significance of creative play (e.g., hobbies) when so much time in retirement is devoted to leisure, but also the significance of mature creative phenomena such as Verdi's *Falstaff* and Thomas Mann's *Felix Krull*. Both are products of old age and both are their creators' most playful works. Similarly, Picasso, Matisse, Klee, and Kandinsky all turned to playful work in their later years.

The creative play of hobbies and the playful creativity of many mature artists reflect the subjective and objective aspects of creativity. The retired businessman who has completed a paint-by-the-numbers picture has a subjective feeling of creativity, even though there is no originality involved. Objective creativity requires a new synthesis (Freud, 1928; Rothenberg, 1976b). The hobbyist reaffirms old pleasures or defenses, while the artist creates new solutions to conflicts. Popular art confirms prejudices, while great art gives new insights. Hobbies, of course, are play, albeit not pure play; there is no sense of responsibility involved. The artist is working, even though it be a playful creation. The frequency of playful works among mature artists suggests that play in older age is not just the result of more leisure, but that play has an increased importance in later life.

Far from being abandoned in adulthood (as Freud described it), play becomes more ritualized, structured, and controlled by the mature ego and coexists alongside of fantasy life. Here I disagree with Freud (1908) who argues that an exchange of fantasy for active play occurs in adults.

> As people grow up, then, they cease to play, and they seem to give up the yield of pleasure which they gained from playing. But whoever understands the human mind knows that hardly anything is harder for a man than to give up a pleasure which he has once experienced. Actually, we can never give anything up; we only exchange one thing for another. What appears to be a renunciation is really the formation of a substitute or surrogate. In the same way, the growing child, when he stops playing, gives up nothing but the link with real objects; instead of *playing*, he now *phantasies*. He builds castles in the air and

creates what are called *day-dreams*. I believe that most people construct phantasies at times in their lives. This is a fact which has long been overlooked and whose importance has therefore not been sufficiently appreciated.

People's phantasies are less easy to observe than the play of children. The child, it is true, plays by himself or forms a closed psychical system with other children for the purposes of a game; but even though he may not play his game in front of the grownups, he does not, on the other hand, conceal it from them. The adult, on the contrary, is ashamed of his phantasies and hides them from other people. He cherishes his phantasies as his most intimate possessions, and as a rule he would rather confess his misdeeds than tell anyone his phantasies. It may come about that for that reason he believes he is the only person who invents such phantasies and has no idea that creations of this kind are widespread among other people. This difference in the behaviour of a person who plays and a person who phantasies is accounted for by the motives of these two activities, which are nevertheless adjuncts to each other [p. 145].

In keeping with the Freudian dictum that nothing disappears from mental life, it is more accurate to say that both the capacity to fantasy and the capacity to play coexist in human mental life, from infancy through old age, and their functions, genetically and dynamically linked, continue throughout life.

At the beginning of my comments, I touched upon the relationship between the neglect of play and nineteenth-century puritanism (which rejected the pleasurable) and nineteenth-century industrial capitalism (which physically separated play from work and rejected the intrinsically complete and noninstrumental elements of play altogether). Before that time, the farmer, the artisan, and the small shopkeeper not only played with his children during working hours, but also retained a playful aspect to his work. To this day, the small shopkeeper in the Middle East considers playful bartering with a customer an essential part of his working life. Few workers in Western industrialized societies have that opportunity. When play occurs in the industrialized workplace, it is generally either totally separated from work and confined to breaks, or it is grafted onto the work in order to relieve boredom, often in a way that undermines the work.

The dichotomy that play is for children and work is for adults came out of the nineteenth century and was accentuated in the twentieth century by our reactions to the abuses of child labor. Since then, in addition to excluding play from adulthood, we have also excluded work from childhood. The fashionable educational theory of the past half century has been based on the concept that pleasurable, freely chosen activities lead to optimal learning. Prevailing psychological views supported that thesis. It is no coincidence that at a time when educators are questioning this thesis, we are also reevaluating the role of work in childhood.

Other forces in our society are also causing us to reevaluate the role of play. As increasing pollution, diminishing resources, and vanishing frontiers lead us to question our focus on the instrumental, we become more interested in less instrumental cultures such as the oriental. As more leisure time becomes available, we are beginning to reevaluate the value and meaning of both work and play. A revision of our theory of play also affords new opportunities for relating psychoanalytic theory to sociology, ethology, and anthropology.

Conclusion

In psychoanalytic theory, play has been assumed to have a subordinate role, with the exception of early childhood play. In the past 70 years much evidence has accumulated that play is of central importance throughout life.

Freud's formulation of psychological health: "the freedom to love and work," could be revised to: "the freedom to love, work, and play." Such a reformulation can serve as a bridge concept between our conflict-based psychology and our psychology of adaptation and health. It will be fruitful to assume that love, work, and play are ideal types of action whose major sources of energy are found in the sexual, aggressive, and ego instincts. Play has its own lifelong ontogenetic development. The stages are: in infancy, recognition play; in early childhood, discrimination play; in preschool years, symbolic play; in school years, games with rules; in adolescence, playfulness with boundaries; in young adulthood, integrated play; in adulthood, generation play; in maturity, creative play.

BIBLIOGRAPHY

ALTMANN, S. A. (1962), Social Behavior of Anthropoid Primates. In: *Roots of Behavior,* ed. E. L. Bliss. New York: Harper, pp. 277–285.

ARIES, P. (1966), Games, Fashions and Society. In: *The World of Children,* tr. R. Baldick. London: Paul Hanlyn.

BATESON, G. (1955), A Theory of Play and Fantasy. *Psychiat. Res. Rep.,* 2:39–51.

BLOS, P. (1962), *On Adolescence.* Glencoe, Ill.: Free Press.

BÜHLER, K. (1925), *The Mental Development of the Child.* New York: Harcourt, Brace, 1930.

CORBIN, E. I. (1974), The Autonomous Ego Functions in Creativity. *J. Amer. Psychoanal. Assn.,* 22:568–587.

ERIKSON, E.H. (1937), Configurations in Play. *Psychoanal. Quart.,* 6:139–214.

——— (1950), *Childhood and Society.* New York: Norton.

——— (1977), *Toys and Reasons.* New York: Norton.

FENICHEL, O. (1945), *The Psychoanalytic Theory of Neurosis.* New York: Norton.

FORREST, D. V. (1978), Spatial Play. *Psychiatry,* 41:2–23.

FRENCH, T. M. (1952), *The Integration of Behavior,* I. Chicago: Univ. Chicago Press.

FREUD, A. (1965), Normality and Pathology in Childhood. *W.,* 6.

FREUD, S. (1908), Creative Writers and Day-Dreaming. *S.E.,* 9:141–153.

——— (1910a), Five Lectures on Psycho-Analysis. *S.E.,* 11:3–56.

——— (1910b), Leonardo da Vinci and a Memory of His Childhood. *S.E.,* 11:59–137.

——— (1915), Instincts and Their Vicissitudes. *S.E.,* 14:111–140.

——— (1920), Beyond the Pleasure Principle. *S.E.,* 18:3–64.

——— (1928), Dostoevsky and Parricide. *S.E.,* 21:175–196.

——— (1930), Civilization and Its Discontents. *S.E.,* 21:59–145.

GIDDENS, A. (1964), Notes on the Concepts of Play and Leisure. *Sociol. Rev.,* 12:73–87.

GREENACRE, P. (1957), The Childhood of the Artist. *This Annual,* 12:47–72.

——— (1959), Play in Relation to Creative Imagination. *This Annual,* 14:61–80.

GROOS, K. (1898), *The Play of Animals.* New York: Appleton.

——— (1901), *The Play of Man.* New York: Appleton.

HARTMANN, H. (1964), *Essays in Ego Psychology.* New York: Int. Univ. Press.

——— KRIS, E., & LOEWENSTEIN, R. M. (1949), Notes on the Theory of Aggression. *This Annual,* 3/4:9–36.

HENDRICK, I. (1943), The Discussion of the "Instinct to Master." *Psychoanal. Quart.,* 12:561–565.

KARDINER, A. & SPIEGEL, H. (1947), *War Stress and Neurotic Illness.* New York: Hoeber.

KRIS, E. (1950), On Preconscious Mental Processes. *Psychoanal. Quart.*, 9:540–560.

———— (1952), *Psychoanalytic Explorations in Art.* New York: Int. Univ. Press.

LOEWALD, H. W. (1971), On Motivation and Instinct Theory. *This Annual,* 26:91–128.

LORENZ, K. Z. (1952), *King Solomon's Ring.* New York: Crowell.

MARCUSE, H. (1969), *An Essay on Liberation.* Boston: Beacon Press.

MARX, K. (1939), *The Grundrisse,* ed. D. McLellan. New York: Harper & Row, 1971.

MILLAR, S. (1973), Ends, Means and Galumphing. *Amer. Anthropologist,* 75: 87–98.

MITTELMANN, B. (1954), Motility in Infants, Children, and Adults. *This Annual,* 9:142–177.

MURRAY, H. A. & KLUCKHOHN, C. (1953), Outline of a Conception of Personality. In: *Personality in Nature, Society, and Culture,* ed. H. A. Murray, C. Kluckhohn, & K. M. Schneider. New York: Knopf, pp. 3–49.

PARSONS, T. (1949), *The Structure of Social Action.* Glencoe, Ill.: Free Press.

PELLER, L. E. (1954), Libidinal Phases, Ego Development, and Play. *This Annual,* 9:178–198.

PIAGET, J. (1951), *Play, Dreams and Imitation in Childhood.* New York: Norton, pp. 110–113.

RIESMAN, D. (1954), *Individualism Reconsidered.* Glencoe, Ill.: Free Press.

ROSEN, V. H. (1960), Some Aspects of the Role of Imagination in the Analytic Process. *J. Amer. Psychoanal. Assn.*, 8:229–251.

ROTHENBERG, A. (1976a), Janusian Thinking and Creativity. In: *The Psychoanalytic Study of Society,* ed. W. Muenstenberger et al. New Haven: Yale Univ. Press, pp. 1–30.

———— (1976b), Homospatial Thinking in Creativity. *Arch. Gen. Psychiat.*, 33:17–26.

SCHAFER, R. (1973), Action. In: *The Annual of Psychoanalysis,* 1:159–196. New York: Int. Univ. Press.

SCHROGER, T. (1970), Marx and Habermas. *Continuum,* 8:52–64.

SHAPIRO, J. (1970), From Marcuse to Habermas. *Continuum,* 8:65–76.

SPOCK, B. (1976), *Baby and Child Care.* New York: Pocket Books.

WAELDER, R. (1932), The Psychoanalytic Theory of Play. In: *Psychoanalysis,* ed. S. A. Guttman. New York: Int. Univ. Press, 1976, pp. 84–100.

WEBER, M. (1925), *Economy and Society.* New York: Bedminster Press, 1968.

WHITE, R. W. (1959), Motivation Reconsidered. *Psychoanal. Rev.,* 66:297–333.

———— (1963), *Ego and Reality in Psychoanalytic Theory* [*Psychol. Issues,* Monogr. 11]. New York: Int. Univ. Press.

WINNICOTT, D. W. (1971), *Playing and Reality.* New York: Basic Books.

CLINICAL CONTRIBUTIONS

Memory, Reconstruction, and Mourning in the Analysis of a 4-Year-Old Child

Maternal Bereavement in the Second Year of Life

THOMAS LOPEZ, Ph.D. AND GILBERT W. KLIMAN, M.D.

WHEN DIANE WAS 19 MONTHS OLD, HER MOTHER JUMPED FROM A cliff, to her death. Though the facts of the suicide were repeatedly explained to her, and though she verbally acknowledged them, for the first two weeks after it, she inquired into her mother's whereabouts and when she would return. Then she began overeating, became very clingy, tentative, unhappy, and prone to spells of crying. Increasingly she feared that people she loved would either be hurt or die, and often she herself fell. At first, her falls resulted in little more than scrapes and bruises, but by the time her analysis began, at age 4, they were placing her in considerable danger. At

Dr. Lopez is on the staff of The Center for Preventive Psychiatry, White Plains, N. Y., and on the child analysis faculty of the New York Freudian Society.

Dr. Kliman is Medical Director of The Center For Preventive Psychiatry and a member of the New York Psychoanalytic Society.

The authors gratefully acknowledge Ann S. Kliman's generous help in providing information and discussing the material presented in this paper.

This paper was presented at a scientific meeting of the New York Freudian Society on December 8, 1978.

that time she also had spells of diarrhea and terrifying dreams of being kidnapped by a witch.

This paper attempts to describe how analysis enabled Diane to mourn the death of her mother and overcome the symptoms and interferences with development which resulted from it. Its principal contribution is intended to be the vivid picture of her mourning which Diane, with her gift for communicating, was able to convey. Clinical material has been selected and is presented in detail to provide evidence that young children, given adequate help, are capable of profound mourning—an issue that has been extensively debated in the literature (for an excellent review, see Furman, 1974).

CASE REPORT

BACKGROUND

Diane's mother was a talented and successful artist. Her father, who remarried about one year after her death, was and is successful in business. Both were of oriental extraction. Diane had three sisters who were 2, 6, and 8 years older. Despite their mother's death, the children had an unbroken relationship to a maternal figure in the person of a housekeeper—a somewhat unreflective and rigid, but very caring black woman who had been with the family since prior to their births. Then their father's new wife, a kind, well-functioning woman, very actively and adequately assumed the principal maternal role, though the housekeeper remained.

His wife's death came as a surprise to Diane's father. She killed herself within an hour of having bade him an uneventful farewell when he left for work. Others who knew her, however, reported that she was obviously withdrawn and depressed, especially in the period just before the suicide. Though he was by no means psychologically disordered, it seems likely that Diane's father had strong proclivities to deny psychic pain in himself and in those close to him.

Nevertheless, immediately after his wife's death, he sought psychological help for his children. For one year, he and his girls had psychotherapy focused on the children's bereavement. The treatment, conducted by Ann S. Kliman, included one weekly session with the children and their father, one weekly session with the father alone, and a number of sessions with the housekeeper. The therapist also made several visits to the home. At the end of the year, when the 2-year-older sister developed night terrors (fearing that a witch would enter her room), she too was seen twice a week for about 9 months. Throughout, the father was very conscientious, supporting the children and providing relevant information about them. However, true to his character style, he refused intensive treatment for himself, although analysis was recommended, and remained quite uncommunicative (with himself, we suspect, as well as with the therapist) about his relationship with Diane's mother and hers with the children. Very little is therefore known about these areas. To date, the older children are symptom-free and apparently progressing well.

Diane, however, required additional help because her symptoms and unhappiness worsened. Mrs. Kliman reported that she had had little therapeutic impact on Diane, even though the latter related extremely well and was capable of quite advanced language. Therefore, some 2½ years after her mother's death, Diane entered analysis. She was seen five times a week during the first year, and three times a week during the second year.[1]

THE FIRST YEAR OF ANALYSIS

At age 4, Diane was enchanting: small, even for her age, her hair jet black, and very intelligent. She had a shy pleading quality about her, and a hard-to-describe, distant otherworldliness.

She was very desirous of a relationship and immediately formed an intense one with her analyst. She said that she wished to be relieved of her fears and unhappiness, and from the beginning produced rich, moving material. She expressed longings to be loved in a number of stories. In one, she was a flower, her analyst the sun and rain sustaining her; in another, a flower died of sadness because it had not been picked; in another, a beautiful fairy chose some but not others from among a group of eager children to accompany her to fairyland; in yet another, clay which had grown

1. The analysis was conducted by T.L., supervised by G.W.K.

hard and dry was discarded as useless, despite its protests, while clay which was still soft and could be used was retained. She conveyed receptive sexual longings by dramatizing stories of men trying energetically to enter a dollhouse through its every opening, and of kindly men who presented gifts of small tame animals to little girls. She conveyed oral longings and aggression. In one story, a small dog chased a cow in order to bite it. In another, oral strivings were blended with heterosexual strivings: a male farmer and a cow developed a relationship in which each needed the other. The farmer needed the cow for milk. The cow needed the farmer to relieve the pressure on its udders ("its tummy").

Themes associated with death moved into the forefront within the first 4 weeks. Diane's imagery increasingly became populated with dead people and dead animals, and with people or things lost or otherwise out of sight. Children bereaved of their parents began to appear in her stories, and in one a fairy brought a dead little girl back to life. Diane became preoccupied with minor bruises and deformities on her own body and that of others. Increasingly she would drop breakable things—toy dishes and cups. Often she herself fell, at times hurting herself to the point of tears.

In her weekly interviews, the stepmother told the analyst that since the beginning of Diane's analysis, Diane increasingly had asked about her mother's suicide, and about life and death in general. She had expressed a special interest in the condition of her mother's body after it had struck the ground. She was told, as before, that her mother had jumped to her death because she had become so unhappy, she no longer wished to live, and had died when many of her bones had been broken.[2]

In her analysis, Diane explicitly acknowledged her mother's death only in its 5th week. Although a toy Diane wanted to use was in plain view, she was unable to find it. When finally she did, she jokingly played at "losing" a number of others by dropping them so that they would roll under a table. The analyst linked her

2. In the earlier treatment, Mrs. Kliman thought it best to present Diane with specific detail for two reasons: (1) the manner in which her mother died quickly became common knowledge in the family, and was freely discussed, especially by the sisters; (2) Diane herself let it be known that she knew of it, by falling repeatedly in her first therapy session with Mrs. Kliman.

activity to what sometimes happens with painful thoughts: we try "losing" them by pretending they don't exist.

Just then, Mrs. Kliman's dog was heard barking (the therapy room was in the basement of her house). Diane said that she and her family knew both the dog and Mrs. Kliman, but—as if she had let slip something she wished she hadn't—refused to reveal how this had come about. The analyst took the opportunity to explain that he already knew that her mother's suicide had been the reason for their acquaintance.

Diane sobered and began searching intently for a doll she had been using to represent a fairy who traveled back and forth between this world and fairyland. The analyst remarked that her search reminded him of a question often asked about a person who had died: where is that person? "I know about my Mommy," Diane replied. "Don't talk about her. I get scared." Thoughts about dead people can be frightening, the analyst said, but more so when we try to push them away. Diane found the fairy, and with a number of dolls representing children "buried it" under the removable top of a small plastic table. "What is it like for your mother under the ground?" the analyst reflected, "is she with other children?" "I know what it's like," Diane replied. "Sad." "Our mother's death so saddens us," the analyst commented, "it is hard to believe only the living feel sad."

In the next session, reversal of affect enabled Diane to arrive in a buoyant mood. Gleefully, she climbed onto a knee-high ledge at one end of the room and jumped off in an obvious enactment of the suicide. She then tooted a harmonica, mimicking the sound of the car that regularly fetched her; threw a ball about with reckless abandon; and hid behind furniture only to reappear amid peals of laughter. Furthermore, she enacted the role of a highly competent mother taking care of her baby. She also had the analyst play the role of a suitor she could permit to enter her home or ostentatiously order to leave.

Then, as if to give the ideas she had been warding off opportunity for expression, she drew a picture of a witch, complete with broom, pointed hat, and malevolent grin, on the very spot on the ledge from which she had jumped. Next, in what seemed an affirmation of her confidence in their relationship, she engaged the analyst in a game in which they stood at opposite ends of the room, ran toward each other, and touched hands when they met. The analyst remarked only that Diane was bringing up many ideas having to do with loss and with her mother's death, and that she and he were getting on with the task of learning about them.

Diane's involvement in the analysis intensified. Dreamlike imagery, at times of near-hallucinatory vividness, emerged: Diane insisted she smelled vanilla pudding while presenting the analyst with the gift of a bracelet. In her doll play she introduced a little girl who loudly complained that she did not want a "skeleton in her closet." In response to the analyst's linking her frequent jumping from the ledge to the manner in which her mother had died, she offered what seemed a denial of her helplessness at the time. She stated, but would not amplify, "I almost told Dad Mom would die before she [actually] did." After the analyst read her a story at her request (*Bongo the Bear*), in which the chief protagonist is thought dead after having fallen over a waterfall, Diane seemed lost in reverie. She lay on her back on an easy chair next to the analyst's, rubbed her genitals, looked up at him, and commented that his head seemed to be floating. Then, in sequence, she asked him if her own leg was full of blood; cautioned him against leaning forward in his chair lest he fall; responded with anxiety at the distortion of his features produced by his resting his chin in his hand; lifted his trouser to see whether his leg was hairy like a man's or shaven like a woman's; and told him she remembered having diarrhea during a session with Mrs. Kliman (a real event).

It appeared that the analytic process and especially the developing transference relationship intensified in Diane the cathexis of ideas, memories, imagery, fantasies, and ego states associatively linked to her mother's death and promoted their entering the analytic work.

During the next 10 weeks themes of Diane searching for her mother, mingled with themes of sexuality and death, emerged in the following order:

1. A vivid illustration of the degree to which Diane at times experienced her mother as "present." Using dolls, she dramatized children preparing to journey to a far-off land in a vehicle capable of traveling on land or water. Abruptly, however, she interrupted

what she was doing, placed the fairy under the removable top of the table, and, while sitting on the table, told of a deer that had been killed in a nearby wood. As she spoke, uncannily a doll fell off the table. Diane was shocked. Trying to jest, she suggested that the doll's fall was caused by the fairy's anger at having been placed in the table. Then, quickly, she assured the analyst that she did not believe in ghosts. The latter commented that perhaps at times she did.

As the week progressed, an eerie atmosphere took hold. Once the children set off on a journey they had to go on "forever." They made several visits to fairyland, wherein resided a "kind fairy." Dolls and other objects fell off tables—apparently unconsciously placed by Diane so that they would—and she herself fell a number of times. She developed a story about a child who frequently became dizzy and fell off high places; and one about children who went up chimneys with Mary Poppins and traveled with her to far-off lands. Sounds from above produced ideas that they had been made by Mrs. Kliman—not unreasonable, since the latter did reside directly above the therapy room. Diane's intense longing look and questioning about her whereabouts suggested a displacement of feeling from her mother onto the woman (approximately her mother's age) who had become involved with her just after the former's death. The analyst underscored that her mother and Diane's hopes for being reunited with her were still very much alive in her mind.

2. The idea that her mother had died as a result of her sexuality. Diane brought two dolls from home, one, old and battered, representing a young woman; the other new, representing a beautiful princess. She fetched a cardboard cylinder, some 3 feet in height, and called it a "tower." Then she dropped the battered doll she called "the prince" on top of it, face to face, in coital position. Laughing sadistically, she proceeded to knock the tower over, causing its occupants to tumble to the ground. The analyst pointed out that she was causing the dolls to fall just as her mother had fallen, and that she seemed to be linking lovemaking, on the one hand, falling and death, on the other. Diane responded by placing the old battered doll on the tower and knocking it off several times. She said that the doll "loved" falling. Later Diane

had the fairy teach some children to fly, assuring them it was possible to fall in love without actually falling. The analyst commented that Diane was not totally certain of this.

3. The idea that in dying her mother had actually gone to have sexual relations. Diane enacted a picture of sadistic sexuality: a stick placed children on the tower and kissed them tenderly, only to knock them off and hit them about the floor amid derisive laughter. The analyst took this up in terms of the weekend separation—of Diane feeling uplifted at the beginning of the week only to feel let down at its end. Diane responded by lifting her blouse and skirt to show her underwear, requesting that the analyst show her his underwear, lying on her back and masturbating with a blanket squeezed between her thighs.

In a short time, however, she was on her feet proclaiming that she possessed a magic wand, which conferred upon her the power to transform people she liked into royal personages; those she didn't, into frogs. Exercising this power, she made herself a princess, the analyst a prince, and pretended they were riding about in a toy car. Presently she had the car go off a cliff, killing its occupants. The analyst took up her guilt over sexual feelings for him—the punishment of death follows their emergence—and suggested a similar sequence with regard to her sexual feelings for her father.

Diane listened carefully and added another element. She timidly volunteered the idea that her mother lived under the ground with "hairy monsters." To encourage her to elaborate, the analyst "drilled" an imaginary hole in the floor so that they might look in on them. His efforts were rewarded. Diane jocularly described *him* in the very terms she had used to describe the monsters, adding that she nevertheless thought he was quite nice. The analyst suggested that children often thought of men as monsters, especially if they heard them breathing heavily at night when making love. Perhaps she had had the thought: "There goes my mother leaving me alone to be with that monster, my father." Perhaps this was how she arrived at the idea that her mother was with men— "monsters"—with whom she made love underground. Diane seemed interested, but denied having heard her parents making love.

Yet, she then placed a mother and a father doll sleeping together in a house she had constructed of blocks. After a time she placed the sleeping mother in a small, transparent plastic box, which she first called "Mommy's bed," but which she then likened to Snow White's glass coffin (a picture of which she had often seen in a book in the therapy room). Again, the analyst drew Diane's attention to her pondering over the consequences for a woman of loving a man: does it kill her? Or, as in the story of *Snow White*, does it bring her to life?

Looking moved, Diane sat next to the analyst and related a story she had heard of an evil man who had stolen Christmas with all its joy from the children of the world. The analyst suggested that she might be asking whether a man had caused Diane to lose her mother and all the happiness she might have known with her either by killing her, or by giving her so much pleasure, she abandoned Diane for him?

4. *Orally and anally rooted ideas regarding her mother's death.* These ideas often reflected ego states prevalent during the oral and anal phases. Diane had children prepare for a journey, while one child who was excluded complained bitterly about being left out. Diane's back was to the analyst, and she loudly passed wind. Embarrassed, she rose to go to the toilet, but asked that the door to the therapy room be left open in her absence. When she returned, she had the children travel over waters teeming with biting fish in a flimsy boat, in constant danger of sinking. They were traveling to Florida, to visit her own maternal grandparents. As it was a Friday session, the analyst first linked the lonely endangered travelers to Diane's feelings of being alone and endangered during the impending weekend break. He then used her references to toilets, water, biting fish, and her maternal grandparents to draw her attention to a possible revival, in the transference, of feelings concerning the loss of her mother. In her mind she seemed to link the weekend separation with being flushed down the toilet, and then being alone and vulnerable in its vast waters. Did she experience her mother's death as mother having gotten rid of her as one might get rid of feces? Did she also have the idea that her mother had gone through the waters, perhaps to visit her own parents, and might well be there now?

In the first session of the following week, Diane engaged the analyst in a dialogue in which he was instructed to say "behind the tree," following each of a number of statements she made. Finally she described a woman undressing behind a tree and asked him where he was at the time. After answering the question as instructed, the analyst reflected on how difficult it was to be a little girl. When grown men and women like each other, they often undress in each other's presence. But alas, grown men don't do that with little girls. "I knew you would say that!" Diane replied sharply. Soon her attitude became one of coy, smiling superiority, however. She declared her hands smelled. They smelled in the same way her stepmother's and father's, her sisters', and the analyst's did. Assuming she was hinting at masturbation, the analyst remarked, "When we have the feelings we've been discussing, we do get the urge to rub ourselves between our legs, and if we do, our hands do smell."

With striking suddenness Diane's coy superiority became transformed into desperate repulsion. She claimed the room reeked of a "doo doo" smell emanating from her shoe, on which there actually was a barely discernible speck of dog's feces. She declared that she was about to vomit, lay on the floor, kicked, writhed, and screamed, much as a toddler would, and insisted that the analyst do away with the speck. He did no more than focus on the discrepancy between her great repugnance and the barely noticeable nature of the odor. He suggested that this must represent a revival of ideas and feelings she had had when she was a much smaller girl; and underscored that the regression seemed triggered by their discussing adult sex.

Diane quickly calmed down and proposed a riddle: "What is black and blue and red all over?" The answer: "A skunk with a diaper rash." So was her mother's body when it struck the ground, the analyst pointed out. Perhaps, Diane thought it had been the odor of her feces that had made her die and go away. At the time Diane was not yet 2, and in the midst of toilet training. Her mother's abandoning her must have made her feel like a malodorous skunk. Perhaps she now was retaliating, calling her mother a skunk.

Diane listened intently, and then expressed a fear that the car taking her home might crash with her in it, causing her to die. She must feel that her mother exists somewhere, the analyst suggested, and is able and likely to punish her, on the one hand for being angry at her, on the other for enjoying her work with him.

Diane asked the analyst to show her pictures in a book, but not read the words. He did, and reflected that her mother had died at a time when Diane was the age when children are shown pictures in books by their mothers. One day, hers simply wasn't there to do it anymore. How painful and sad that thought is. While she was waiting to be fetched, the analyst heard Diane sobbing softly in the waiting room.

Connections between genital sexuality, anality, and falling from heights were further explored. Genital and anal sexuality were linked by a common element—*falling* from a height, the *falling* of feces from the body, and *falling* in love. In one sequence, Diane first depicted a female doll, its legs wrapped around a broomstick, sliding up and down in a clearly sexual manner, then as screaming and falling. Next, with a mischievous grin, she dropped blocks of wood and a female doll from the area of her buttocks.

Considerable work was also done on anxiety associated with her feminine sexual desires, and on her fear of men's sexuality.

By the 20th week, Diane's expressions of love toward living and available objects, the analyst included, had become more open and intense. For example, the family hastily arranged a trip to Florida for a reunion with Diane's three sets of grandparents (the analyst was told of it only two days in advance). Though at first elated at the prospect of it, Diane soon saddened and commented on drawings by other children hanging on the walls. The analyst suggested that despite being happy about leaving, she was not happy he would be seeing other children.

Diane responded with vivid imagery and with wishes to identify with the analyst in drawing, an area in which her mother had been extremely talented. She first drew "three sisters," each on a separate sheet. She then laid out three paths for them to travel and provided them with a shoe, a barrel, and an old box as vehicles. After moving them along their paths for a time, she said that her own sisters would not accompany her because they had to attend school. She then asked the analyst to draw a picture of a little girl.

As he worked, Diane with great seriousness admired his effort, and wished she would someday be able to do as well. Then she switched off the lights, placed a ring on the analyst's ring finger, removed it, and placed it on hers. She ordered him to remain silent and described a number of endearing characteristics of her grandparents: one grandfather's snoring, another's playing with her; one grandmother's cooking, another's liking to take her to shops. The analyst interpreted that she seemed to fear that her enjoying and loving others might prompt him to do likewise and abandon her. She seemed intent on keeping him under control— if necessary, by marrying him.

Diane verified the interpretation by relating a story, partly borrowed from television, of a man married to a witch, angry at her flying about with her witch friends. When the parallel between the interpretation and the theme of her story was pointed out to her, she laughed and responded with erotic feelings. She related that her father had carried her to bed the previous night in the manner she had seen him carry her stepmother, and Diane jovially suggested that the analyst pull his trousers down to show her his penis. As the session drew to an end, however, Diane became very sad, allowing the analyst to take up depressive as well as heightened erotic feelings in reaction to the imminent separation.

In the final session of the week, Diane depicted a little girl who wished to marry not only her boyfriend, but also her three grandfathers and several uncles. The analyst focused on her deep desire to give her loving feelings free rein.

After her trip Diane continued to elaborate thoughts connected with her mother. She depicted a fairy (who this time she bluntly called "my first Mommy") as flying off with a boy and a girl. She then turned off the lights and had the doll explain to the children that the darkness of the room was like that of the grave. Diane developed the idea that the fairy was forced to sleep alone, felt lonely, and therefore tried to get children to come and sleep with her. The analyst interpreted that Diane was projecting her own loneliness and longing onto her mother, imagined her to be alive somewhere, and wished to join her. Diane verified this interpretation by telling a story of a little girl who lived on an island, totally alone and very lonely. An entourage of dolls representing children visited her, expressed their sympathies, and offered to keep her company.

In another sequence a "barrier" between the living and the dead was prominent. Diane set up a game in which she and the analyst were each to stand in a "base"—one of two rectangles, drawn on the floor with chalk, at opposite ends of the room. While standing in them, they were to throw a ball to one another. An inviolable rule was that they were not to cross a "barrier," a line placed halfway between the bases. Diane was elated each time she succeeded in throwing the ball accurately to the analyst. In the next session, Diane made the fairy and a group of dolls she called the "fairy's children" residents of fairyland. A small boy entered the scene, and asked the fairy to be his mother because his own was dead. He was refused since he was not a fairy; only fairies may have fairies as parents. The boy, deeply disappointed, continued to plead. Suddenly the fairy grasped him and flew off with him. Diane made him witness her murdering his father, brother, and sister. Then, with him, she flew back to fairyland, and now permitted him to join the family of fairies.

The analyst interpreted the sequence as representing suicide more than murder. Fairyland, like heaven, seemed to be a land where the dead go. If there were such a land, one could reach it only by dying oneself, not by killing others. Diane responded by having the fairy travel to the land of mortals. She singled out two female dolls as "dead mothers," made them come alive, calling one "bad" and the other "good," and then promptly and brutally killed the "bad" one again. The analyst focused on the hatred she harbored toward her mother for having abandoned her, and on her attempt to separate the image created by this hatred (the "bad" mother from that of the loved and "good" one).

Another sequence of stories emerged around the third anniversary of her mother's death, in early spring. She constructed a train of boxes, on which she placed dolls representing two kinds of beings: ordinary people and immortal "fairies." The former were attacked time and again by toy soldiers, called "bad guys," who were determined to kill the ordinary people. These were protected by the fairies and an assortment of magic rings, necklaces, and bracelets, which each time succeeded in repulsing the "bad guys." As the story unfolded, a mother and her daughter were pursued by "bad guys" intent on devouring them. The mother, however, was able to fly and, carrying her daughter, took to the air to escape. But the "bad guys" also could fly, and they set off in hot pursuit. To save her daughter, the mother dropped her, offering herself as a sacrifice. The analyst focused on Diane's effort to defend against the anger she felt toward her mother for having abandoned her, an anger she had displaced onto the "bad guys." She was reversing what had actually happened: instead of an abandonment, she was depicting her mother's suicide as an act performed for her daughter's sake.

Diane listened quietly and went on to enact a commentary on the cruel unpredictability of death. She had a toy garbage truck arrive at totally unexpected times and surprise sometimes a child, sometimes a mother or father, sometimes "just anyone," by removing them and taking them to their deaths. When in the process of controlling the truck she became increasingly sadistic in demeanor, the analyst took the opportunity to verbalize her view of death as a sadist who comes without warning.

In the next session—after she had fallen when the analyst turned his back, and hurt herself to the point of crying—first the ravenous "bad guys" and then the truck of death reentered the scene. This time, however, they were forced into retreat by a most unusual defender: an Easter bunny doll! Then, with great determination, Diane set herself to draw one flower after another on the white top of a small table, until it was thickly populated. Each flower had human characteristics—face, limbs, genitals. The analyst commented that her mother had died in early spring, 3 years ago. Death must have seemed omnipresent, and she must have feared that not only her mother, but others she loved and needed, and even she herself, might die. However, then as now spring arrived. Nature, accompanied by the Easter bunny, came to life and countered death. It must have been very reassuring.

In the following weeks (32 to 36), Diane further elaborated ideas concerning her mother's death. In one story, a garbage truck abducted Burt and Ernie of *Sesame Street* and took them to a far-off land. There storms and monsters abounded, and night and day alternated irregularly. When the analyst verbalized the turmoil depicted, Diane blurted out that she preferred her "first" mother to her "second," then quickly reversed her position. The analyst suggested that the turmoil she was depicting reflected the turmoil caused in her by her mother's death and by her feeling compelled to choose between her love for two mothers. Diane sadly said she remembered her "first" mother carrying her out to the lawn and playing with her. She then asked the analyst to lift her so that she might look into the space created by the room's lowered ceiling. The analyst again focused on her continuing search for her mother.

In another story, repair of the destruction caused by her mother's death was central. A woman represented by a yellow marble flew down from an unspecified place to marry a man also represented by a yellow marble. They went to live in a house made of blocks. Soon, however, it was rent asunder by convulsive rocking (produced by Diane). The woman flew out from the rubble to return to whence she had come. However, she was replaced by a woman, represented by a dark marble (Diane's housekeeper was black; her stepmother, dark), who married the man and together with a small child set about to rebuild the house. The analyst verbalized the obvious parallels between her story and the history of her life. He also suggested that because her mother had voluntarily ended her life, perhaps Diane believed that she had a unique relationship to life and death—one in which she was able to travel between them at will.

In a very striking, longer sequence, Diane depicted her efforts to reconstruct the situation as it had been just prior to her mother's suicide. Diane had the analyst take the role of herself as a baby, while she took that of her mother, energetically cleaning and ostentatiously ignoring her daughter (the analyst). She explained that "Jane" and "Thomas"—her stepmother's and the analyst's names—were coming to dinner. After participating for a time, the analyst interjected that since their arrival was imminent, the time for her mother to die must also be imminent. "Everyone knows she's going to die except her," Diane replied crisply. "Why doesn't she know?" the analyst asked. "Because she doesn't want to hear about it," Diane answered.

Diane then depicted how her father and housekeeper had cared for her after her mother's death. And she continued to show her mother compulsively cleaning and emotionally indifferent. No simple repetition of overheard conversation seemed involved, for neither father, nor stepmother, nor housekeeper could recall having articulated the picture Diane was conveying, either in her presence or outside of it. Rather, what seemed to be involved was an active effort at reconstruction, based perhaps on memories and things overheard, however vague.[3]

She began the next session on the same tack, but soon lost interest, appeared gradually to become frightened, and said she wished to play outside. Sensing that she was attempting to take flight from anxiety, the analyst interpreted her request as defensive, and suggested that they stay in the room. Diane, looking frightened now, tripped, fell and got up, "accidentally" knocked over a house of blocks, and again tried to get the analyst to go out with her. He stood his ground. Suddenly Diane noticed the presence of an electric heater. Her anxiety was quickly replaced by elation. She announced that she would turn it on in order to roast the analyst, and now urged *him* to try to escape while she stood her ground, barring the exit. The analyst followed her lead, whereupon Diane cheerfully went through the motions of roasting, carving, and eating various of his parts. Soon, however, her demeanor again betrayed anxiety. She lay on the stairs leading out of the room, rubbed her genitals, sucked her thumb, and asked what the analyst had eaten for breakfast. In answer to his question, she guessed it had been eggs and added, "Mommies have babies in their tummies. That's why they're so fat." She then climbed to the top of the stairs, and proceeded to step in and out of the door leading to the outside of the building, simultaneously forcing saliva in and out of her mouth through tight lips.

Attempting to elicit further what seemed to the analyst to be

---

3. In response to the material as a whole, Mrs. Dorothy Burlingham stated: "I wondered how a child of that age could have such an amazing verbal memory. I think she must in some way have reexperienced the event, not as a 2-year-old, but as an older child, even older than her years, and that she must have absorbed the content of overheard conversations and used them in the present."

oral-incorporative fantasies, he pointed to the parallel between her actions at the door and those with her saliva. Diane immediately saw the link, and proceeded to engage in both with greater vigor. If the door is like a mouth, the analyst suggested, perhaps the room is like a tummy, and perhaps she had wanted to leave to avoid being in a tummy like the babies in pregnant women's tummies about which she had spoken. Diane stopped, looked serious, glanced about, and proposed that the stairs might be teeth. After a feeble attempt to be jocular, Diane again looked very scared. To make the ideas more understandable to her, the analyst tried placing them in genetic perspective. Employing a large baby doll, he illustrated how central the mouth is in a baby's relationship to her mother, and how natural it is for a baby to wish to eat and be eaten by her mother (Lewin, 1950). He underscored how intense, hard to outgrow, and frightening these ideas can become if the baby loses her mother, as she had lost hers.

In the next session, at her suggestion the room became the inside of a whale's body. To the mouth, teeth, and tummy of the previous session she added a place where feces goes prior to being expelled. As she and the analyst sat in this place at her invitation, she made shrill noises which she called "ghost sounds." The analyst reflected on her linking feces to death. Pointing to recent material in which she had linked a garbage truck to death, and death to being disposed of, he suggested that she might have had many ideas concerning feces at the time of her mother's suicide: her mother's body had been disposed of like feces, and she herself must have felt disposed of by her mother, causing her to feel unloved and without value—like feces. The analyst's comments seemed meaningful to Diane.

Additional work on her experience of herself as devalued, in the week that followed, shed further light on Diane's reaction to the loss of her mother. She told a story involving three houses. In one lived a hungry child; in another, a black child whose mother had died; in the third, an oriental child whose mother also had died. The second child was cared for by a black housekeeper and a black doctor. In the course of the session, the three children were readily identified as representations of herself; the black housekeeper and doctor, as the woman who cared for her and the analyst; and the blackness of the second child, as her sense of having been rejected by her light-skinned mother.

That evening Diane's stepmother phoned the analyst and told him that Diane was demanding that her analysis be stopped. She claimed she no longer needed it. Her bad dreams had ceased. The analyst didn't play with her enough, and he talked about her mother far too much. When she came to her next session (following mild coercion by her stepmother), she sat for a time, looking very sad. Finally she removed a doll representing a black baby from a bag she had brought with her and fondled it tenderly. Again, she reached in her bag, and this time removed a doll representing a white little girl-angel and another representing its mother. Haltingly, Diane told a story in which the mother rejected the child-angel for being too dirty. The latter set up her own home; but because she felt unworthy, she had no friends. The analyst focused on the angel's turning aggression against herself; instead of thinking her mother unworthy, she thought of herself as such. Diane responded by angrily shouting at him to be quiet, and vehemently insisted she wished to terminate analysis. While shouting, however, she fell backward from the stool on which she was seated and hurt herself painfully. The analyst simply verbalized how deeply her pain actually went: she was hurt not only on the surface of her body, but also well within. For more than 10 minutes she cried inconsolably.

As the first year of analysis came to an end (weeks 37 to 45), feelings of great vulnerability associated with ideas of being alone and unprotected came to the fore. Oral-sadistic themes involving wishes to devour and be devoured again became prominent, as did depictions of cataclysmic upheaval—of earthquakes and storms which destroyed people and homes. Throughout, the analyst related Diane's reactions to separating from him for the summer to her as yet unmastered feelings about the loss of her mother. It should be added, however, that Diane also presented material indicating that she experienced the holiday separation in positive oedipal terms.

Diane's home situation, overall, seemed a very good one. The atmosphere was one of warmth, stability, and liveliness among very attractive people. The stepmother, solidly invested in her maternal attitude toward Diane and her sisters, appeared to exert an especially empathic and positive influence. She was intelligently sensitive, receptive to and tolerant of Diane's pain. In addition to attending at first weekly and then bimonthly meetings with the analyst (the father attended about once a month), she often phoned him to report observations she thought might be of value. Diane's father, while more aloof characterologically, continued to be essentially supportive. The housekeeper remained loving and involved, and seemed an uplifting influence by way of her buoyant spirit. As the year progressed, both parents reported that Diane had become more confident and assertive. Her distant look gradually disappeared.

Nevertheless, they felt that she was still an unhappy little girl; more fearful than the average child, more prone to teariness, more lacking in comfort and ease with herself than she ought be, and very definitely in need of further treatment. The only negative note was contained in her father's insistence that she attend three, rather than five, sessions a week in the coming year. In his opinion, she (one would suspect, he) was in need of "relief" from the intensity of her involvement in analysis.

THE SECOND YEAR OF ANALYSIS

Analysis resumed on a dramatic, though puzzling note. Diane's parents reported that on the evening prior to its resumption, and just before they were to go out to dinner, her father reprimanded her for some minor matter, the exact nature of which escaped his recall. Diane became extremely angry at him and refused to kiss him good-bye. Then suddenly, and for nearly a half hour, she behaved as if "possessed." She refused to move from the staircase on which she was seated, stared blankly into space, and, when approached, kicked and thrashed about in an uncanny manner. Just as suddenly she became composed and returned to normal. The analyst was unable to detect any references to this event in Diane's material, so its meaning must remain a matter of conjecture. However, if it was triggered by the impending resumption of analysis, it indicates the intensity of her involvement in it and, as with her falling, her tendency to respond with global symbolic action to material relating to loss of, and reunion with, a loved object.

Once underway again, the analysis moved very well (weeks 46

to 56). At first oedipal themes were in the forefront as Diane initiated husband-and-wife games, depicted children in search of "overnight dates" (a term used by local children for an invitation to sleep at a friend's home), and masturbated in a clearly sexual manner. Then anally colored sexual ideas of how her mother had died emerged.

Diane told a story in which a mother and a father, with much ado, wash up after having gotten dirty from "riding horses." Then she had the analyst, on hands and knees, play the part of a horse on which she rode; and while doing so, she rubbed her genitals. Finally, she enacted a suicidal leap from what she called "a cliff" (the ledge) into "water" (a large cushion). The analyst focused on how ideas (rooted in the anal phase), such as becoming dirty, and falling into water, were intruding into her thinking of what it was like for a woman to make love to a man. Diane responded to his comments by intently questioning the analyst about how her mother had managed to get to the top of the cliff from which she jumped: was it along its interior or exterior? Were there elevators or did she climb stairs? The analyst answered realistically, but stressed that her questioning must have other meanings which he did not yet understand.

"Bad" angry representations of herself, isolated from "good" pleasant ones, and then a disinhibition of pleasure in smearing (paint and ink) next came to the fore. These themes were followed by the emergence of depressive affect, a period during which feelings of having been rejected as worthless permeated her material. Now, however, there was no threat of stopping analysis. Diane referred to her mother explicitly, and for the first time in realistically positive terms. She proudly reminded the analyst of her mother's artistic talents, and sadly reflected on how she wished mother were still alive to help her with her own drawing and painting (her drawing was remarkably good for a child of her age).

Oedipal material again became dominant. However, in contrast to the way in which it had emerged earlier, it was much less infiltrated by preoedipal themes and much more solidly anchored in the present. It centered on ideas that there were too many females at home (five) and too few males (one, her father); being excluded from the sexual activities of adults; and envy of women's procreative capacities.

What proved to be an important turning point occurred during the 57th week. In her stories, Diane increasingly displayed a self concept more of an adequate, competent, caring woman rather than of a needy little girl. In one she enacted a woman who had adopted a baby and was taking care of it. The baby had been rejected by its mother for biting and scratching. In others she played the part of a wife and mother caring for her husband and children; and of a woman who gave generous banquets and had many guests. Diane's verbalizations became more direct and open. She berated the analyst if he was late in starting a session; she punched him, threw things at him, and proclaimed her hatred for him when she disapproved of something he said or did; but on a number of occasions she openly asserted her wish that he were her father. She also gave clearer expression to mixed feelings regarding her mother. While she continued to express longings for reunion with her, she now also revealed wishes to be free of her.

In the course of weeks 57 to 65, Diane's relationship to the family's housekeeper came more clearly into focus. Diane elaborated her conception of the housekeeper as a degraded "anal" mother to whom she had been demoted by her own mother, on the one hand, and as the loyal, caring woman she was, on the other. For example, in one session, Diane assigned to the analyst the role of child; to herself, that of the housekeeper. Then she went to the toilet and returned with a "meal" for the analyst; the "meal" was made of soap and water and looked very much like urine. Then she loudly passed wind, and absent-mindedly hurled a doll representing a baby to the floor. When the analyst focused on her low opinion of what the housekeeper did for her, Diane righted the balance. She gave many details of how good and caring this woman had been.

Diane's thoughts turned to conditions under which her mother might still be alive. She enacted stories in which:

it had been her father and not her mother who had died;

her parents had been divorced, but her father had moved out, while her mother had stayed and remained alive;

her mother had had a son, either as an only child, or in addition to the four daughters she did have (the implication was that though she and her sisters had not been able to, a male child might have made her mother think it worthwhile to remain alive);

the home was kept fastidiously clean and orderly, causing her mother to feel so pleased, she did not leave;

a sibling who bit and scratched was expelled, while her mother remained at home to care for the remaining, mechanically compliant children.

Diane developed an insightful hypothesis—that at the time of her suicide mother had been unable to love herself. She brought in a doll representing a little girl whose name also was "Diane" with whom she played "being with Mommy." She took the role of mother, and assigned to the doll and the analyst the roles of daughter and son. She fixed an elaborate dinner and comported herself as a somewhat overly conscientious housewife. Then she turned to her doll and enacted the part of a tenderly loving mother. "Diane loves Diane," the analyst commented, adding, "When people we love are not available, we must be able to rely on and love ourselves." Diane immediately responded. She proposed that the analyst ought to have a "Lopez doll," just as she had a "Diane doll," to love when he was lonely. In a jocular mood, she wished that each member of her family, as well as the analyst's cat, had namesake dolls. Then, very seriously, she wondered: would her mother have killed herself if she had possessed such a doll? The analyst added that she seemed to understand that for a person to kill herself she must have very little self-love and must feel terribly alone. Soon thereafter Diane composed lyrics which she sang to the tune of *Shoo Fly Shoo*. Their gist was that though she had lost her mother, someday she would be a mother herself, but one who would care for and not abandon her baby.

In the session that followed her use of the namesake dolls, Diane herself spontaneously and sadly introduced the termination of her analysis. (Her parents denied having brought up the matter with her.) She unashamedly declared her love for the analyst and remarked on how sad it would be in autumn when she would be in first grade in school, a big girl, and no longer meeting with him. In the final session of that week, she cried at the idea of the weekend separation, but stuck her tongue out at the analyst and punched him when it was over. The analyst interpreted that on separating from someone we love, anger as well as sadness is immobilized.

The analyst followed Diane's lead and agreed that termination should tentatively be set for that summer—still nearly 6 months off. Diane seemed ready for it and worked it over in her play (weeks 66 to 71). She developed stories of people forced to travel different roads after having traveled the same one. In another story, a little girl's father had gone away. The ground quaked, but in a short time it became steady again. The implication seemed clear, and the analyst focused on it: their separation would be upsetting. But Diane was confident the upset would be only temporary. Diane's positive oedipal declarations of love for the analyst became strikingly direct, but also restrained by a good sense for the limits of reality. For example, she played at being his wife and mother of their child. After a time, however, she lost interest, asserting that in fact they would never marry one another; the analyst was much too old for her (in guessing his age, she overestimated by 10 years) and he already was married. Often she played the part of a mother caring for a baby and embellished her enactments with rich fantasies.

Her comfort with sexual matters became impressive. In one session she had the analyst carry her about, while she hung by her hands from a broomstick. The activity led to a very detailed discussion of male and female genitalia. Her anxiety that penetration in sexual intercourse might result in pain or injury to the woman was taken up. She illustrated her understanding of how the vagina functions by stretching the lips of her mouth. She expressed confidence that by the time she was grown up her vagina would be adequate to accommodate a penis. In another session, after the analyst had taken up her obvious sadness over the coming weekend separation, Diane initiated a game of catching a ball, in which sharing and mutuality were strikingly prominent. Then she built a house, at one side of which she made an entrance that she called a "hidden tunnel." She invited the analyst to kick the ball gently into it. Whenever he missed, she generously consoled and encouraged him, much like an understanding woman helping a sexually not too adept man. In a different game Diane urged the analyst to shove her. When he did, she would fall onto a cushion. Then she shoved him and urged him to fall, which he did—all amid much hilarity. The buoyancy of her self-esteem was underscored by the following interchange: the analyst focused on how she had moved from experiencing herself as a frightened, needy little girl, to one oriented to the future, to loving men, and to becoming beautiful. Diane snapped: "I already am beautiful!"

Stimulated, it seemed, by the approach of spring which marked the fourth anniversary of her mother's death, as well as by the imminence of termination, themes having to do with her mother and with separation again came to the fore in the final weeks of analysis (weeks 72 to 89).

The shift in material was ushered in when Diane, very sadly and without explanation, drew a woman, every part of whose body was either broken or disfigured. She then drew a mound of earth on a grassy lawn, shaped somewhat like a breast. On it she drew some flowers that she called a "family of flowers," and at its base a "little flower" that was between 1 and 2 years old. The sun was shining on them all. After she informed the analyst that she had no story to accompany her drawings, he suggested they might have to do with her mother's death; with her crushed body, her grave, and the family and little girl who had lost her. He added that the approach of the anniversary of her mother's death might be stimulating these ideas. (According to her parents, no mention of it had been made at home. However, they were now urged to discuss it by the analyst.) In the next session Diane spontaneously said that she remembered Mrs. Kliman having met not only with her, but also with her sisters at that time. She then remarked on the gloomy cloudiness of the present day, and very sadly dropped her drawing of the mangled woman to the floor. The analyst said, simply, "She's gone."

Diane then drew a girl in a picture, one side of which was made to look springlike and sunny, the other wintry and full of snow. Next came a drawing of a house similar in appearance to the one in which she and the analyst had met during the first year of their work (they had moved to a different office at the beginning of the second). When again Diane offered no associations, the analyst suggested she was continuing to remember. He pointed to the similarity of the house she had drawn and the house in which they had first met; and he reminded her that her mother had died just as winter was turning to spring. After tinkering absent-mindedly for a time, Diane tenderly snuggled with the analyst's pet cat and remarked on how warm it felt. He commented that life was so much more appealing than the terrible cold of death.

Similar imagery emerged some 5 weeks later (and 2 weeks after the anniversary of her mother's death). Diane asked the analyst to draw bushes, a tall tree, four little trees, and then another tall tree that had fallen. She asked of the latter, "Is that my Mommy?" The analyst said that her ideas were the important ones. Diane asked him to draw tearful eyes on the standing trees. He commented that just when nature had begun to come alive, in spring, 4 years ago, her mother had died. She, her sisters, and her father, like the trees, had been very sad indeed.

As termination approached Diane explicitly equated the analyst with a mother. In one of Diane's stories a group of children played and picnicked on the lawn of a house in which lived a woman they called "Mom." "Mom" chose now one, now another, but never more than one at a time to enter and stay with her—a privilege highly desired by all of the children. The analyst did no more than point to the parallel between "Mom" seeing one child at a time in her house, and his seeing one at a time in his.

On another occasion Diane expressed pity and tenderness for her mother, and a sense of helplessness in the face of her death. Wandering about the room aimlessly, she picked up the "Mom" doll and, looking very serious, held it tenderly, much as a mother would hold a baby. She was dissatisfied with its slightly tattered dress and asked if the analyst could provide a better one. He gave her some half dozen which were at hand. Diane tried each one of them. With much care she chose the one she considered prettiest, and again held the doll tenderly. The analyst commented that she was showing such touching tenderness; she seemed to understand how terribly alone, even babylike, her mother must have felt when she killed herself. Diane responded by grimly tearing the limbs from the doll, and then unsuccessfully attempting to force them back on. "How you wish you had the power to take your mother apart and put her together again," the analyst interjected. Abruptly, relieving the intensity of the moment, she put the dismantled doll aside.

Then she drew a girl wearing a "party dress," volunteered that today was her "new Mom's" birthday, and that she, Diane, would be wearing a "party dress" for the occasion. The analyst under-scored her wanting to give up the futile effort to put her dead mother together again, to bring her back to life; and her wanting to turn more fully to the living, loving mother she did have.

In the final weeks, longings for reunion with her mother alternated with a defiant celebration of life, her own youthfulness, and her future. In a sequence of several sessions, Diane darkened the therapy room, and enacted going underground and entering her mother's grave. In the course of it, she elaborated on her longings to see her mother again, her anger at her mother for being dead, and her own refusal to give up living as the price of joining her.

The final two sessions illustrate something of what Diane had gained from analysis. In the next to last session, she drew a man and woman joined at the head. They were from outer space and since they already were inseparable, they had no need ever to marry one another. The analyst interpreted her conveying that people can continue relationships in their imaginations—in their heads—even if they cease to see each other in reality. Diane responded by playing at cutting and combing the analyst's hair as a barber would. As she did, she mimicked the sounds of scissors by clicking her teeth. The analyst verbalized the implied incorporative strivings. Diane laughed and immediately reminded him of something he had said earlier: people can imagine other people within them. It is not necessary actually to eat the other person.

In the final session, following the analyst's interpretation of efforts to suppress her feelings, Diane vehemently proclaimed her hate for him and angrily kicked the "Mom" doll about. She insisted that the therapy room was her home, and challenged the analyst's right to prevent her from coming. His statement that the strength of her feelings was testimony to how well they had worked for the past 2 years was enough to allow her to calm down. At the end of the session she sadly bade him farewell *and, as she had done on a number of occasions, in the final 3 to 4 weeks, also bade her mother farewell*. The experience was not one of equating the analyst with her mother, but conveyed recognition that feelings for her mother had become vividly revived in the analytic relationship and somehow existed within its essence.

On the way out, Diane commented on how well a number of young trees on the lawn were growing.

DISCUSSION

The preceding material documents the reactions of a young child to her mother's death. We believe that these constituted a profound work of mourning, a process that was facilitated by psychoanalysis.

THE NATURE OF MOURNING

In Anna Freud's (1960) words: "The process of mourning . . . taken in its analytic sense means . . . the individual's effort to accept a fact in the external world (the loss of the cathected object) and to effect corresponding changes in the inner world (withdrawal of libido from the lost object, identification with the lost object)" (p. 58). Freud (1917) formulated "the work which mourning performs" as follows:

> Reality-testing has shown that the loved object no longer exists, and it proceeds to demand that all libido shall be withdrawn from its attachments to that object. This demand arouses understandable opposition—it is a matter of general observation that people never willingly abandon a libidinal position, not even, indeed, when a substitute is already beckoning to them. This opposition can be so intense that a turning away from reality takes place and a clinging to the object through the medium of hallucinatory wishful psychosis. Normally, respect for reality gains the day. Nevertheless its orders cannot be obeyed at once. They are carried out bit by bit, at great expense of time and cathectic energy, and in the meantime the existence of the lost object is psychically prolonged [p. 244f.]. Each single one of the memories and situations of expectancy which demonstrate the libido's attachment to the lost object is met by the verdict of reality that the object no longer exists; and the ego, confronted as it were with the question whether it shall share this fate, is persuaded by the sum of narcissistic satisfactions it derives from being alive to sever its attachment to the object that has been abolished [p. 255]. . . . when the work of mourning is completed the ego becomes free and uninhibited again [p. 245].

The "memories and situations of expectancy" which enter the bereaved's consciousness do so as a result of their cathexes being intensified by *longing* for the lost object. The ego's severing "its attachment to the lost object" constitutes a partial withdrawal of libido from its unconscious representation (Freud, 1917; Furman, 1974).

Identification with the lost object, perhaps "the sole condition under which the id can give up its objects" (Freud, 1923, p. 29), plays an important role in all mourning. It acts to "preserve" the lost object psychically, both in the form of an "introject"—an internal substitute for it (Fenichel, 1945, p. 394ff.)—and in the form of an identification proper—an alteration of the representation of the self so that it more closely resembles the lost object's representation. As formulated by Furman (1974, p. 61ff.), identification may play either a positive or a negative role in the bereaved's adaptation to loss. It plays a positive role to the extent that it facilitates mourning by helping to bridge the gap between the loss of the object and the time required to effect the necessary "corresponding changes in the inner world"; and to the extent that identification itself, as a central aspect of those changes, acts to enrich the personality of the bereaved. It plays a negative role to the extent that it becomes an end in itself, thereby impoverishing the life of the bereaved. Identifications which are rooted in relatively advanced developmental phases (oedipal and postoedipal) lend themselves, because they are partial and selective, to being integrated within the personality and to enriching it. They thus tend to play a positive role. Identifications rooted in developmentally earlier phases (preoedipal), are "magic by nature, . . . founded on . . . mechanisms of introjection or projection, corresponding to fusions of self- and object-images which disregard the realistic differences between the self and the object. They will find expression in illusory fantasies of the child that he is part of the object or can become the object by pretending to be or behaving as if he were it" (Jacobson, 1954, p. 102). These identifications therefore do not lend themselves to promoting a bereaved child's development or to being integrated within a bereaved adult's mature personality. They tend to diminish the ego's freedom, to impoverish life, and thus to play a negative, unhealthily regressive or fixating role.

Mourning draws motive force from at least three sources. One stems from strivings to preserve reality testing, which requires that, however painful, the fact of object loss be acknowledged.

The second derives from strivings emanating from "the sum of narcissistic satisfactions . . . [derived] from being alive" (Freud, 1917). The bereaved's wish to remain alive and to live as fully and richly as possible motivates efforts to separate, to differentiate, from the dead object—in a word, to mourn.

A third motive force of mourning derives from strivings to cope with and master the painful "flood" of affect to which the psychic apparatus of the bereaved is subjected. The sources of the flood include: (a) intense longing for specific transactions with the lost object (Freud, 1926, pp. 169–172); (b) affects "reactive" to the loss. These comprise narcissistic pain, rage, despair, guilt, the full range of anxieties triggered by the intensification of drive tension and grief. Grief is a painful " 'taming' of the primitive violent discharge affect, characterized by fear and self-destruction, to be seen in mourning savages" (Fenichel, 1945, p. 395) or "in a child's panic upon the disappearance of his mother" (p. 162), or, in Rapaport's (1959) terms, a tamed state of helplessness activated by the loss of the object. The work of mourning accomplishes a mastery of this "flood" by regulating its rate of discharge, so that the ego may come to terms with it, in a piecemeal and gradual manner (Deutsch, 1939; Mahler, 1961).

DIANE'S INABILITY TO MOURN UNAIDED

When her mother died, Diane, 19 months old, had not yet reached the stage in her psychological development at which she could mourn unaided.[4]

Her reality testing had developed to the point at which she could verbally acknowledge, but could not fully appreciate, the fact of her mother's death. Much like the 10-year-old boy who following the death of his father remarked, "I know father's dead, but what I can't understand is why he doesn't come for supper" (Freud, 1900, p. 254), Diane at first repeatedly asked where her mother was and when she would return. Later, her analytic material showed that she continued to entertain ideas that her mother had not ceased to exist but had only gone away. It also showed a

---

4. Furman (1974), A. Kliman (1978), G. W. Kliman (1965, 1968, 1979), Mendelson (1974), Miller (1971), Nagera (1970), and Wolfenstein (1966, 1969) offer thorough discussions of children's capacities to mourn.

prominence of magical ideas that somehow she herself had been the cause of her mother's disappearance, and grandiose wishful ideas that she could somehow cause her mother to return.

Her identificatory processes were still at primitive levels of development, cognitively and in the continuum of part versus whole objects. She was therefore unable flexibly to perceive and identify with many specific characteristics of her mother. Instead, she identified with her mother as the person who fell, jumped, or was discarded as feces.

Her ego was unable to tame the "flood" of affect which followed her mother's death, and could not yet express it in a modulated, piecemeal manner, and master it. Instead, there occurred global blocking of affect on the one hand, and frequent breakthroughs in the form of anxiety attacks and tearful crying on the other. Her unhappy demeanor at the outset of treatment reflected narcissistic depletion, feelings of helplessness and depression (Bibring, 1953), and lack of emotional vitality, rather than the depressive state of mourning itself.

At the time of her mother's death Diane's drive development had reached the oral and anal-sadistic phases, with their heightened ambivalence. With regard to object relations, she probably was in the late rapprochement subphase of the separation-individuation process, characterized by acutely painful awareness of separateness from mother (Mahler et al., 1975), and great dependence on her for maintenance of narcissistic equilibrium, including self-esteem regulation (Kohut, 1971). Therefore, Diane reacted to the loss of her mother in a "catastrophic" manner—by globally blocking affect discharge to stem her sense of personal disintegration. This supposition is supported by the analytic material which indicated that: (a) Diane had a sense of the entire world, of existence itself, being in disorder and upheaval; (b) she "split" the presumably unmanageable ambivalence, a process resulting in coexisting images of her mother as a "good" fairy and a "bad" witch, each of which she expected to materialize; (c) she suffered from profound narcissistic injury, feeling dirty, smelly, worthless, and discardable like feces; and (d) she reacted with impotent narcissistic rage in a context of magical thinking and prominence of projective mechanisms, as a result of which she also feared being attacked, viewing aggression as omnipotently powerful.

MOURNING AIDED BY ANALYSIS

In the course of her analysis, however, Diane experienced a process that did not in principle differ from what Freud (1917) called the work of mourning. On the one hand, much material organized around longings for her mother emerged. It included the revival of fantasies, ideas, and affects stimulated by her death, but not mastered by Diane at the time. On the other hand, it became possible for Diane to submit this material to "reality's verdict" that her mother no longer existed. This process enabled Diane to withdraw a good deal of libido from her mother's inner representation, vague, painful, and terrifying as it was, and shift it to her stepmother, who increasingly became Diane's "psychological mother" (Goldstein et al., 1973)—perhaps her first reliable one since infancy. Further, important identifications with the more positive aspects of her mother, undoubtedly supplemented by what she perceived in living mothers in her environment, took place: a wish to become a mother herself, but to care for and not abandon her children; and a predilection for communicating by way of drawing, as her mother had communicated.

Analysis aided Diane's mourning, in several ways. The transference acted to organize "the memories and situations of expectancy which demonstrate the libido's attachment to the lost object" (Freud, 1917) by providing it with an object on whom it could be focused, and around whom it could crystallize. Freud's (1912) words are apt:

> If someone's need for love is not entirely satisfied by reality, he is bound to approach every new person whom he meets with libidinal anticipatory ideas. . . . Thus it is a perfectly normal and intelligible thing that the libidinal cathexis of someone who is partly unsatisfied, a cathexis which is held ready in anticipation, should be directed as well to the figure of the doctor [p. 100].

Persons who have suffered the loss of an important object, as Diane did, are of course in a state of unsatisfied libido, as well as of aggression (Hartmann et al., 1949). How they deal with this state depends on their developmental status, characterological makeup, especially on their defensive style; on the attitudes of important people in their family and environment; on cultural and other factors; and, in relation to the analyst, frequently on the initial impressions made by him or her. It has been our experience, however, that bereaved patients—be they children or adults—will deal with this state in one of two ways. Either they will take flight from forming a new relationship, or they will turn to the analyst in the hope of filling the void and thereby establish an intense transference (G. W. Kliman, 1979). The first alternative has often been described as typical of the bereaved person.[5] The second alternative clearly describes what Diane did. From the very outset, she was intensely attached to the analyst and longed to be accepted by him. At first, the analyst, as her mother in the transference, served as a person around whom Diane could crystallize her wishes for reunion. As she resolved to break the tie, he could serve as a person around whom she could crystallize her wishes to separate.

However, it was the context provided by the analytic relationship as a whole that made mourning possible for Diane. The therapeutic alliance (Greenson, 1967); the analyst's remaining alive and loyal to her; the relationship extending over a period of time; the consistent, organized, verbal mode of communication—all contributed to providing Diane's immature and beleaguered ego with the assistance it needed to carry out the piecemeal process of working through that is characteristic of mourning. Furthermore, the substantial pleasure she derived from her relationship to the analyst as a "real" object, one who worked with and cared for her, enhanced the "narcissistic satisfactions" she derived from being alive, and thus gave impetus to her motivation to mourn.

At the time of her mother's death Diane had been in the preoedipal phase of development, to which she remained fixated prior to analysis. The mourning accomplished in analysis loosened her tie to the inner representation of her mother and thus was one of the factors enabling her to move to the position of oedipal domi-

---

5. The opposite is depicted in the movie *Last Tango in Paris,* in which intense mourning is shown to take place very much within an equally intense, though initially self-centered relationship with another person.

nance. In addition to providing her with the opportunity for identifying with her mother in a more positive way, this move also allowed her to experience life in a more complex, future-oriented manner. It freed her from repetitive and compulsive preoccupation with loss, death, and self-destruction, giving her a more sustaining range of object relationships and interests. The positive triangular relationship including her stepmother, her father, and herself played an important role in furthering this development. It provided Diane with a situation in which she no longer had to be the little girl, who after having been abandoned by her own mother was relegated to the housekeeper—a "mother" whom father devalued by rejecting her sexually. Rather she could become an active member of a lively oedipal triangle, competing with an attractive, desired woman for an attractive man. Furthermore, this woman also loved Diane and was one with whom she could readily identify. Diane could now more easily think of herself as attractive, valued, and valuable (Kohut, 1977). Of course, these factors, by providing Diane with a foothold in a world removed from and far more exhilarating than the preoedipal world of her dead mother, made an important contribution in their own right to the impetus to mourn.

We wish to underscore two special problems which the mother's suicide created in Diane's narcissistic line of development, problems which we believe generally exist in young children in similar circumstances. First, the fact of having had a mother who discarded herself provided Diane's developing self with a pathogenic, mirroring self-object (Kohut, 1971). Mirroring her mother, she clearly experienced herself as discardable, disposable garbage. This mirroring often was demonstrated explicitly, for example, in the recurrent themes containing precise mirror images of self and mother concepts: a dead girl with a dead mother; a sad girl with a sad mother; a lonely girl with a lonely mother. Second, the material indicated that loss of her mother, so very early in life, became a powerful stimulator of narcissistic rage (Kohut, 1977). The latter, in turn, activated the repetition compulsion, interfering with reality testing and a number of executive functions. Diane repeated her mother's fall over and over again, and at such times was literally unable to use her own labyrinthine, proprioceptive, and kinesthetic perceptions and related executive functions. The experiences of repeating her mother's fall had a frightening quality, similar to repetitive night terrors of shell-shocked soldiers whose buddies have been blown up while they themselves stood by helplessly. In Diane, the repetition appeared not in dream form but in a waking state, with a prominent, concrete, motor identificatory component. The analysis allowed a more abstract and muted form of day-terror to emerge, leading to a working backward and through of the narcissistic rage and the preceding narcissistic injury. Diane made grandiose efforts to feel powerful in the face of helplessness concerning her mother's mortality and her own mirrored mortality. The analyst needed considerable tact in order gradually and very gently to deflate her identification with her mother as the one who fell and was dead but could fly and was immortal.

The process of working through the narcissistic injury permitted Diane to invest more libido in herself, increasing her sense of vitality and well-being, and diminishing her sense of aloneness. All of these contributed to Diane's ability to differentiate her self concept from that of her mother at the time of and after her death—a concept that was essentially hating and self-hating, narcissistically depleted, alone, unloved and unloving, rejecting and rejected, fecal and pitiful. The working through of narcissistic injury, by reducing narcissistic rage, also reduced Diane's conflict over aggression and helped her to neutralize the pathogenic qualities of her tie to her dead mother's mental representation (Lampl-de Groot, 1976). She came to see her mother's death as not reflective of her own, Diane's worth, but rather of her mother's despair, aloneness, and inability to love. Idealization of her dead mother and a turning of aggression against herself in the form of self-deprecation, in the service of maintaining a libidinal tie to her, were replaced by empathy, pity, and undisguised anger toward her mother and empathy and sympathy toward herself.

Once the narcissistic problems had been dealt with forthrightly, the ready availability of affect in Diane was most impressive. It is our hypothesis that the crystallization of the transference neurosis allowed the archaic narcissistic injury and the archaic self concepts to be reviewed and reworked.[6] A gradual heightening of self-esteem occurred as Diane brought into a more up-to-date perspective what had become a predominantly anal-sadistic, devalued, dirty, malignant, and omnipotent self—one that had murdered her mother. Diane came to see herself as a lovable, phallic-oedipal child who could charm her analyst, but not seduce him. She was powerful, but not omnipotent and grandiose. The analyst, as well as Diane's parents, acted as a self-object in another sense. The dawning cognitive and creative functions of the child needed attention, esteem, and auxiliary ego functions of adults to progress to adequate levels. These self-object functions were amply supplied in and out of the analysis, more than compensating for the child's maternal bereavement. Concomitantly, motor forms of repetition compulsion, particularly falling, were obliterated.

Kohut's (1977) concept of transmutation via working through in the transference is valuable here. A corrective experience occurred, not in Alexander's (1925) sense of it, but via interpretation of transference, which permitted working through of archaic narcissistic injuries.

It is, of course, prudent to be cautious about prognosis, a caution that is reflected in the arrangements we made to follow up Diane and her sisters at regular intervals for an indefinite period. However, it was our impression that at the end of the 2 years of analysis, Diane emerged with an unusual capacity for acknowledging and tolerating the grimness of life, while at the same time finding joy in it. As often happens, successful mourning led to a constructive outcome (G. W. Kliman, 1968). Diane seemed more the pleased master of herself than the majority of children her age. She was vital, thriving, and symptom-free. We judged her prognosis to be good. In the 4 years since the end of her analysis— admittedly a short time—nothing has happened to dampen this optimism.

The effectiveness of the treatment may have owed a great deal to a special quality of the psychological environment in which the

6. See G. W. Kliman (1976) for an earlier essay illustrating the feasibility and value of childhood mourning in a well-established transference neurosis in a 4-year-old boy who was paternally bereaved.

analyst, supervisor, and the first therapist were working. It was one committed to the proposition that mourning in childhood is feasible. The opposite attitude, we believe, is all too common among psychotherapists and psychoanalysts, resulting all too often in a less vigorous or absent mourning.

Treatment may paradoxically have been aided by the loss Diane experienced when it was decided that she should be treated by an analyst instead of by her family therapist. This imposed a bereavement at a "low dose"; one which included occasional unplanned meetings between her and her previous therapist and which could readily be taken up and worked through in the analysis. We suspect that the far less formidable work of mourning the loss of her first therapist produced something of a "desensitizing" effect on Diane, which contributed importantly to setting in motion the far more formidable work of mourning the loss of her mother.

BIBLIOGRAPHY

ALEXANDER, F. (1925), A Metapsychological Description of the Process of Cure. *Int. J. Psycho-Anal.*, 6:13–34.

BIBRING, E. (1953), The Mechanism of Depression. In: *Affective Disorders*, ed. P. Greenacre. New York: Int. Univ. Press, pp. 13–48.

DEUTSCH, H. (1937), Absence of Grief. *Psychoanal. Quart.*, 6:12–22.

FENICHEL, O. (1945), *The Psychoanalytic Theory of Neurosis*. New York: Norton.

FREUD, A. (1960), Discussion of Dr. John Bowlby's Paper. *This Annual*, 15:53–62.

FREUD, S. (1900), The Interpretation of Dreams. *S.E.*, 4 & 5.

——— (1912), The Dynamics of Transference. *S.E.*, 97–108.

——— (1917), Mourning and Melancholia. *S.E.*, 14:237–258.

——— (1920), Beyond the Pleasure Principle. *S.E.*, 18:3–64.

——— (1923), The Ego and the Id. *S.E.*, 19:3–66.

——— (1926), Inhibitions, Symptoms and Anxiety. *S.E.*, 20:77–175.

FURMAN, E. (1974), *A Child's Parent Dies*. New Haven & London: Yale Univ Press.

GOLDSTEIN, J., FREUD, A., & SOLNIT, A. J. (1973), *Beyond the Best Interests of the Child*. New York: Free Press.

GREENSON, R. R. (1967), *The Technique and Practice of Psychoanalysis*. New York: Int. Univ. Press.

HARTMANN, H., KRIS, E., & LOEWENSTEIN, R. M. (1949), Notes on the Theor of Aggression. *This Annual*, 3/4:9–36.

JACOBSON, E. (1954), The Self and the Object World. *This Annual,* 9:75–127.

KLIMAN, A. S. (1978), *Crisis.* New York: Holt, Rinehart & Winston.

KLIMAN, G. W. (1965), Oedipal Themes in Children's Reactions to the Assassination. In: *Children and the Death of a President,* ed. M. Wolfenstein & G. W. Kliman. New York: Doubleday, pp. 107–134.

——— (1968), *Psychological Emergencies of Childhood.* New York: Grune & Stratton.

——— (1976), Analyst in the Nursery. *This Annual,* 30:477–510.

——— (1979), Facilitation of Mourning during Childhood. In: *Perspectives on Bereavement,* ed. D. Peretz. New York: Charles Thomas, in press.

KOHUT, H. (1971), *The Analysis of the Self.* New York: Int. Univ. Press.

——— (1977), *The Restoration of the Self.* New York: Int. Univ. Press.

LAMPL- DE GROOT, J. (1976), Mourning in a 6-Year-Old Girl. *This Annual,* 31: 273–282.

LEWIN, B. D. (1950), *The Psychoanalysis of Elation.* New York: Norton.

MAHLER, M. S. (1961), On Sadness and Grief in Infancy and Childhood. *This Annual,* 16:332–351.

——— PINE, F., & BERGMAN, A. (1975), *The Psychological Birth of the Human Infant.* New York: Basic Books.

MENDELSON, M. (1974), *Psychoanalytic Concepts of Depression.* New York: Halsted Press.

MILLER, J. B. M. (1971), Children's Reactions to the Death of a Parent. *J. Amer. Psychoanal. Assn.,* 19:697–719.

NAGERA, H. (1970), Children's Reactions to the Death of Important Objects. *This Annual,* 25:360–400.

RAPAPORT, D. (1959), Edward Bibring's Theory of Depression. In: *The Collected Papers of David Rapaport,* ed. M. M. Gill. New York & London: Basic Books, 1967, pp. 758–773.

WOLFENSTEIN, M. (1966), How Is Mourning Possible? *This Annual,* 21:93–123.

——— (1969), Loss, Rage, and Repetition. *This Annual,* 24:432–460.

The World of Disguises

Unusual Defenses in a Latency Girl

LAURIE LEVINSON, M.Sc.

THIS PAPER IS ABOUT A CHILD WHO, IN ORDER TO FORM A RELATION-
ship with her mother, developed a personality characterized by a
striking lack of certain real feelings. The search for these feelings
and the reasons for their absence constituted a major task of treatment. I shall present material from the analysis of Amy, focusing
on her rigid and unusual defenses against particular affects.

The theoretical issue I would like to raise concerns the nature
of Amy's character structure. Anna Freud, in discussing this case,
commented that when environmentally caused damage produces
a developmental disturbance, the ensuing conflicts are not neurotic, but rather constitute character pathology. This sort of
skewed development would represent an adaptive, yet insuffi-
ciently successful attempt at coping. On one level, Amy's personality was an adaptation to her mother's needs—both in reality and
in Amy's perception of them. However, at the same time she was
at odds with her mother—unable to obtain the kind of relationship she really needed.

One might describe Amy's initial picture as having had ele-

The author did this work at the Hampstead Child-Therapy Clinic, and is
now a member of the Association for Child Psychoanalysis.

Revised version of a paper presented at the Wednesday meeting of the
Hampstead Child-Therapy Clinic, July 21, 1976.

I wish to express my indebtedness to Mrs. Anne-Marie Sandler for her
supervision of this case; and to Dr. Marianne Kris for her invaluable comments and discussion.

ments comparable in appearance to those of the "as if" personality described by H. Deutsch (1942). Yet there were enough differences to make it clear that she was not at all a fully developed "as if" character, although she did at times *simulate* affects. Thus, certain questions posed themselves. If Amy did not fit Deutsch's description of adults, could it be that there exists in childhood a precursor to this later form of pathology? If so, what would be the *form* in childhood for the later emergence of an "as if" disorder? If, on the other hand, Amy only presented similar characteristics, would her disturbance be based on different sources and represent a different entity?

CASE PRESENTATION

Amy R. was referred to the Hampstead Clinic at the age of 6 by her mother, whose therapist had convinced her that "Amy was not just a naughty child, but an unhappy child." Mrs. R.'s main complaint was that her daughter was stubborn, intensely argumentative, and particularly provocative with her, a state of affairs which she found highly irritating.

In her diagnostic interviews Amy gave a good picture of her defensive use of charm and cheerfulness as well as of her underlying confusion. The diagnostician reported:

> Amy is an attractive, feminine-looking, little girl with long dark hair. Her most striking feature is her large deep blue eyes. Her manner was friendly and rather happy. She talked easily, smiling and laughing frequently, but almost too readily. At once I had the impression of an attention-seeking quality and wish to please. At times she would talk in a somewhat silly voice; at other times her manner would seem inappropriately excited.

HISTORY

Amy's parents married when the mother was 18. She immediately became pregnant with Mark, the first child. Mrs. R. had already had one abortion when she was 16. In addition to working part-time as an actress in television, she seemed to have spent the years between 18 and 24 almost continually pregnant. Simon was born

18 months after Mark; Mrs. R. then became pregnant again and had another son, Jonathan. Amy was born 2 years after Jonathan. When Amy was 3 years old, Mrs. R had a miscarriage. Another pregnancy was terminated when Amy was 5; following this, Mrs. R. had a depressive episode necessitating hospitalization for a month.

The R.'s marriage was from the beginning a stormy one. Each parent would torment the other with accusations of infidelity and neglect, and each frequently walked out on the other. At the time of the initial referral, the parents had been separated for a year. Mrs. R. was living with Robert; and Mr. R., with a woman called Alice. Mr. R.'s attitude toward treatment was one of uninvolvement—an attitude which paralleled his relationship with his children. His visits were few and were always marked by inconsistency. He often failed to turn up at the appointed time, came when the children were out, and repeatedly forgot birthdays.

During the last years she lived with her husband, Mrs. R. was completely self-absorbed. She described herself as being "like a zombie"—taking 15 tranquilizers a day. She had no memories of her children during this time, except to feel that they must have been "freaked out" by her state. She had been confused, anxious, and constantly crying. She also remembered moving from flat to flat, burdened with shopping bags and four children. One can perhaps view her many pregnancies as a last attempt at warding off her depression. Yet, the abortions and miscarriages also pointed to her conflicting feelings about herself as a woman and mother. A few months before Amy's referral to the clinic, Mrs. R. took an overdose of sleeping pills and was hospitalized for two days. At this point she sought psychotherapy for herself.

Altogether, Mrs. R. had remarkably few recollections of Amy's first 3 years. Due to her depression, she allowed the children to be cared for by a succession of *au pairs* and friends. In view of the mother's state of distress, one may assume that it was difficult, if not impossible, for her to provide the secure holding environment her small daughter longed for.

Amy's birth was normal; and Mrs. R. described her as having been a happy baby. Feeding was never a problem and remained one of Amy's main areas of pleasure. She was bottle-fed from birth and had a bottle on going to bed until the age of 3. Thumb-sucking and hair-twisting were present as long as the mother could remember.

Amy's entry into nursery school at the age of 3½ was a disaster. She reacted with tears and many battles, the ultimate result being that her mother gave up. School, which Amy started at 4½, seemed to have been welcomed; Amy always enjoyed school and did well academically. Rather than transferring her conflict-ridden relationship with her mother to her teachers, Amy was able to respond positively. Her school reports indicated that she was valued for her charm, good intelligence, and outstanding verbal abilities.

At the time of referral, Mrs. R. was bitterly resentful that Amy behaved so well at school. She would have preferred her to have shown her "bad side" to the teachers, so they would appreciate the extent of the mother's suffering. She felt no one believed her.

This theme of Mrs. R. wishing that others would witness Amy at her worst persisted; it reflected her worry that Amy's problems were her fault. She often asked hopefully whether Amy had been difficult with me and spoke angrily of the fact that her husband felt Amy was fine and not in need of treatment. Interviews with Mrs. R. were characterized by lengthy descriptions of Amy's stubbornness, provocation, and inability to enjoy anything at home. Mrs. R. found herself unable to remove herself from the battleground. Later it became clear that for her it was easier to fight with her daughter than to acknowledge what lay under Amy's provocativeness. Amy's depression and withdrawal were always unacceptable to her mother. When the mother would see Amy sit for hours staring into space and sucking her thumb, she would be swamped with guilt and frustration at not being able to reach her. Just as she had to run from her own depression, whether to pregnancies or to a passing relationship with a man, so Mrs. R. had to avoid making contact with these painful feelings in her daughter. She also felt hurt and left out by Amy's withdrawal, experiencing it as confirmation of the fact that she was a bad mother; that Amy didn't want her.

TREATMENT

Amy's analysis lasted 3 years and dealt with many areas of conflict. There were, however, certain themes which provided the focus for our work. All of these centered on Amy's unsatisfied longings for a close relationship, in which she could feel special and favored. Due to her lack of trust, she consistently expected to meet with disappointment and rejection, as she had in the past.

The beginning months of treatment were characterized by Amy's attempts to ward off her feelings of not having enough and of being worthless. In the transference, I represented the depriving and critical mother who could not possibly care about such a needy and horrid child. For weeks Amy began every session with the announcement: "I only need a few things today!" In fact, she needed me to procure an enormous amount of extra supplies. At the end of the first month, I voiced Amy's feeling of being needy. She screamed at me desperately: "What do I come here for? To *get things!*" At that point, Amy was able to deal with her deep sense of helplessness only by ordering me about. Her panic and rage when I did not comply were seen as a repetition of what had transpired with her mother—neither of us was able to understand what she was really missing. Throughout much of the analysis Amy equated proof of my caring with her ability to make me do things. In the third year, she said to me, "If you walk me to the corner, then I'll *know* you care." Such a verbalization was impossible in the early months; instead Amy would resort to highly provocative behavior in pursuit of punishment. Her guilt that she had gone too far needed to be appeased.

Feelings of guilt were prominent in Amy's analysis and were often connected to her conviction that she was full of bad and greedy wishes. There was a circle, which began with her sense of emptiness and longing to be special. From there, she would take a provocative and demanding stance, positive that unless I were driven to irritation by her nagging insistence, she would never get what she wanted. Then, believing that I was angry and fed up with her, Amy would be full of guilt. She knew she had been awful. How could I possibly like a girl who needed so much? Surely I would contrive some way to get rid of her. Did I really like her? And so the demands for more and more would start anew.

In the fourth month of analysis, prior to the Christmas break, I took up Amy's having to write on the walls as demonstrating her anger with me for going away and her fear that I would not come back. Amy screamed that she didn't care and did not like me one bit. Suddenly she yelled, "You look allergic to me. You don't want to come near me. You hate me and think I'm disgusting! I know it!" Amy then did many drawings, each of which had to be thrown away because it was not good enough. I noted how hard she was on herself, to which she replied, "I can't do anything without you bringing in something bad. Why are you always criticizing me?"

Fear and panic about being deserted were highlighted in the week directly preceding the holiday. To fend off her feelings of helplessness and anxiety, she became a competent and independent Amy who could do everything for herself, even trying symbolically to hold herself together. She sewed many containers, bags, and purses which she intended to fill up and take home. Amy's wishes to be held in safety, to be able to contain herself, were too frightening to talk about. She actually had to make the containers. At one point, Amy sang quietly in a babyish voice, "Sometimes I think I'm one year old and that all of life is just a dream." I remarked that it must be nice to pretend to be a baby, because then people would stay with you and keep you safe. Amy laughed and said, "You bet!" She spoke incessantly of presents, informing me that she "needed" one from me—something that I would buy specially. When I told her I would be giving her something, she wanted to know why. Was it because she wanted one? Because I liked her? Or because she nagged me so?

My gift of a calendar was of course, not enough. Nothing could fill the inner void she felt; and Amy needed to take home with her all sorts of special things she had been saving in her locker. She still asked for more, becoming provocative. She gave me a box of chocolates and wanted to eat them all herself; she tried to open other lockers, screaming that she wanted to take everything home with her.

Giving and receiving gifts, a major theme in the first year of analysis, had many meanings for Amy. One function of the gift-giving was to placate all those involved in Amy's intensely conflicting loyalties. For months she spent every session making something for someone, usually her mother, Robert, or me. We all had to receive the same number and type of drawings. If Amy showed any favoritism, she feared hurting or neglecting the others, who would then retaliate by withdrawing their already questionable love. She could take no chances. Amy's drawings were remarkably age-inadequate and unoriginal, always of a smiling sun in a perfectly blue sky. While making them, she would sing merrily to herself of her marvelous and perfect family. It was clear that Amy hoped to please both me and her mother with these glossy versions of herself. The mother habitually responded with indifference or irritation, complaining to me that the pictures were on the level of a 4-year-old.

Thus, it was logical that Amy would denigrate anything I gave her. At one point, I provided a much desired dollhouse, but Amy found any number of things wrong with it. When I said that perhaps she felt she did not deserve to be given it, Amy asked me why I had. "Was it because you didn't want it? I know! It was just lying around." She always found it difficult to believe I might like her; and when I spoke of her needing to cover up her wish that I would, Amy experienced my comment as teasing—a trick to make her vulnerable and to undermine her enormous defense against her wish to be significant to me.

At the beginning of the second term of treatment, Amy found out that her mother as well as her father's girlfriend were pregnant. Typically, she showed nothing but the greatest pleasure for quite a while, but her conflict over trusting me was accentuated. How *could* she trust me? Would I be like the other ladies, who always let her down, did not care about her, or left her for another child? In our sessions we had innumerable contests and games. Amy would test me on the facts of her life, who was in her family, where she lived, and what she liked to do. In one session, she was preoccupied with promises. I had to promise to tell her what I said to her mother; what her mother said to me when we met. In fact, she made me write "I promise" after everything I said, and then sign my name. At the end of the session I wondered what she really wanted me to promise. Did she want to make sure I would not forget her, either when I was with Mummy or over the weekend? Amy sighed, and said softly, "And to come home with you. I've never seen your house." She then immediately asked me the time, saying, "I know. It's because I hate it when you tell me, so I have to leave first." Thus, we saw how any open acknowledgment of her wish for closeness had to be followed by some maneuver to protect herself from the disappointment and rejection she always felt to be imminent.

Amy's lack of trust was closely linked with her intense feelings of being excluded. She felt left out of everything, ignored, and completely powerless. In the sixth month of treatment, Amy developed the pattern of spending a few minutes of every session out of the room. Ostensibly she was in the lavatory, but in reality she wandered around the clinic, listening at different doors, and finally knocking on the door of a room which she knew was occupied by a female therapist and a male patient. Occasionally I found her sitting outside the room, quietly sucking her thumb and staring dreamily into space. Amy was enacting something which was actually going on at home at the time—she would wander around the house at night, ending up in her mother's bedroom, where she sat silently watching the couple sleep. Mrs. R. reported waking up suddenly to find Amy sitting there and angrily sending her off to her room. During that phase of treatment, we were playing many hide-and-seek games and Amy was preoccupied with peeking and being secretive. She gleefully agreed that she would indeed like to interrupt the two people behind the closed door, but had to deny her anxiety. This enactment also represented a repetition of what must have happened during parental rows: Amy would wake up and go to her parents. On reaching their room, she heard them arguing, which made her feel terrified, helpless, and unprotected. Later Amy herself described this: "When they shut their door, I felt like they were shutting *me* out, even though I knew it wasn't true. I felt like I was falling apart."

Amy's enactment of the nighttime wandering was, of course, also linked with sexual preoccupations. Her feeling of having been excluded by everyone also related to her exclusion from parental sexual activities, which in her mind were closely connected with fighting and arguing. Throughout treatment, Amy tended to use all sorts of sexual material defensively—almost as if she were trying to divert my attention by calling out, "Look at this! Aren't you interested?" Everyone talked about sex in her house; and Amy probably saw more of it than most children her age. Thus, it was quite easy for her to tell me with delight of her pleasure in interrupting the other therapist and patient. She could even admit how left out she felt when Mummy preferred Robert or Robert preferred Mummy, but she could *not* own up to feeling terrified and panicky, needing to be comforted, and feeling all alone. These feelings remained inaccessible until late in the second year of treatment. Since Amy used sexual material defensively, it was usually taken up as a shield behind which were hidden very painful and frightening affects.

Amy did find ways to get the comforting and caring she wanted; and in spite of the pretense involved, it was virtually the only means at her disposal: Amy pretended to be ill or hurt, concocting all sorts of imaginary ailments. At the time of her referral, we heard of a limp which had lasted for three weeks; and of a day when she had pretended to be blind. In sessions, she often complained of various ills, usually before a separation. In the first month of analysis Amy laughingly agreed that her wish for a "big bandage" for her sore shoulder was a way of ensuring that people would feel sorry for her and give her lots of attention. On one Friday, Amy spent much time enumerating her aches and pains. I spoke of another child called Emma, who also had aches and pains. In Emma, these pains usually covered up other worries; and what *she* really wanted on Fridays was for me to stay with her and take care of her. Amy heartily sympathized with Emma's plight. At the end of the session, after having wished me a nice weekend, Amy came running back to whisper, "Emma also wants you to have a nice time."

My description of Amy may convey the impression that rather than being a child who was out of touch with her feelings, Amy was very much aware of her inner state—or at least that she responded well to interpretations. I certainly found myself believing she was the perfect child patient. However, I gradually began to feel that something was missing. It was as if somehow Amy had figured out how to be a good patient. She had learned what sort of feelings I was after; and she did her best to please me. On the conscious level, she most likely believed that she was working hard and coming to terms with her worries, but her real anxieties were as yet untouched. What made it so difficult was that, for the most part, Amy had no idea what she was feeling, save perhaps a vague state of tension or unhappiness. Thus, when I offered an interpretation, Amy would latch onto it, hoping to put some label to the limbo in which she lived.

A typical example of Amy's behavior can be seen in the way she acted after a weekend with her father. She arrived for her session ten minutes late, asking blandly, "Was I late today?" When I wondered why she had asked me, Amy launched into a description of the most wonderful visit with her father. Everything was superlative. She had had not one, but two horses to ride. Daddy gave her lots of gifts; Alice had made the *most* wonderful meals. Amy then began prancing around the room, showing me ballet steps— obviously enjoying it and pretending not to. I said that Amy often seemed to do that with her real feelings—cover them up with pretend feelings. Then she ended up confused, not knowing what she felt. Amy glanced at me, and asked, "Do even you do that sometimes? Does it make me bad?" I said that when certain feelings were unpleasant for some reason, she had to push them away, putting pretend ones in their place. Amy was perfectly oblivious, singing gaily to herself as she prepared a doll for one of the babies soon to be born. Suddenly Amy turned to me and said in an extremely artificial and imperious voice, *"You* do the sewing please." I wondered why she had to act so much of the time; and why it was so hard to speak in her own voice. Amy replied, "I like speaking in this voice!" I noted that the voice was not her real one, and spoke of another child I knew who was so confused about her own feelings that she had to get rid of them and pretend to act like someone else. This other child was particularly worried about her sad and angry feelings and often felt that she did not deserve to be given anything. Amy looked at me quizzically and asked whatever was I talking about.

In the same week in which Mrs. R. was taken to the hospital for what turned out to be false labor, Amy was behaving in her most unreal manner. Our sessions were full of commands, given in her superior tones. When I did not instantly obey her, Amy screamed at me that I was stupid, and that she was the boss. I commented that she must feel very small and bossed around, by herself and others; therefore she pretended to be the opposite. To my surprise, Amy calmed down, but not for long. Soon we were having more contests, this time with Amy casually informing me how much more she knew than I. She wanted to play the game Hangman, and I wrote the word "pretend." After having all the letters but one, Amy refused to say the last one and asked me for a clue. I said it was what some children did when they felt worried or upset about something. "Oh, . . . they pretend." This was said as if she had just realized the answer. But Amy could laughingly admit she had known all along what the word was. Only then was she able to show her real feelings of concern and worry about her mother being in the hospital. She had been too frightened to mention her worry about who would take care of her. She smiled genuinely when I verbalized what a relief it must be to see things as they really were.

Amy continued to work hard in the treatment, perhaps spurred on by her strong feelings about the new baby. In addition, she found it a relief that I was not fooled by her. While Mrs. R. was still in the hospital, there were difficulties about getting Amy to her sessions; and twice she was unable to come. On both occasions I phoned her; and on both occasions she sounded mature and reasonable, with not a care in the world. Although we both knew she had not come because Robert had been unable to bring her, Amy acted as if it had been her fault; she had simply forgotten to come. When I noted this contradiction and connected it to her confusion about what was going on at home, Amy began throwing things around the room. I said that we knew that when she behaved like that she was upset about something; and maybe she was not sure what was worrying her. Thus she had to act some part—either of the girl who forgot to come to the clinic, or the girl who threw things. Amy then acknowledged for the first time that she was acting, saying in her "saccharine" voice: "But this *is* the real Amy." I wondered whether at times she was not sure who the real Amy was and therefore acted the way she thought people expected her to act. When I added that we could wait until the real Amy felt safe enough to come out, Amy looked quite serious and asked, "But how do you know who she is?"

Another way that Amy dealt with her affects was to present her real feelings as if they were fakes. She would adopt a self-mocking and self-deprecating voice, as if imitating someone making fun of her. At one point, when she was actually feeling terribly distraught about her mother being in the hospital and my absence over the weekend, Amy said, "Poor me! Isn't it awful!" I noted how hard it must be for her to face the frightened little girl feelings, so she had to make fun of herself in case I too would laugh. For a moment, Amy caught herself, saying sadly, "We've lost the real Amy, haven't we?" I said we could find her if we looked.

In our search for this hidden child, it was important to Amy that I should not allow her to repeat earlier situations of rejection. Time and again she tried to get me to allow her to miss sessions— always for the most sensible reasons. There would be a birthday party or an invitation to her father's or a dentist's appointment. When I checked, there invariably was no such event. On one occasion, Amy almost convinced me that she had been invited to her father's for her half-term break. Although the clinic remained open during that week, I felt it would be important for Amy to be with her father. At the last minute I discovered that there never had been an invitation; but in her disappointment Amy convinced herself that it would come. Amy's wish to be with her father was also a displacement from her wish to be with me—because we had just had a four-day break. She could tell me that she had wanted to get back at me for going away and leaving her. Amy spent that session leaning against me and holding my hand, unusually open in her expression of her affection. I said that she must be glad that I had not let her stay away because she really did not want me or the other grownups to be tricked by her. Amy nodded silently, and then decided to read my palm. She told me that I lived alone in a flat, having as my only companion a little girl pussycat. I would live in London until I would be 85 years old. Amy then asked me, "Will I have left here when I'm 14?" She went on to say that she was just fine and didn't need to come anymore. I noted that she was testing me to see if I wanted her; and that in reality we both knew she did not always feel so fine. Amy said with genuine wistfulness, "I don't want to leave." We then set off on a trip to Mars. She was the captain and I was the cook, first-aid person, and passenger.

Amy was slowly beginning to tolerate the coming to awareness of her hitherto hidden longings. We saw more and more the extent to which she had had to shut away the lonely and panicky little girl feelings in the hope that without them she would be more acceptable—to mother, and later to me. Now she could tell me in the midst of her pretending, "Well, the real Amy is underneath, you know."

I once asked Amy what her mother did when Amy was feeling bad. She replied, "Oh, she doesn't know what I'm feeling. Even if she asks, I just say nothing is bothering me." I wondered whether she thought her mother knew she was pretending. Amy said no, but then added, "But I want her to notice, really!" She agreed that at the very moments when she was confused or worried and wanted her mother's help, she was convinced that her mother would not be able to help her.

When Mrs. R. finally gave birth to a baby girl, Amy was superficially pleased, but spent the session singing the song, "Bye-bye baby." When I commented on her letting us know how she felt about the new baby, Amy laughed and sang, "Hello, children!" Yet her affect of sadness belied her cheerful song. When I noted that now there was another girl in the family, Amy said with resignation, "I was never special." She then proceeded to hurt herself in all sorts of accidents. First she showed me her scraped chin; then she tripped on the stool, causing it to fall on her; and finally she caught her finger in the door. For the first time in treatment, Amy allowed herself to cry in front of me. I spoke of how sometimes, if people feel sad or frightened, they think it's bad to have such feelings; then they do something accidental which hurts them. Amy listened intently and said, "But I don't do it on purpose. It just happens . . . freely!" I remarked that she was right. Freely meant that something happened and she did not know why; but there were reasons for it. She grinned, pleased with herself and her new word. In this instance, *I* was taken in. Amy had managed by the end of the session to get rid of her sadness and jealousy by superimposing a cerebral formulation. She *was* right that she hurt herself for unconscious reasons, but she used her insight defensively.

Amy always reacted to holidays with great distress. To deal with her anxiety about my well-being and hers, Amy acted as if she were in control, did not need me, and was eager to part. Often, before or after a holiday, Amy had to take a day or two off—to prove to us both how independent she was. In the weeks preceding the summer break, Amy said to me, "Well, if I get lonely, I can just ring you up and ask for an appointment!" When I told her that I would be away, she replied, "That's all right. I can send you a post-card saying I'm worried; and you can send me one back telling me why." I agreed that I would send her a postcard to keep in touch, but added that she too could figure out why she might be worried. Amy said, "The worst thing about being worried is not knowing why. Sometimes I can tell you and sometimes I can't." She then be-gan to draw messy paint splatters, getting paint all over us. I said she seemed to be showing us her messy and confused feelings. Amy looked up brightly, saying, "Well, it's quite a good way, isn't it?" She told me that certain colors were happy and others were sad— and that was how she felt about the holiday. During our last ses-sion, Amy was engrossed in making out of felt the picture of a girl. At the end she wrote on it, "My image" and handed it to me. I verbalized her concern that I might forget her over the summer, adding that she knew I did not really need the picture to remem-ber her. Amy asked, "Do you like your job?" She could smile when I asked, "And do I like Amy?"

By the end of the first year of work, Amy was beginning to show some signs of trust in me and to feel safe enough to share some of her feelings of worthlessness and loneliness. Her real fear of panic remained to be dealt with.

Amy arrived one day in the autumn, announcing that she would try a "very hard task." She would attempt to draw a picture—not of her usual smiling sun, and not to be given away! While she drew, Amy delivered a long monologue on giving gifts. "Well, sometimes when I've had an argument with someone, I want to say I'm sorry. With Robert, I can tell by the expression on his face. So that's when I give him a present. With Mummy, I either give her something or make her a cup of tea." I said it sounded as if she often worried that we were all cross with her. "Not a lot, but some of the time." Amy continued, telling me of a school friend. Someone else had told Amy that this girl did not like her. Though Amy didn't believe this, she was worried and had given many gifts to this girl. She said, "Isn't it awful the way people say they will be your friend if you do something for them? It doesn't make any sense, but I know I do it myself!" I remarked that it seemed some people felt friends could be bought with presents. Amy looked at me for reassurance, asking, "But they can't, can they?" Noting her uncertainty, I wondered if she ever felt that the only way to make someone like her would be to give them a present. "Yes, that's it! Just don't say it again, okay?" She then asked shyly, "Miss L., you know how sometimes we say I'm pretending? Well, was I pretending today?" I said she could answer that herself. Amy was quiet for a moment and then said in a whisper, "Real?" I agreed, and voiced her difficulty in sorting it out.

In the next session Amy indicated how she used her insight to try to gain my approval. She sounded like a mature adult when she said, "You know yesterday's session? Well, you know how sometimes people like to get away from painful feelings? That it's embarrassing to talk about them. You know how it is when someone, like a therapist, reveals the truth that you hadn't known before? I didn't want to leave yesterday because you made the painful feelings go away." I commented that she had understood *herself* that she often pretended when she was embarrassed. Amy came close to me and said, "You know how I talked about my worries yesterday? Well, was I as good as adults? If I stop pretending, will I be the winner?" I said it sounded as if she felt there was a contest going on among my patients. "Yes, I want to be the best!" I noted how hard she tried to please me, sometimes saying what she hoped I wanted to hear.

Amy usually responded to my pointing to her frequently simulated feelings with shame, humiliation, and anger. Several days before a holiday, Amy delivered a speech on the naughtiness of her friend Sara, who apparently had been stealing from other children and making herself a general nuisance. Amy said, "Sara walks around with a guilty look on her face—as if she wants to be found out. She will be awful to Jane and then Jane will be cross with her. She will lose her friends! Maybe Sara does it because people are always saying she's fat; and she feels hurt and angry. But then that makes her bossy and she gangs up on the other kids. Sara probably wants to be punished because she feels so guilty about being bad." Amy readily agreed that she was talking about aspects of herself, namely, her belief that no one thought she was important. This led her to angry demandingness—the only way she felt she could get attention. Then she felt so bad about it she needed to be punished. When I said that it all sounded a bit empty of feelings, she retorted angrily, "I was only talking about it!"

Later in the same week, Amy told me proudly that she had given up her bottle at 4 months of age. I remarked that even then she had tried hard to be grown up. I wondered what had happened to her baby feelings, as she so often separated the thoughts from the feelings. Referring to her formulation about Sara, Amy asked, "But weren't you proud of me the other day?" I said that she certainly had wanted me to be impressed with how well she had understood Sara's naughtiness. Amy reacted as if I had attacked her, "So! You weren't proud!" I said that we could see how very hard she tried to be the good girl—the kind of grown-up patient she thought I would prefer. Amy looked hurt and said accusingly, "You are always criticizing me!" I replied that it was Amy criticizing herself—that with the coming holiday she did not like having such sad and angry feelings about me. She would much prefer to leave thinking I was proud of her, and did not know about her crossness. I asked Amy how she thought another child might feel if someone the child really cared about was going away. Amy asked in her grown-up voice, "Unhappy? Sad? Guilty? Guilty because maybe the child thinks the person is leaving because he is naughty." I said that *if* Amy felt angry with me for leaving, then I would know why she had to pretend not to care—because people she loved had left her in the past. Amy asked, "Like who?" I said like her father. Amy fell silent for a moment and then said in a desperate voice, "You would still like me? Sure? Honest?" I said it seemed she felt she could be liked only if she acted happy all the time. Of course I could like the sad and angry Amy as well as the happy one. After all, they were really different parts of the same person. Amy wanted to know if I had ever heard of the saying: "When you're happy, the whole world laughs with you; and when you weep, you weep alone." I wondered what she thought it meant. Amy replied, "You are saying that it's not true. That you can be sad and people will still love you." I verbalized how doubtful she sounded, as if she could hardly believe it was true; and I spoke of how Amy had to try to be happy in order to be with Mummy and not all alone.

For Amy, to feel excluded, all alone, and having less than others was to feel vulnerable and weak—at the mercy of an inconsistent adult world. Thus, she had to defend against such humiliating affects by becoming independent, not caring, and grown up. Being a girl in a family where the three boys were obviously preferred was another humiliation; and there were various moments in treatment when Amy expressed her belief that things might be better if she at least had a penis. Rather than seeing Amy's wish for a penis in libidinal terms, I usually interpreted her feelings about not having one in the context of a penis being one more thing that *she* didn't have which others did. No matter what she did, or how good she was at things, she felt she would never get the attention and love her brothers received. Amy arrived one day for her session in a most demanding mood. She wanted a balsa-wood knife. She knew we had some because she had seen a male therapist give one to his adolescent boy patient. Actually, there were none left; and I told this to Amy. She reacted with rage, screaming that she knew there were knives, but that I just didn't want to give her one. I said that she seemed to feel I would give a balsa-wood knife to other children and not to her. Perhaps she believed I would give it to a boy. Amy said angrily, "Oh yes, boys do get more! They get more of everything!" Amy went to the blackboard and drew a penis. She then collapsed on the floor, saying sadly, "It's Simon's birthday today and Dad's tomorrow. I thought that if I could go home and say you'd given me a balsa knife, then I wouldn't feel so bad." Amy was able to talk of how left out she felt on her brother's birthday; and how this birthday reminded her of other times when she felt that being a boy would get her more attention.

Another maneuver which Amy used to hide her low self-esteem from both mother and me was a rather precocious pseudosexuality. She acted flirtatiously, talked about sex in an exhibitionistic manner, and when really in a panic sought out sexually exciting situations. One wonders if this escape from depression was an identification with her mother, who also had sought an outlet for her longings in a spurious sexuality.

During a long break from analysis, when Mrs. R. was very depressed over the death of a friend, Amy behaved in her most provocative manner. She was aware of her mother's distress; and she panicked. She nagged and whined and picked fights with everyone until finally her mother threatened her with boarding school—the very thing Amy feared most. Though clearly distraught, Amy feigned indifference, telling her mother that what she really wanted was to live with her father. Feeling abandoned and frightened, Amy thus had to actualize her fantasy of being sent away by a withdrawn and disapproving mother.

At the same time, Amy was staying away from home all day and not letting anyone know where she was. Mrs. R. told me she feared Amy was going to a local fair, where, in her opinion, Amy was easy prey for any stranger. It turned out that Mrs. R. was correct. In our first session after the break, Amy told me that she and a friend had gone to the fair and had asked people for tenpence, saying they had lost it. One woman gave them the money, but suggested they stop asking other people. The excitement and danger were too tempting. The girls went up to a man whom Amy described as having "curly blond hair—American probably." They asked him for the money and he replied that he would take them on all the rides if they would do something nice for him. What he wanted was for them to play with his penis. Though Amy sounded as if she had been disgusted by this, she told me jokingly that she had said she would play with it with a stick. She said she then got scared and started for home, where she was told off for being so late. Amy pretended not to have known this was a dangerous thing to do, and made me promise I would not tell her mother. Amy wanted to know why I thought the man had asked her to play with his penis. Was it because he wanted comforting? This was why she played with her genitals. I said that although that might be the reason, what was missing were her feelings about the incident. I added that though she appeared to be disgusted, she didn't sound it. Amy went on to talk about being kidnapped, her voice having an excited tone. I noted this and linked it to the event at the fair. Wasn't she really seeking from this nice American man something she felt she needed so as not to be lonely or empty inside? Since I was not around, she found another American who she hoped would make her feel better. But then she saw that the sexy man was scary and did not provide the comforting she wanted.

Amy responded with more acting, behaving as if she were a provocative sexy adolescent. She told me she had three boyfriends with whom she was in love and how sexy they thought she was. She danced around the room showing off her figure and asking me whether she was sexy. I took up this grown-up and sexy talk as hiding her little girl feelings. How could an 8-year-old not feel left out when she did not feel special? How could she not worry if she felt I had left her never to return? And on top of everything, Mummy was worried and sad herself—something which must have caused Amy to worry too. In the end, she had nagged and been naughty, perhaps just to get some attention, but really she had been very sad. Amy was quiet and seemed to be in touch with her feelings for the first time that week. She said miserably, "Well, the baby doesn't get much attention if she cries." I said maybe that was why Amy was so frightened of showing her own tears.

In the last week of our second year of work, Amy was able to relive in the transference some of the traumatic experiences surrounding past separation. She finally could permit herself to feel the pain and express with real tears her early longings for her mother, together with the panic she felt when her mother had not been there for her. It became clear that Amy's need for such rigid defenses had been in direct proportion to the intensity of her feelings of worthlessness and self-hatred. Her misery was profound.

Following a weekend when her mother had been away, Amy arrived on the Monday in an exceedingly manic mood. She herself had spent the weekend at a friend's, and she related histrionically how "fab" it had been. As Amy ran about the room, exclaiming dramatically about all the wonderful things she had done, I remained totally silent. Her anxiety increased, as did the histrionics. Finally, she stopped, looked directly at me, and asked, "What time did you take me today?" (She had arrived early.) I said she knew I had taken her at her usual time. At this Amy became enraged, screaming, "Well, if we are both here, WHAT is the point of waiting?" She continued to yell at me until I said that the real issue was not whether or not I was free, but rather why she was distraught that I had not taken her when she wanted to be seen.

Now I could understand why she had had to pretend to be so marvelously happy. When I had not taken her early, it reminded her of the small Amy feelings of wanting her mother to be there when Amy needed her. Instead she had felt that Mother and I ignored her and paid more attention to other people. No wonder she had to try so hard to be grown up and controlled; it must have felt awful when she thought I didn't want her! Amy lapsed into silence for five minutes. Finally, she said tearfully, "But why do I have to feel these feelings? They are so awful." Amy cried and cried. She then said thoughtfully, "I wanted to be home when Mummy got back; but I couldn't. I was afraid I'd be in a bad mood because she went away; then we'd get in a row—and I hate that. Why couldn't she take me with her? Do you know?" I wondered whether Amy was certain her mother would not understand how cross she had been at her leaving. Amy sadly shook her head, "No, I'd be cross and Mummy would just yell at me. She just wants me to be nice." I said that we could see why Amy had had to be away when her mother returned—to protect Mummy from her angry and hurt feelings. She then *had* to pretend to be happy because that was the only way the small Amy could think of to be close to her mother or me. How hard for her to imagine that grownups might be able to accept a child's sadness and anger. Amy continued to weep, asking pathetically, "But how will feeling like this make anything better? I just want somebody to be near to, you or Mummy." I remarked that by understanding where these feelings originally came from, and putting them into perspective, she could use words to express herself—and might even be able to tell Mummy how she had felt, rather than having to push her away. Amy left the session still crying.

The remainder of that last week before the summer holiday was characterized by much crying, which took on a whining and somewhat overdramatic flavor. Amy presented the main problem as her terror of being tyrannized by her friend Sara. She had been invited to this child's house and was totally unable to say no. Amy pleaded with me to intercede; she begged me to ask her mother to tell Sara no; and she wept copiously, wanting to stay with me. Amy's anger toward and fear of Sara clearly were displaced from her mother. She said at one point, "But I can't say no to Sara or she won't be my friend." It was then that I verbalized for Amy that her feelings of panic had very little to do with Sara. Rather, they represented the panic Amy must have felt as a little girl, when she had feared her mother would stop loving her if she discovered Amy's angry feelings. Therefore Amy had had to pull away from her mother, feeling hurt, and believing her mother didn't love her. Her mother, not having understood Amy's reasons for rejecting her, had also pulled away in anger and disappointment. Thus, they had ended up always fighting with each other. Amy asked, "But why *do* we fight?" I replied that sometimes when people felt very hurt inside and believed that the other person didn't care about them, they were afraid to show loving feelings. Amy finally calmed down as we were able to make sense of what had happened in the past and how it was affecting her present life. The reconstruction of past experiences was crucial in enabling Amy to gain control over her maladaptive defensive behavior.

The transference of Amy's longings for closeness was intense, as was her expectation of rejection. It was in relation to me that Amy first verbalized the original reason for her need to behave in an unnaturally cheerful manner. At the end of that week, Amy arrived for her session looking dejected and waiflike. She spoke at length: "Miss L., I have something to ask. It's babyish. But you know how babies like being held in someone's arms? Well, would you hold me? You're like part of my family: actually, I love you. I want to be with you. Do you like me? Do you love me? I don't want you to go away or for school to end. I'm sorry. I'm making you unhappy, aren't I? I can't write to you because it would make you upset." I wondered why. Amy went on, "Well, I don't want to write a whole bunch of pretend. And what if I'm having a horrible time?" I took up Amy's feelings in relation to her baby feelings about not wanting to upset her mother. She replied, "When I was five, Mummy used to cry a lot; I did too. Mummy would try to comfort me, but I worried that she might do something silly—like kill herself. Then I'd be left all alone." Amy wept, saying over and over, "I need comforting. I feel like I'm falling apart. The Sara thing reminds me of this. I don't want you to go away. At least if you were in London, I could have an extra session. I would know where you were. Miss L., you *can't* come

back late. DO you care about me? I want to be close to you. When
I was little, I felt shut out of everyone's lives. Mummy was probably upset about fights with Dad; and Dad was always leaving. I
thought it was all my fault. I'm just no good—useless. Nobody
can love me." I linked Amy's current hopelessness and longing
toward me to her early childhood. Then she had felt she was the
cause of her mother's depression—a situation resulting in Amy's
conviction that she was a bad and unlovable girl. In fact, we knew
now that the real reasons for her mother's unhappiness had had
nothing to do with Amy. Amy listened and then whispered, "I
want you to walk to the corner with me. Nobody ever does things
because *I* want them to. It would be proof that you care about
me." I explained that Amy's feelings of being unlovable were
inside her; and that my doing an outside thing—like going to the
corner with her—would not change how she felt about herself.
She continued to weep, telling me how hopeless her life was and
that no one could ever care about her.

At this point, I compared my leaving for the summer with her
parents' having so often left her, both emotionally and physically.
Amy seemed to feel that I, too, was leaving because of her. Amy
calmed down considerably, again asking if I would hold her. She
drew her chair right up to mine and held my hand. I said that if I
held her, it might make her feel better for a minute, but that I did
not think it would last. If we could together understand these old
feelings, then she might not even need me to hold her. Amy told me
how left out she felt at home, in the present as well as in the past.
She described being sent to bed when everyone else was awake.
She would call and call for her mother, who never came. "They
always had better things to do." I told Amy that she knew her
mother was at present not depressed; that she often did spend
time with her; and that the small Amy feelings of being no good
had been the little girl's way of trying to make sense out of something she could not understand. Amy said, "I never want therapy
to be over. I will never be able to try things on my own. I need
you." I agreed that she still felt frightened of being without
therapy, but that some day she would want to stop treatment—
and, in fact, did not have to lose me to do it. Amy wanted to know
if her terrible feelings would ever go away for good. I said that in

time she would be able to say to herself, "Look, Amy, you may feel bad right now; but you know where these feelings come from. When you were little, you thought your mother's worries were your fault, and that she didn't love you. So instead of showing your real feelings of anger, sadness, and fear, you tried very hard to be the perfect little girl—always cheerful and happy. That was the only way you knew of then to make Mummy pay attention to you. Now you are older and can trust your mother more. And now you can use words to say what you really feel." We sat together for a while, with Amy silently holding my arm. Just as it was time to leave, she asked if I really thought she could tell her mother how she felt; and if she did, whether I would be impressed. I said I would be impressed if she could drop her pretending with her mother. Amy looked a bit skeptical, "You think I can do it?" I said we both knew the answer to that question.

Mrs. R. came to see me at the end of the second year of treatment. Her visit coincided with the week just described. She was unusually in touch with her real feelings and was able to acknowledge herself for the first time how *she* had yearned for caring as a child. She spoke of her own need to disguise this longing, in her belief that her mother had emotionally abandoned her. Amy's mother, in conjunction with the change in her daughter, could thus begin to relate more positively to Amy. Her ability to see Amy as a separate person had increased; and she described how until recently Amy had only reminded her of the bad, demanding parts of herself. She was now even able to enjoy Amy! The day after our meeting, Amy—who always came to the clinic on her own—was amazed and delighted to find her mother waiting for her.

Although Amy's analysis lasted another year, the breakdown of her rigid defenses against depressive affects marked the turning point in her treatment. The first two years of her analysis had consisted for the most part of the struggle to trust me with her real feelings, the loosening of a defensive style of relating designed both to protect her from her own and her mother's depression and to be close to mother. Her achievement was impressive and freed her to use real insight to work through the remaining conflicts. The process of helping Amy to establish more adaptive mechanisms had been set in motion when she allowed herself to confront the terror and helplessness of the past. In one sense, I represented for her a new object, to whom she could bring the old feelings and later work out new ways of responding. The fact that at the end of the third year I would be leaving the country triggered an intense reaction to me as a real object and in the transference.

In view of Amy's past history and persistent fears of loss, it was important that she be told of my departure almost a year in advance. Despite the fact that her family would be moving to another city at exactly the same time, my news was felt as a severe blow. Amy asked, "Are you going forever? I always hoped that therapy would never be over. When you don't want something to end, it goes too fast. I don't have mixed feelings like I do about holidays; all of me doesn't want you to go." For days, Amy played the game of "Solitaire," becoming very proficient at "doing things by herself."

The theme of dealing with my leaving by becoming independent and pseudosophisticated was a recurrent one throughout the year. Amy experienced the loss of me as a repetition of earlier losses; father deserting her; mother abandoning her in favor of other men and her three brothers. Thus, it was natural for her to attempt the same old solution—only this time with a different twist. Rather than just pretending to be carefree and unaffected, Amy turned to boys in a precocious sexuality. At first she was convinced that if she were a boy, I would not leave and desperately tried to find a way to make me stay. She came in one day with a bag from which she pulled out all sorts of trinkets, saying in a pleading voice, "There must be something you haven't seen yet!" When I interpreted her need to show me her possessions as indicating her concern about whether I liked her or preferred boys, who had extra possessions, Amy looked startled. "Do boys ever wish they could have babies?" I said yes; at times they did. Amy looked sad, telling me, "Well, then I guess it isn't worth it to be jealous."

At last we seemed to be reaching Amy's oedipal conflicts, which until then had been overshadowed by her preoedipal difficulties as well as the realities of her extremely confusing set of parents and stepparents. My leaving brought about a revival of her preoedipal struggles with her mother—struggles which in turn ushered in the wish to deprive me of all the good things and have them for herself. At the beginning, Amy railed at me for seeing a boy patient after her: "I hate him because he sees you! You belong to me; you are MY Miss L." But this material was rapidly followed by tales of chasing boys at school, sleep-over parties with boys, and various kissing games. In her sessions, Amy presented herself either as the knowledgeable woman of the world or as Cinderella, whose mother wanted to deprive her of everything, including the prince. It was particularly interesting that Amy clearly seemed to have perceived and identified with her mother's former methods of dealing with her own loneliness—acting out sexually, getting pregnant, chasing men. Thus, for Amy, the only way to get caring was either to be a boy or to have one all to herself. On the eve of a sleep-over party at a boy's house, Amy was beside herself with excitement and delight. Five boys had "confessed" that Amy was their true love. I commented that Amy was in a great hurry to grow up and have the reassurance of being liked by boys. She thought for a moment: "You know, it's a lot easier for other people to like you than it is to like yourself. After all, you're the only person who knows your feelings!" When I wondered what those unlikable feelings were, Amy replied, "The angry ones—when I want everyone to be jealous of me!" She then asked me to ask her a question: did she feel lonely because the weekend was coming? When Amy quickly changed the subject back to the exciting party, I said, "And since I can't be the good and caring Mummy over the weekend, you'll show me by doing exciting things with all the boys." Amy put her thumb in her mouth, "Yes. There is so much to talk about and so little time left." She left the session telling me that no matter how unhappy she might be in the future, she would never go back to therapy. She would feel too guilty about excluding me.

Amy's oedipal conflicts were complicated by her torn loyalties. The difference between her relationship with Robert and that with her father was particularly striking. The former appeared to be at an age-adequate latency level, with much enjoyment of Robert's attention, praise, and admiration. The relationship with her father was characterized either by an identification with her mother's negative attitude or by a secret longing. Amy's wish to be close to her father was certainly conflictual—his conspicuous absence from her life only making it more so. In one session she told me with assurance that Robert "belonged" to her. He had taught her to do the "jive" and she adored to dance with him. She then told me that her father had bought her eldest brother a fancy tape recorder; she felt her father tried to buy their love with expensive presents. Robert, however, gave them his real time and attention. When I noted that she must also have had some positive feelings for her father, Amy could agree. She said with sadness that lack of money had never bothered her as much as it did her mother.

Amy's identification with her mother was stronger than she knew. Both of them saw being rich as the equivalent of being safe. Amy described her father's "rich office" with pride; and she told me, "I hate being poor." In her father's office was a large refrigerator and Amy frequently took food from it and brought it home to her mother and Robert. When I remarked that to enjoy the good things with her father made her feel she was leaving out Mummy and Robert, Amy reacted with rage, saying that her father had much more money than he needed. I pointed out how difficult it was for her—when she was at home, she felt that her mother had Robert and she had nothing; when she was with her father, she feared her mother would be jealous and angry if Amy had a good time. She was able to say that the worst feelings for her were the jealous ones, when she felt she had nothing and no one; and that everyone else did. Thus, she would indulge in wonderful, wish-fulfilling fantasies. In one, Robert was her chauffeur and boyfriend. Amy exulted in the envious stares of children at school when he would collect her. She described how she would lounge in the back of the car, saying, "Jeeves, take me home!" Amy immediately informed me that she was "a fat greedy pig." I connected this comment to her feeling that wishing to be rich and to take her mother's place made her a bad and greedy girl.

In the last week of analysis, Amy continued to express her belief that "Grownups have everything better!" She complained bitterly that her mother would not buy her the new shoes she needed. Her clothes were falling apart; nobody was noticing.

I said she sounded like Cinderella. Amy was not pleased with my remark and yelled, "Well, if I'm Cinderella, then you are the wicked stepsister!! I only get hand-me-downs!" Here Amy had to laugh at herself, but added, "You know, I *was* Cinderella." I agreed that when she had been small, she had felt very left out and neglected; but perhaps she now was ready to say, "Amy, you are not really Cinderella anymore."

Amy could acknowledge the changes which had taken place during the 3 years of our work together. In one of the last sessions, she told me a story about the "World of Disguises," where no one could be recognized, and everyone had amazing powers. She drew a picture of a person covered with weapons. Suddenly she looked up and said, with a slight hesitation, "You know, even though this person has all these weapons, he's really . . . unprotected underneath." I sympathized with the plight of someone who felt so frightened. Amy agreed: that was why he had needed his disguises. The problem was that the disguises no longer worked. Underneath he was just an ordinary person. Amy was very serious: "The disguises used to work; but they weren't very . . . realistic."

Our last session was full of feeling—Amy being too uncomfortable and nervous about the end. She was excited about the family's move to the new town and enthusiastically expressed her wish to enjoy her new life. She now even believed I would answer her letters, and that our relationship would not be over for good. Her feelings were aptly conveyed in the Beatles' songs she sang throughout the session. She started with "I'll write home every day, and while I'm away, I'll send all my loving to you." She talked of her much-improved relationship with her mother, who was collecting her that day: "She's getting better all the time!" And finally she sang: "Sergeant Pepper's Lonely Hearts Club Band." Amy said she would not leave the room unless I gave her a kiss. I did; and with a very flushed face she turned abruptly and walked away from me.

DISCUSSION

Amy's treatment terminated in part because of environmental circumstances, but also because I felt—and Amy agreed—she was ready to stop. She had accomplished a great deal in her analysis and in many ways appeared a changed child. Her battling with her mother had ceased—a situation which gave great pleasure to them both. Amy no longer acted the "perfect person" she had sought to be; she could say to me, "I'm happier now that I don't have to be perfect." Her disguise was gone, as was the quality of brittleness described at the diagnostic stage.

The treatment material clearly indicated that Amy's disturbance of affect was at the core of her pathology. She had built a personality based on the suppression of certain very frightening feelings. The protective mechanisms Amy employed to avoid contact with these feelings became habitual and necessary for her to elicit a response from her surroundings.

The analysis focused on how to understand what we called her "pretending" or "acting." Her brittle and artificial qualities and her consistently spurious affects brought to mind both H. Deutsch's "as if" personality and Winnicott's concept of the "false self." Both Deutsch and Winnicott postulate that the basis of these disturbances lies in the lack of a secure infant-mother relationship, often one where there is a succession of caretakers. This had certainly been true for Amy as a small child. Amy closely resembled some of Deutsch's descriptions of the "as if" personality; "the individual's whole relationship to life has something about it which is lacking in genuineness and yet outwardly it runs along 'as if' it were complete" (p. 263). Deutsch also speaks of this type of patient as "intellectually intact, gifted, and [able to] bring great understanding to intellectual and emotional problems" (p. 264). However, when they try to be creative, their results tend to lack any originality. In respect to all of these characteristics, Amy was similar.

Early in treatment I thought Amy was the ideal insightful child patient. As time progressed, however, it became clear that she would agree to almost any interpretation, often making them herself in a glib and facile manner. Her excessive compliance and imitation of the analytic activity mirrored her early attitude toward her mother. "Total sharing" represented the only avenue to closeness, and it was in this area that Amy differed greatly from Deutsch's cases. Amy did not accept just any object for this kind of

closeness, but rather chose people who in reality presented the opportunity for genuine trust. Here her "object hunger" was served
by what I think was a preconscious awareness of her real needs and
feelings. Although at times obscured, Amy's capacity to trust was
obviously still intact.

As our knowledge deepened, it became evident that Amy's "as
if" qualities could be seen as her defense against overwhelming
anxiety, lest she find herself in a position of total unsafety. Her
underlying conviction of being unlovable and thus quite expend-
able was at the root of her anxiety, causing her to experience
enormous panic as she approached awareness of such feelings.
Winnicott (1960) sees the origins of the "false self" in the lack of
synchrony between mother and infant:

> The mother who is not good enough is not able to implement
> the infant's omnipotence, and so she repeatedly fails to meet the
> infant's gesture; instead she substitutes her own gesture, which
> is to be given sense by the compliance of the infant. This com-
> pliance . . . is the earliest stage of the False Self, and belongs
> to the mother's inability to sense her infant's needs.
> . . . where the mother cannot adapt well enough, the infant
> gets seduced into a compliance, and a compliant False Self reacts
> to environmental demands and the infant seems to accept them.
> Through this False Self the infant builds up a false set of rela-
> tionships, and by means of introjections even attains a show of
> being real. . . . The False Self has one positive and very im-
> portant function: to hide the True Self, which it does by com-
> pliance [p. 145ff.].

Winnicott's emphasis on adaptation to the environment is
especially pertinent because Amy had made an adaptive, yet unsuccessful attempt to cope.

Amy's need to construct her "disguise" originated in her early
relationship with her mother, who in her depressed and agitated
state had been unable to pick up Amy's signs and signals, causing
Amy to experience constant disappointment and frustration. Due
to the mother's difficulties, she could respond positively only to a
happy and undemanding baby. Amy's real needs and wishes—to
be held, to be reassured that her mother could protect her and
keep her safe—were experienced by the mother as insistent de-

mands she could not meet. She sensed in her small daughter her own unsatisfied longing for nurturance—detested in herself and therefore either denied or denigrated in Amy. Amy's real self and real feelings were not in harmony with what her mother was able to offer; Amy's development of a "disguised" personality was her way of trying to establish some sort of relationship with her mother, even if it had to be on an unreal basis. The battling relationship was defensive on both parts, each believing the other didn't love or want her. In their disappointment and guilt they had constantly to push each other away. When Amy told me late in the treatment that the "disguise" had been comprised of weapons, she showed her awareness of having felt in need of protection. The weapons at her disposal were fortunately not totally successful in eliminating either the dissonance she experienced with her environment or her intrapsychic conflicts.

Had Amy not come into analysis, she might well have gone on to become a person completely out of touch with her inner life, one whose object relations would be based upon identifications of the most superficial sort. In Deutsch's framework: she would never have had "occasion to complain of lack of affect for she would never have been conscious of it" (p. 269). This solution would have led Amy as an adult to be almost a caricature of her mother's artificiality. The basis for such a disturbance lay in Amy's identification with the mother's pathology.

Insofar as the mother had externalized the bad, angry, demanding, and uncared-for aspects of herself, she could respond to these aspects in her daughter only with loathing. At the same time, the mother maintained an idealized fantasy object—both of herself as she should have been, and of Amy as she wanted her to be. It was this fantasy object of the good, cheerful, grown-up little girl with which Amy identified in her attempt to get love from her mother. If Amy acted as if she were the charming little girl mother wanted, maybe mother would provide what she wanted. But of course, the mother's idealized fantasy object was just that; and on some level the mother was aware of its artificiality. Mrs. R.'s disappointment with Amy intensified as she saw in Amy more of the aspects she most hated in herself—feelings of helplessness, worthlessness, and anxiety about being abandoned. As her disappointment deepened, she became more rejecting and hence more guilty. Though designed to make a relationship with her mother, Amy's complaint behavior only put them farther apart. Mrs. R. once said to me: "I know Amy is me; and I feel paralyzed with her. Just the sight of her makes me furious. I'm afraid of battering her and so I'm frozen. I feel so helpless with her; and can't reach her at all."

Amy's awareness of what her environment expected resulted in the formation of a personality based on a defensive identification with her mother's idealized fantasy and her mother's actual artificial style of relating. According to Deutsch, "the tendency to mold oneself and one's behavior" is accompanied by the facility for "identification with what people are thinking and feeling" (p. 265), traits she considers to be characteristic of the "as if" personality. What Deutsch does not make explicit is that for the small child, this type of identificatory process represents the only means of achieving closeness and love from the object. Amy's feelings of worthlessness and emptiness were in part borrowed from, and in part a reaction to, her mother's direct criticism. Once internalized, however, the affects of her mother met Amy's own conviction that it was on her account that mother was withdrawn, depressed, and did not love her. The panic and primitive feelings of falling apart which Amy experienced at the end of the second year of analysis indicated that her disturbance dated back to her very early childhood, when the lack of feeling safe was predominant.

It may be questioned whether Amy's character was not simply based on the excessive use of denial and reversal of affect. Deutsch believes that the "as if" character tries to *simulate* affective experience. Amy did simulate affects at times of stress, but would do so in order to block a real feeling. In this, she was different from Deutsch's patients, where there was not a blocking of real affect. Deutsch also says that all real inner experience is unavailable to these people. Amy excluded only the *specific* affects relating to her early panic engendered by her mother's inability to provide a safe and holding environment. The feelings of helplessness, frustration, and depression were intolerable. Amy was aware that she had to respond with some affect to different situations and was able to discern cues coming from the environment as to what the appropriate feelings might be. This reaction represented the inhibition of her real feelings, but not their elimination.

In the early phase of analysis, after Amy had spent a weekend with her father, she arrived in a mood of great happiness, although in fact she had not enjoyed herself. When a holiday was coming up, she seemed appropriately ambivalent, telling me, "Well, it's 50/50—I'm happy and sad." Her words sounded apt, but they were empty of feelings. Obviously, Amy had to make use of both denial and reversal of affect to build up her style of relating; but once established as habitual, it took on a life of its own having an all-pervasive quality to it. For example, when Amy was sad, I would find myself asking, "Is she really sad? Or is she, by acting sad, defending against some other feeling?" Amy's sadness tended to have a dramatic flavor, as if she were acting the role of the queen of tragedy. I would find myself questioning her histrionic quality. Yet, her words and even her analytic formulations were invariably correct.

Amy once came to a session and immediately began to cry. Her friend Jane had fallen and broken her arm at school. Amy said, "I'm so sad. Now Jane will be a cripple for life. I feel so guilty, because maybe I made it happen by being nasty to her." Sensing that Amy's tears were not quite genuine, I wondered aloud whether Amy was really upset about something else, perhaps a recent phone call from her mother to me, in which Mrs. R. had mentioned that Amy had been coming to her bedroom at 6 in the morning to wake her up. At this, Amy became truly enraged, yelling, "Well, it's not nice to be chucked out of their room!" Thus, rather than reversal of affect, Amy had used one feeling to defend against another. She had not really been very sad at all; she felt rejected and humiliated when her mother sent her away.

At the beginning of her analysis, Amy's friendships, her manner at school, her helpfulness in the clinic waiting room were too good to be true. What emerged later was that Amy would rather have any feeling than experience the panic at not being wanted. She was terrified of showing her mother or me her real longings and then being spurned—a situation which would revive the old feelings of worthlessness and danger to her very existence. Amy once wrote a poem to describe how she felt at times of separation:

Holidays come and go
Bringing worries from long ago.
People were always coming and going.

Returning to the question posed at the beginning of this paper, I would conclude that Amy did not present as an "as if" personality, with the likelihood of becoming fragmented, but rather as someone prone to depression. She appeared to have an established self, with "as if" aspects superimposed upon it. In this sense Amy differed from other cases which presented pseudoidentificatory aspects, but lacked an established "real self." What had saved Amy was her ability to maintain her "object hunger" and her analysis at an early age.

FOLLOW-UP NOTE

I saw Amy a year after her analysis had ended. She and her mother came to London for a few days, and I met with each of them. Amy had just had her eleventh birthday and had grown a great deal. She looked almost like a teen-ager. In addition to wanting to see me just for a reunion, Amy also had certain problems on her mind. Her capacity to make use of two sessions was very impressive. She said that she was having trouble with some of her new friends who she felt were bullying her. In addition, she had recently been fighting with her mother again, always feeling her mother was singling her out for criticism.[1] Lastly, Amy complained of her father, who she felt treated her "like one of the boys." When he gave her presents, he chose things like skateboards or football shirts—not the pretty dresses she really would have liked.

I understood Amy's difficulties as stemming from her own conflicts regarding her developing body. She was definitely prepubertal, and unsure herself whether she wanted to be one of the boys or a feminine girl. The resurgence of her oedipal impulses was causing her guilt in relation to her mother and thus the need to provoke her mother to punish her. The problems with friends represented displacements from mother. In addition, although

1. I discovered that the fighting with her mother had begun soon after Amy received the news that they would visit me.

Mrs. R. had changed in many ways and was much more accepting of Amy's feelings, she was still somewhat ambivalent about Amy's sexuality. She feared Amy would repeat her own past—of growing up too fast and becoming promiscuous. Thus, she had not been able to help Amy deal with the normal conflicts of that phase of development.

I discussed these issues with Amy and her mother. Amy could see at once that the difficulties were "the same as the old ones"— her own anger with her mother and with me for having left her was experienced as coming back at her through the friends' bullying and her picking fights with her parents. I was struck both by Amy's use of previously gained insight to understand the current problems and by the total absence of any need to pretend that all had been perfect since the family's move and my departure. Mrs. R. also responded quickly and, in fact, told me that the reasons she was worried were connected to her own anxiety about Amy suffering her fate.

I received a letter from both a month later. Amy reported that everything was going well, and that school was much better. Mrs. R. wrote, requesting the name of a therapist, in case she ever felt the need to discuss the problem of her own identification with Amy's development. I was pleased that she could acknowledge her own difficulty and that she wanted to clear the way for Amy by getting some help for herself.

BIBLIOGRAPHY

DEUTSCH, H. (1942), Some Forms of Emotional Disturbance and Their Relationship to Schizophrenia. In: *Neuroses and Character Types*. New York: Int. Univ. Press, 1965, pp. 262–281.
FREUD, A. (1936), The Ego and the Mechanism of Defense. *W.*, 2.
——— (1965), Normality and Pathology in Childhood. *W.*, 6.
WINNICOTT, D. W. (1960), Ego Distortion in Terms of True and False Self. In: *The Maturational Processes and the Facilitating Environment*. London: Hogarth Press, 1965, pp. 140–152.

A Screen Memory in a Child's Analysis

MARLENE ROBINSON

THE SCREEN MEMORY DISCUSSED IN THIS PAPER EMERGED IN THE
second year of the analysis of an 8-year-old boy. Like all screen
memories, it involved a seemingly unimportant event in the life
of a young child. It was remembered with unusual detail, in contrast with the rather ordinary quality of the content and with the
way in which it was related. The child remembered and related
the event as if he were an interested onlooker, rather than the
main participant. The repressed, significant events covered by this
apparently indifferent memory were early seductions which occurred when he was about 2½ years old. The uncovering of these
seductions was, of course, extremely important and became a
major part of the analytic work. However, just as important, and
striking for me, was the way in which the screen memory became
a "tool" and a reference point throughout the analysis, facilitating
the general understanding of this case and highlighting the multiple uses of one piece of material recovered in the course of
treatment.

The author is on the staff of the Hampstead Child-Therapy Clinic and
the Walthamstow Child and Adolescent Psychiatric Service, London.

This child was seen at the Hampstead Child-Therapy Clinic, an organiza-
tion which at present is maintained by the G. G. Bunzl Fund, London; the
Field Foundation; the Freud Centenary Fund, London; Mr. Paul Mellon; the
New-Land Foundation; the Leo Oppenheimer and Flora Oppenheimer Haas
Trust; W. Clement and Jessie V. Stone Foundation; the Wolfson Foundation;
the Anna Freud Foundation.

A version of this paper was read at the Clinic in March 1976.

CASE PRESENTATION

David was referred by his parents at the age of 7 for aggressive behavior following a separation from his mother, who had to be hospitalized. He destroyed toys, became uncontrollable with rage at home, and tried to hurt himself. Once he put his hands around his throat as if to strangle himself, saying, "I am awful." He also attempted to strangle animals. He had a history of placing himself in dangerous situations, such as walking in front of moving cars. He restricted his food quite severely and refused to eat with the family at the table. A long-standing sleeping difficulty became more severe, and he had frequent nightmares. He usually ended up spending the night in his mother's bed.

David shied away from any contact with girls or women and formed intense, passionate relationships with boys, often embracing and kissing them in public. He had little contact with his father and seemed frightened of him. He was clumsy and so uncoordinated that he could not join in any games or play with the few friends he managed to find. He was very slow and quite incapable of coping with the basic tasks at school.

David was described as an "odd" child by most adults because he showed a marked preoccupation with horror, sadism, and violence. His fantasies about such things were overt.

In view of his difficulties and disturbances in almost every area of life, David's parents wondered if there had been brain damage at birth. They harbored this fear for several years, supported in part by medical reports and observations.

David was not a planned baby, and to some extent was an unwanted child, his mother having had three difficult pregnancies which seriously taxed her health. Consequently, this pregnancy was a tiring one, and Mrs. Jones continued to suffer from many illnesses and anxieties after his birth. However, in spite of these difficulties, she seemed to cope well with him when he was a baby. She remembered her pleasure in him even though she found him a "handful"—he was a large and active baby. Breast feeding had been uneventful, except that David was an avid, quick, and, according to the mother, "greedy" feeder. Nonetheless, she commented that he loved being cuddled and held, and the feeding experiences appeared to have been enjoyable for both.

Until the age of 2 David seemed to have been a content, thriving baby. Then difficulties in the mother-child relationship developed. Because of her growing concern about the health of a close relative, the mother withdrew from David. A long separation followed, and after David refused to recognize her when she returned, she began to express disappointment in and unhappiness with her young son. She now considered him to be a difficult, demanding, irritating child who wept and clung to her. Sleep disturbances emerged; toilet training, introduced at 2 years, had to be abandoned because David screamed and ran away at the sight of the pot.

At the same time that David was experiencing these problems, he was participating in highly stimulating sexual play with a 5-year-older sister. Mrs. Jones reported that David bathed with his father and played with father's penis. She was obviously distressed by this, but was unable to stop it.

ANALYSIS PRIOR TO THE EMERGENCE OF THE SCREEN MEMORY

During the first 18 months of treatment David appeared to be a highly disturbed boy with few defenses, little impulse control, and no hints of a capacity to form a treatment alliance. His sessions were flooded by barely disguised id material and threats to hurt me, the room, or himself. During this period, much of my work consisted in siding with his weakened ego in the battle against his impulses. Therefore, I was acting in the capacity of an auxiliary ego for much of the time.

The intensely sadomasochistic nature of the transference pervaded sessions. I was continually under threat of attack from David, for I was seen as a dangerous, uncaring, and potentially overstimulating woman who rejected him at every level of development. Slowly, David began to understand this, and signs of a change in the analysis emerged. He expressed positive, libidinal feelings toward me as a helper and an ally. This led to a growing ability to distinguish more clearly between the real and the transference aspects of treatment and me. There seemed to be indications that a binding of aggressive drives might be supported and that a treatment alliance could be fostered. For the first time, David began to work with me, rather than against me.

THE SCREEN MEMORY

The screen memory emerged during a period in which oedipal material dominated our work. In fact, the first importance of the screen memory lay in its relevance to David's oedipal conflicts, and for that reason I shall give a short account of this period in the analysis.

A holiday, which coincided with my marriage, became a link to oedipal material in the transference. David was sullen and uncommunicative before the holiday, and after an angry outburst agreed that he felt worried about the holiday and my marriage. (He had "guessed" that I was to marry, he said.) He thought that I would rather be with the "other man" than with him. When this was linked to his feeling of being left for the preferred man, he sang a song about a man who wanted to be with a girl, but he couldn't. David felt that he had "lost." After the holiday, David became very curious about my husband and me. When I related his many questions to the preholiday theme, he responded that I was cold, never gave him anything, and that what we needed was a "relationship." But, he added, he couldn't marry me anyway, because I was too old. The interpretation of his anxiety, sadness, and feeling left behind for another, when he wished he could have the older married women in a special (sexual) relationship, led to a memory of when he had been left by his mother who went away on a trip with his father. He had been left with a horrible, cruel nanny. I was able to take up his feeling of being abandoned because mother really preferred father and did not care about what happened to David. Although it meant many things in the analysis, at this stage the cruel nanny memory represented David's feeling that he had been left to a cruel fate—never to have mother, never to be chosen as the preferred one. Added to this was the idea that he had been pushed aside because he was angry, dirty, greedy, and unlovable. He concluded that "we don't like David" feelings took over inside of him, and his only way to counter them was to become angrier and more powerful than the fearful people who did not want him. He felt trapped in a vicious circle, a circle of feelings which were of course relevant to more than just the oedipal phase.

The wish to steal his father's penis and replace him had been hinted at much earlier when David became exceedingly anxious about being accused of stealing a wooden pole. In fact, he had not stolen it, but his guilt was so great that he felt he had done it. This theme was elaborated on now when David complained about his sports teacher who considered himself great and tried to boss David around. It was unfair, he said, that such an idiot should have such power. He had privileges he did not deserve, and David had none. His feelings about the teacher were soon linked to the privileged father at home who had such power, in the form of such a big penis. His rivalry was intense, and he told me that he couldn't stand it when his parents were alone together in the evenings. He wanted to "break it up" and always interrupted them. The danger, of course, was father's retaliation in the form of castration. David described this as his revenge, and asked me to close the window when we discussed his anger, rivalry, and wish to castrate father "in case anyone [like father] hears."

The memory emerged about this time, released, it would seem, by work which dealt with the time he felt frightened by father's retaliation for David's wishes in the phallic-oedipal conflict. He said that he remembered something from when he was little. (His dating of this varied from 2½ to 3 years.) The memory was vivid, and he was struck by how clear it was. He went for a walk with his parents in a large wood. (He still remembered the name of this wood.) He began to walk very near the edge of a lake in the wood. His mother said she thought he should come away, because it was not a good idea for him to walk so close to the edge. His father said this was silly, and that it was all right for David to walk near the edge. David thought that the lily pads in the lake were stepping stones and stepped on one. He fell into the cold water, was pulled out, and he cried on the train ride home. As a result of falling into the lake, he had an ear infection. He added that ever since this time, he had had recurrent ear infections. (In fact, during the course of treatment he suffered from several ear infections. In the last 2 years of treatment, he did not report having any.)

At first the emphasis was on his mother's "abandoning him." She had, in the end, sided with his father. This fit in with the oedipal material we had been dealing with. At this stage the significance of the ear infection was "father's revenge"—that is, castration, displaced upward from the penis to the damaged ear.

Underneath this was his feeling that his mother had not helped enough. She tried, but it was not good enough, and she had not protected him. She was weak, and had given in. Their early relationship seemed condensed, in part, in this bit of the memory for David. Starting from this feeling, we were able to bring in bits of of his view of her as the inadequate and inconsistent protector from internal and external dangers throughout his development. He felt that the reason she "failed" him was the "we don't like David" idea. This culminated at the oedipal stage in the fantasy that she did not want him and saw him as a poor (castrated) pet dog, rather than a masculine, admired boy.

His remembering the helplessness of the little David in the lake at the mercy of such frightening things resulted in a change in the transference, in which he attempted to fool and trick me into confusion. He devised clever plots to see if I would collude with his "baby feelings," as he put it, which really often led to frightening things. He was totally convincing and persuasive in his tricks and arguments. He was testing me, but more cleverly than in the initial phase of treatment. He noted that he would not be fooled because *he* was the tricker now. He was really worried that I would trick him, just when he had begun to trust me and believe that I would help. His mother, he said, fell for his tricks every time, and he realized that he was really frightened of being fooled by her. With the aid of the screen memory, I made the reconstruction of the little boy who had trusted mother to protect him, but then felt tricked by her—"betrayed," so to speak. He had fallen into the lake because she was too weak to help or to care about him. This seemed to point not only to his feeling of being let down, but also to his feelings that once he had been loved, cared for, and protected. He told me about a movie star who once had been appreciated and loved, but who now was a "nothing." He commented that this was how he felt. Although the wish to be the loved, cherished, all-important baby was evident, this story also indicated his feelings that things had changed (e.g., that he was a dirty, stubborn, aggressive boy in the anal phase whose products were valueless) as well as the reality of the change in his relationship with his mother. He concluded that the answer to his desperate question "Why didn't she help me?" had been wrong. He "misrecorded," that is, misunderstood, things. She had problems of her own, he said, which he confused with his ideas of why he wasn't liked. Perhaps she wanted to keep him an angry baby at times, and this confused things more, he added. He decided that as a little boy, he could only "misrecord" these things because he was too young to understand.

THE SEDUCTIONS

The screen memory took on another meaning as analysis proceeded and led to a reconstruction of early seductions. David became obsessed by a police film which warned children about the dangers of accepting rides, gifts, or sweets from lurking men who might turn out to be kidnappers. He was frightened by it and had nightmares about being kidnapped. At the same time, he was fascinated and excited by the theme of kidnappers.

In the transference I became the frightening kidnapper who might seize David. He thought that I might make suggestive passes at him and tested to see if I would be excited by and enjoy his sexy language and pornographic pictures. He was terrified that I would be a sexual attacker. After I wondered if these feelings could be linked to other people, he acted out what he called a "family monster play," in which a little boy is being attacked by an angry, raping father. The little boy ran to mother, but she could not help. The child then becomes the "6 million dollar man" who defended himself and won. At first David denied that this had anything to do with his father. "My father isn't like this." However, after telling me his fantasy that Jack the Ripper had chased me down the street, he said that sometimes he had felt his father was like Jack the Ripper. At this point the screen memory reemerged. Father had "lured" him to play too near the lake. This fragment soon was understood as luring him toward something exciting, somewhat forbidden, and, in the end, very dangerous. This insight led to memories that were pieced together to form a picture of young David feeling that his father had tempted him to do "something we shouldn't have done," while his mother, although protesting, had not been able to help him or to stop these frightening events. At this point, memories of stimulating games with his sister emerged. In particular, he remembered one in which she played Dracula and chased the screaming, excited David around the house. He remembered the excited frenzy of being caught by her. He suddenly spoke with disgust about a young girl who was "corrupting a younger girl" by playing sexual games in which she touched and fondled the little one. David then recalled sexual games he had played with his sister. These involved exposing and touching each other's genitals. He later remembered that his father had also played exciting monster games and David felt that "sex things" had happened in these. In one session when we were discussing Jack the Ripper, David said that it seemed that our voices were echoing, as if we were in a small room. He was reminded of being in a dark place where "Jack the Ripper hands" reached out for him. I wondered if this might be a clue to the sexual play with his father. While David was unable to elaborate on this, it seemed to me that the reference to the small room in which voices echoed might point to the bathroom where, as his mother had told me, the bathing and playing with his father had taken place. The relevance of the lake to the bathtub seemed indicated, especially because throughout the treatment water had always been a symbol for overwhelming impulses. Whenever we discussed his fear of being overwhelmed by his drives, David turned on the taps at full force and yelled, "Help! Help! It's a flood!" While David himself never made these associations to the bathtub, the reconstruction seemed "right" to him.

His recurrent ear infections were again related to castration fears, but now appeared to have been aroused at a much earlier time by father's and sister's sexual play in which David's penis had been fondled.

David added to the memory at this point. He said that he could remember crying all the way home on the train after he had fallen into the pond. The misery and vulnerability he had felt throughout that period were crystallized in this; as in the play, in order to counteract these feelings, he had to identify with the aggressor and stimulator and be the "6 million dollar man" from then on.

His behavior outside of treatment began to change considerably during this period. He became calmer, and his sadomasochistic battles with his mother decreased. He became interested in age-appropriate activities. He started flute lessons, played with toys and in games, and made moves toward joining the football team. He began to learn—something thought impossible before this time—and there seemed to be signs that after the reconstruction of the seductions from the screen memory, he was taking a step forward in development and for the first time showed a sublimation potential. At last, at age 10 years, he seemed to be in latency, at least from the ego's side.

David later wondered if he might inherit Jack the Ripper traits from his father. From this we were able to see his identification with the seductive father who he thought was "mad."

CASTRATION FEARS

David's castration fears were not exclusively related to the experiences of seduction, although these undoubtedly aroused them at a very early age. The screen memory became a link to tracing the fate of such fears in other phases of his past. After the reconstruction of the seductions themselves, David developed a praying ritual which persisted over a long period of time and was highly over-determined. He was forced to pray whenever he accidentally or intentionally touched his mouth. At first I was able to link the praying to oedipal fears and masturbation conflicts. He told me a story of a girl who attacked a man in a hospital with a pair of scissors. He was terrified, and constantly repeated this story. I viewed the attack with the scissors as expressing his fear that his penis would be cut off. On one level this castration was carried out by his mother, as mentioned above. However, David also felt that the dangerous, castrating person was an angry father who would seek his "revenge" for oedipal wishes. The obsessional act of touching his mouth was therefore related to a reassurance that his penis was intact. The castration fears were also linked to his father and sister as the seducers. The anxiety aroused by touching his mouth was, however, so great, that he had to undo it by praying. This material led to his masturbation conflicts—his wish to touch his penis, displaced upward to the mouth, and the prohibition against it.

This aspect was further elaborated on when David began to have trouble playing the flute. He had been one of the best players in his group, but suddenly decided to stop. The oedipal significance of this decision came to light in terms of "winning"; if he won and was the best, his father would hate him and David feared the consequences. At the same time, playing the flute was associated with masturbating—"playing the penis," as it were. David said that he would never play his flute again because he had broken it; it was damaged, no good, useless. When the displacement upward was taken up, he said he felt that the flute had become "like a part of my body." He had become "too attached" to it. His flight from it also was his flight from his phallic exhibitionism as the boy who played solo and enjoyed the praise so much.

The praying ritual could soon be understood in the light of fears of damage to his penis because of masturbation. At this point, David said that in his prayer he asked God to make him strong and rich. David's wish to be a strong, masculine boy and not one who had been castrated by father, the angry vengeful rival and the frightening seducer at the lake, or damaged himself by masturbating, was implied in this prayer. After we had talked about masturbation conflicts, the screen memory took on another meaning. David said that he felt extremely attracted to the lake. He wanted to go near it. Falling into the lake was therefore equated with succumbing to drives which resulted in danger. The danger of the drives was great, seemingly because of their intensity which had resulted from prolonged overstimulation at an early age.

CASTRATION WISHES

Underneath these castration fears were intense wishes, aroused by the early seductions which had reinforced passive sexual aims and a feminine identification. Our work and understanding of the memory shifted its emphasis and centered on these passive wishes and his use of aggression as a defense against them and as a reassurance. The uncontrollable tempers and toughness which had been major factors in the parents' referral served to hide his passivity.

One link to castration wishes in the present came when David hurt his foot and went to the hospital to have it bandaged. He worried that it was damaged forever and dwelled on the things he used to be able to do with it. He emphasized his feeling that his foot could never be any good again. Castration fears already touched upon were apparent, but his concern over his foot also indicated his wish to be damaged and worthless as a boy. He himself noted that he sometimes acted as if he wanted to stay hurt and damaged. After the interpretation of the wish to be castrated, David added that his acting the part of a Scotsman in a school play was worrying him because he had to wear a "skirt." Everyone would call him a "poof," he said. Finally, he admitted, "There is just a little part of me that wants to be a homosexual just to keep me worried." The screen memory then became significant in terms of the wish to have father and sister tempt and seduce him. He had been "tempted" to the lake not only by his father, but also by his own wishes for passive stimulation and excitement. He experienced his father's letting him go near the lake as father's agreement to David's passive wishes. Playing near the lake and falling into it were really equivalent to succumbing to passive wishes he expressed in relation to his father. In his words, he wanted to be "father's lover," and thus be castrated.

After the screen memory was used to highlight these wishes, David expressed his conviction that women were castrated. He brought the book *Jaws* and read to me a passage about a woman who while swimming in the ocean has her leg ripped off by a shark. She felt for her leg, but there was nothing there but a wound. He said, quite spontaneously, that for some reason this reminded him of losing a penis. He remembered his sister exposing herself to him. In talking about this, he was very uncomfortable and had a rather painful expression on his face. Eventually I could link his discomfort to the frightened, painful feeling of seeing a castrated, wounded girl.

Another factor determining these feelings was his view of mother as the castrator who could see no good in David because he was a boy. This became important in the transference. David became very angry with me and accused me of being critical of him, never praising him for efforts and achievements and always picking out things which were wrong about him. A long period of resistance followed. Every attempt to interpret this led to an angry outburst and accusations that I was criticizing him again. I never thought he was any good, he said. He then complained bitterly about the attention and praise his mother gave his sister. He was intensely jealous and envious because he felt his mother thought this sister was a "genius" and preferred her to him. His sister also made him feel that in comparison with her, he was nothing. This provided a link from the transference to mother. David felt she could never see him as capable because he was a boy. She thought girls were better, he felt. He recalled feeling like the tolerated, incompetent pet dog at home. He said that when he was little, he used to feel that whenever he tried something, she said he couldn't do it and discouraged him. This made him feel that she thought he was stupid and worthless. At other times, he felt she allowed him to do things too advanced and difficult for him, so he failed, which further reinforced his idea that he was hopeless. "She overestimated and underestimated me," he said. He remembered wanting to put on sister's dress and actually wearing her shoes because he wanted to be the girl who would be loved and praised.

Following more work on David's masturbation conflicts, we began to see that his wish to be "father's lover" also implied that to be loved by father meant to be beaten by him. The masochistic nature of his fantasies became apparent when David first hinted at his torturing himself mentally, as he put it. He would either place himself in, or fantasize about, a situation which aroused nagging anxieties, usually about being beaten, and then go over and over these scenes in his mind. For example, he tore a boy's coat and lived in fear that this boy would come and beat him, and for weeks he was "on the lookout." At the same time, he found himself frequenting places in which this boy regularly appeared. Often, David worked himself up into an excited, anxious state, followed by dramatic relief. He was never actually beaten, but he wished that something dramatic would happen. As he told me this, he touched his penis through his trousers, and I linked this to our talk on masturbation. Now he seemed to be mentally masturbating when he had these thoughts. He referred to the book *Clockwork Orange* and its combination of sex and violence, which led to the masochistic, sexualized nature of his ruminating fantasies. He tried to start a battle with me, noting that such a fight was sexually exciting. He wanted to see if I would beat him in the fight. I related this to his earlier attempts to start fights with his teacher (which inevitably led to punishment).

His anxiety aroused by, and interest in, sex magazines with pictures of women being beaten on the buttocks by men became a further bridge to the wish to be beaten by father, thus gratifying passive sexual aims. He told me that these photographs were frightening, but also "sexy." What was exciting, he said, was the idea of being beaten or punished. At first the person beating David was mother. He remembered masturbating and becoming very excited when he saw Emma Peel, the star of the television program, "The Avengers," beat up men. He then thought of her doing this to him. He was reminded of his fights with mother, and we made the link to his wish to be beaten by her. He noted that he thought this had been confused with his "poofy feelings" when he was little. I referred to the earlier work on the wish to be castrated and "father's lover." The identification with the beaten women was a further link to these wishes. Thus, to be loved by father ultimately meant to be beaten by him.[1]

1. The nature of David's beating fantasy continued to be an important issue up to the time of termination. On the one hand, it seemed to respond to interpretation in that David understood his present wishes and behavior regarding being punished in terms of his past experiences and fantasies. The need to be downtrodden and emasculated made sense to him, and in the last phase of treatment he linked many of his problems with peers to this. When analysis ended, David, then aged 14, was expressing interest in girls and having age-appropriate fantasies about relationships with them. He also recognized that this area could pose great problems for him in the future. On the other hand, there had been a long history of great disturbance for David. His ego and drive development had been disrupted, and there had been a long-standing sadomasochistic relationship with his mother, which, although lessened somewhat, continued after termination. Moreover, his passive sexual

The underpinning of these problems was the fixation to the anal stage, which has been discussed to some extent. Here I would add only that when he dealt with his wish to be beaten, David showed me a poem he had written. Entitled "The Pig," the poem, written in the first person singular, concerned a pig's wish to be left alone as a dirty, nasty pig. "I am a Pig" he shouts from the rooftop. Just leave me alone as one. David's wish to be a passive, dirty, provocative, sadistic, emasculated boy who had retreated from the phallic stance was apparent.

David commented that this wish made sense to him because he had been so confused about sex. It had seemed like a fight to him. The fight was his sadistic intercourse fantasy, arising from early primal scene observations, which enhanced the fixing of the scoptophilic component instinct readily seen throughout treatment. David had always been fascinated by looking at forbidden (usually sexual) things. We called these "Sex-X" things, derived from the "X" ratings given to films. He was quite unable to control his curiosity, which manifested itself in his need to see photographs, drawings, or films depicting sexual activities of all sorts. (This behavior had been prevalent since the age of about 7 when he entered treatment.) This theme had been hinted at in the screen memory; he told me that he had been very curious about the lily pads, which he could not "figure out." He remembered looking at them closely to find out about them, and then ended up in the cold water. I suggested that he might also be remembering other things that he was very curious about, but could not understand, and that these, too, had made him feel he was in a frightening, even dangerous situation. In subsequent sessions he peeked outside our door in order to see what a couple in the hall was doing. I could eventually link his curiosity to his wish to find out what his parents were doing behind the closed living room door in the evenings. He supposed that they were doing "sex things," and he

wishes certainly had received strong reinforcement from several sources. These factors would seem to point to a "fixed beating fantasy" (Novick and Novick, 1972), which remains a relatively permanent part of a child's life, is impervious to years of interpretation, and seems to persist after termination. A more definitive evaluation of the influence of the beating fantasy on David's psychosexual life must wait until he attempts to form a heterosexual relationship.

lurked outside the door until he could no longer tolerate his curiosity and barged in on them. Of course, the wish to barge into the closed parental bedroom to see "sex things" between them was apparent and had resulted in his observing intercourse when he was about 2. To David, it had seemed like a fight, and he commented, "How could a 2-year-old understand sex? No wonder I'm confused; it's sex and violence together." He said that it seemed that the woman was the one hurt in this fight. Therefore he must have regarded the penis as a dangerous weapon, a knife. That was another reason for not wanting to be a man, he concluded. He would be dangerous and could hurt a woman, just like his father who seemed like a Jack the Ripper. Thus, David felt that if he were an active, masculine boy, his penis would either be dangerous or be in danger. In either case, he must retreat from the active, phallic-oedipal position.

David's religious obsessive phase, accompanied by a praying ritual, was then linked to his ambivalence and homosexual wishes toward his father. His full prayer was "Please God, make me rich and strong and make all the poor people in the world rich." During the time that analysis was dealing with this prayer, David had to make frequent visits to the toilet. He told me that each time he had diarrhea, although it did not occur elsewhere. Eventually this was linked to a fantasy of anal birth, in which the stool was equated with the baby. Thus, the eating of sweets, already associated with good, loving feelings, now became linked to the stool which gave anal pleasure. Thus, his passive wishes toward his father could be further related to his wish for anal intercourse and his wish for an anal baby.

"Make all the poor people in the world rich" could be understood in reference to his anxiety at witnessing the primal scene. His idea had been that father was being castrated by mother. His subsequent sympathy for "all the poor people" was therefore really for his "poor father" (whom David also had wished to castrate, of course).

At the time when the praying ritual reached its height, David began to go to church with his father every Sunday. They were the only members of the family to attend. Several months later David expressed a wish to be confirmed. His father took an active part in his religious instruction. Thereby David's passive wish toward father was gratified. He was with father every Sunday. At the same time, his sexual wishes were controlled by religious activities and rules. The return of the repressed wish, however, was manifest in his obsessive praying. He felt compelled to repeat this prayer whenever a door was opened, as well as when he touched his mouth. He had to shut the door, pray, and cross himself. This too was linked to his witnessing of the primal scene when the door to the parental bedroom had been open.[2]

DISCUSSION

Throughout this paper I have referred to David's memory as a screen memory, thus indicating my belief that it differed from the many other childhood recollection seen in the course of treatment. However, the validity of this viewpoint can be questioned because David was 8 when he told me his memory of events that occurred when he was about 2½ years old. Such a short time span may lead one to assume that this memory was not a formed screen memory, but rather one in formation. The view that the analyst adopts will, of course, influence the way in which the memory is dealt with in the treatment.

David's memory conforms to Freud's concept of a screen memory, which he first described in 1899. In later works (1914, 1917) Freud noted that the screen memory could be likened to dreams in that a significant repressed latent content underlies a less important manifest content. He added that processes such as repression, displacement, condensation, and symbolization take part in the formation of the screen memory. Fenichel (1927) emphasized the importance of traumatic experiences, while Greenacre (1949) noted several factors that contribute to the formation of a screen memory, among them: the state and strength of ego development, the intensity of the disturbing experience, the stage of libidinal

2. This phase of the analysis led me to reread the case of the Wolf-Man (Freud, 1918). Similarities between the two cases are striking. Of particular interest in both was the development of a religious phase accompanied by a ritual which served to repress, and at the same time gratify, passive wishes toward the father.

development, the amount of aggression aroused, and the accompanying erotization at the time of the events.

David's ego state and strength at the time of the seduction were weakened, and he had had little available support from his recently ill and depressed mother. Anxiety was already raised when these experiences occurred, and their intensity led to an overwhelming rush of both aggressive and sexual impulses. David was described as "out of control" at that time. The accompanying erotization during the anal-sadistic stage can readily be seen in his beating fantasies and wish to be the castrated dirty "pig" of his poem. The sadomasochistic characteristic of David's personality was certainly in formation at the time of the events.

In a study of the formation of screen memories in a latency child, Kennedy (1950) concluded that although the child's memories have some of the special characteristics of adult screen memories, they cannot be considered as formed screen memories. Rather, they are screen memories in formation. In a later paper (1971), Kennedy added, "Whereas reconstruction from the analysis of adults has led to an understanding of the role of 'screen' or 'cover' memories, direct work with children has focused on the multiplicity of the pathogenic happenings, and the complex distortions and ramifications that occur during development" (p. 389).

However one decides the issue whether David's memory was a formed screen memory or would have undergone further transformations, I can only conclude that in this analysis the memory was used as a fully formed screen memory would be. From it we were able to uncover early traumatic events which had been repressed. The screen memory became a reference point for further associations and memories, leading to further reconstructions and insights. It was a shorthand for several conflicts at various stages in David's life.

I had made certain assumptions regarding this memory which, although correct in the end, were not the significant points at the time the screen memory emerged. On the basis of my previous knowledge of David's developmental history and my understanding of the impact such experiences would have on a child of 2½ years, I had assumed that the significance of the screen memory lay in the covering of these seductions that his mother had told me about earlier. I had assumed, quite wrongly, that once these events had been reconstructed, the memory would lose most of its "value" in the analysis. In other words, we would have a "That's it!" response when it was understood. In fact, David did have this reaction. He said, "We have got it!" but this was not the end of the screen memory.

My assumptions were, therefore, only partially correct. First, the relevance of the screen memory to the emerging oedipal had to be considered. It became a confirmation of interpretations regarding his feelings that his mother had betrayed him for another man. This theme was carried further when the transference shifted and the fantasy of having been fooled into a sense of well-being by an untrustworthy mother emerged. He felt that she had betrayed him by the lake because of her weakness and rejection of him, just as he had felt she had done in the past at various stages of his development.

This piece of work was followed by the uncovering of the seductions. However, the memory continued to play an important part in the analysis, either summarizing, confirming, or leading to material dealing with other conflicts.

Ernst Kris (1956) clarifies the use of childhood memories in analysis. He points out that the recovery of the actual events is not the aim or goal of reconstructive work:

> We are misled if we believe that we are, except in rare instances, able to find the "events" of the afternoon on the staircase when the seduction happened: we are dealing with the whole period in which the seduction played a role—and in some instances this period may be an extended one [p. 73].
>
> . . . reconstructive work . . . cannot aim at such a goal: its purpose is more limited and yet much vaster. The material of actual occurrences, of things as they happen, is constantly subjected to the selective scrutiny of memory under the guide of the inner constellation. What we here call selection is itself a complex process. Not only were the events loaded with meaning when they occurred; each later stage of the conflict pattern may endow part of these events or of their elaboration with added meaning. But these processes are repeated throughout many years of childhood and adolescence and finally integrated into

the structure of the personality. They are molded, as it were, into patterns, and it is with these patterns rather than with the events that the analyst deals [p. 76f.].

The temptation to reconstruct the "actual events" covered by the screen memory was certainly present for me. I became fully aware of how limiting such a viewpoint is only as the work on the screen memory developed and continued long after its recovery. As Anna Freud (1951) noted, the analyst underestimates the telescopic nature of memory if he searches for *the* traumatic experience. "One traumatic prohibition or punishment, remembered or reconstructed, becomes the representative of hundreds of frustrations which had been imposed on the child" (p. 27). The memory was, indeed, "loaded with meaning"—meanings from various periods in David's life and from various conflicts. The screen memory had consolidated into a pattern which seemed to be the core upon which many events and conflicts were built.

The formation of this pattern can be understood in terms of the concept of multiple function. Waelder (1930) notes that according to "this principle, every attempt to solve a task is necessarily, at the same time, an attempt to solve other tasks, even if incompletely" (p. 71). Every psychic act therefore has more than one meaning.

Consequently, my initial tendency to limit work on the memory to reconstruction of early seductions would have taken no account of the multiple function of such a piece of material.

Kennedy (1971) pinpoints this problem of relying on reconstruction of *the* experiences when she notes that "in the process of remembering in any form, the material of past experience is reorganized in a new way, albeit slightly. The new memory structures that are created will reflect the maturational and developmental level of the child's mental apparatus. Interpretations and reconstructions by the analyst inevitably enter into this reorganization as well, so that the child, by establishing causal relations in connection with the memory, *changes the content and structure of the memory*. He will be seeing it in a new way" (p. 396). The screen memory in fact attempted to deal with several problems which had occurred at various stages of David's development; for example, falling into the lake "satisfied" the wish to be castrated through the resulting ear infection, and, at the same time, dealt with the fears of being castrated for oedipal wishes. Father, in the memory, punished David by letting him fall into the lake; but father also tempted him into it, thus stimulating passive wishes.

Waelder further comments "We see . . . that from psychoanalysis there emerges an aspect of the enormous multiplicity of motivations and meanings of psychic occurrences. . . . Because of the multiplicity . . . , it is perhaps fitting to be on one's guard against premature simplification" (p. 82). I can only add that in David's analysis, it was not possible to reconstruct the seductions covered by the screen memory and then assume that work on it was "finished." The memory did not stop being part of the analytic work, and the need for carefully working through the material as it emerged, not according to a preconceived (even if correct) assumption, was apparent.

BIBLIOGRAPHY

FENICHEL, O. (1927), The Economic Function of Screen Memories. In: *Collected Papers,* 1:113–116. New York: Norton.

FREUD, A. (1936), The Ego and Mechanisms of Defense. *W.,* 2.

———— (1951), Observations on Child Development. *This Annual,* 6:18–30.

———— (1965), Normality and Pathology in Childhood. *W.,* 6.

———— (1971), Problems of Psychoanalytic Training, Diagnosis and the Technique of Therapy. *W.,* 7.

FREUD, S. (1899), Screen Memories. *S.E,.* 3:303–322.

———— (1901), Childhood Memories and Screen Memories. *S.E.,* 6:43–52.

———— (1914), Remembering, Repeating and Working-Through *S.E.,* 12:145–156.

———— (1917), A Childhood Recollection from *Dichtung und Wahrheit. S.E.,* 17:145–156.

———— (1918), From the History of an Infantile Neurosis. *S.E.,* 17:7–122.

———— (1919), 'A Child Is Being Beaten.' *S.E.,* 17:179–204.

———— (1924), The Economic Problem of Masochism. *S.E.,* 19:159–170.

———— (1937), Constructions in Analysis. *S.E.,* 23:255–269.

FURMAN, E. (1971), Some Thoughts on Reconstruction in Child Analysis. *This Annual,* 26:372–385.

GLOVER, E. (1929), The Screening Function of Traumatic Memories. *Int. J. Psycho-Anal.,* 10:90–93.

GREENACRE, P. (1949), A Contribution to the Study of Screen Memories. *This Annual,* 3/4:73–84.

JOSEPH, E. (1973), Sense of Conviction, Screen Memories, and Reconstruction. *Bull. Menninger Clin.*, 37:565–580.

KENNEDY, H. E. (1950), Cover Memories in Formation. *This Annual*, 5:275–284.

———— (1971), Problems in Reconstruction in Child Analysis. *This Annual*, 26:386–402.

KRIS, E. (1956), The Recovery of Childhood Memories in Psychoanalysis. *This Annual*, 11:54–88.

NOVICK, J. & NOVICK, K. K. (1972), Beating Fantasies in Children. *Int. J. Psycho-Anal.*, 53:237–242.

WAELDER, R. (1930), The Principle of Multiple Function. In: *Psychoanalysis*, ed. S. A. Guttman. New York: Int. Univ. Press, 1976, pp. 68–83.

The Oral Drive, Clinging, and Equilibrium

LESTER H. FRIEDMAN, M.D.

IN THIS PAPER I SHALL OFFER A NEW EXPLANATION FOR SYMPTOMS of disequilibrium, which occurs when there is a rapid acceleration of the fluid in the semicircular canals. There are a number of interrelated symptoms which involve altered states of consciousness and which could be subsumed under the term disequilibrium: vertigo, dizziness, giddiness, lightheadedness, feeling a sense of imbalance, or a feeling that one is spinning. Such symptoms have previously been attributed to sexual excitement (see Freud [1894] on vertigo as a symptom of actual neurosis; Glenn [1974] on physiological concomitants of sexual excitement), or ego, id, and superego regression to preoedipal states (Isakower, 1936), or a regressive revival of being cast away by an archaic superego agency (Peto, 1970); they have been explained as hysterical or anxiety symptoms or related to physiological factors such as orthostatic hypotension, hypoglycemia, cerebrovascular malfunction, general anesthesia, and vestibular-cerebellar disorders. My clinical observations impelled me to reconstruct a particular experience in infancy

Faculty, New York Psychoanalytic Institute.

The hypothesis presented in this manuscript was stimulated by a discussion with Harold Levitan, M.D. I want to thank a number of colleagues who made invaluable suggestions: Drs. Charles Brenner, Manuel Furer, Jules Glenn, Ernest Kafka, Norman Margolis, Wayne Myers, Henry Nunberg, Henri Parens, Andrew Peto, Arnold Richards, Jay Shorr, John Sours, and Nicholas Young.

An earlier version of this paper was presented at the Annual Meeting of the American Psychoanalytic Association, May 1974, Denver, Colorado.

which, as a result of regression, played a significant role in the occurrence of symptoms of disequilibrium.

I shall attempt to show how transient disturbances in equilibrium in childhood and adulthood may have their roots in the feeding/clinging situation in infancy. I believe that the universal experience of an abruptly interrupted feeding/clinging is a significant factor in determining the later symptomatology of dizziness or disequilibrium in some patients. I view this genetic experience as one of the determinants, in addition to others that vary according to the individual's life history. The first experiences of disequilibrium occur when an infant's feeding/clinging is interrupted or terminated and the infant, often in a drowsy state, is *moved abruptly and rapidly*. When a feeding is interrupted in infancy, I postulate that the wish to suck and cling is given added impetus. Since clinging and sucking initially form a single unit (Schilder, 1939), later one may stand for the other. That is, when sucking occurs, the wish for clinging is evoked, or the reverse, on an unconscious level. There are several possible dynamic constellations. If there is repression or conscious inhibition of one of the two functions, the other may become more prominent. I shall describe how in one patient when clinging was consciously inhibited, the wish to suck was intensified. A separation which involved an interruption of clinging could revive the early experience of an interrupted clinging and/or the accompanying infantile disequilibrium. If there is repression of the wish to cling and suck, and the wish is increased in force, disequilibrium may result. And if there is an increased wish to cling and suck, together or separately, when an object is unavailable, either actually or potentially, some form of disequilibrium could appear. The end of an analytic hour or an approaching holiday, which interrupts treatment, or the termination of an analysis, all could revive the disequilibrium that occurred in infancy when feeding/clinging was abruptly interrupted.

I want to emphasize that feeding is the earliest situation in which the infant's capacity for mastery begins to develop. An interrupted feeding followed by transient disequilibrium would make additional demands on the infant's capacity for mastery. Any later situation requiring mastery could contribute to a partial regression to the original situation requiring mastery and thereby revive the disequilibrium that occurred during an early feeding.

I shall first present a clinical example in order to show how this patient's material could be more fully understood by using my hypothesis. I shall then review the relevant literature and give additional clinical illustrations.

CLINICAL EXAMPLE

Mr. R. was a short, stocky, 30-year-old Midwesterner, who looked lost at his initial consultation. At first he described his mother as aggressively controlling and later as depriving and seductive. Although he was breast-fed for several weeks and bottle-fed for a few months, his mother did not like holding babies. His father liked holding him as an infant. One of Mr. R.'s early memories from age 1 to 3 years was holding his father's hand at a time of distress. Age 2 to 3 years was the time of one of the major organizing memories of his early childhood: his mother left him for about a week when she went to California with his father. He was subsequently left several times for a week when his parents were away on trips. At age 4 years a paternal substitute played a game with him in which he was thrown in the air. He recalled getting lost in early latency; and later on, in early adolescence, he tried to make himself sick in order to force his mother to stay home with him. The atmosphere in his home was excessively stimulating both sexually and aggressively.

Initially Mr. R. wanted to please me (he recalled wanting to please his mother beginning at age 2 years). Much later in his analysis he revealed his disappointment when in the first year he had arrived early for his hour, expecting me to be ready with milk and cookies, and I had not been ready to see him until the appointed time. There was an intense, desperate longing for closeness with me. This appeared in part as a regressive response to his marked castration anxiety, and in part as a strong, positive, maternal transference. He wanted to be the only one I cared about, fantasied my holding and rocking him like a baby, and his crawling in bed next to me. When he felt rejected by a woman, he thought of being in his mother's arms and her breast being near.

When his supervising teacher reminded him that they would finish their work in several months, he woke during the night with a "blocked ear" and feared losing his balance. He felt extremely threatened by the first summer interruption, which occurred several months after he had begun his analysis. He had many fantasies in which he kept me with him in a substitute way in an attempt to cope with the impending interruption. The threat of loss in the transference gave extra impetus to his sexual fantasies and activity; these increased his castration anxiety, which in turn was regressively expressed and experienced as a threat of the loss of the object. When he tried to be closer to his parents in reality, they were both unavailable and needed him to take care of them.

After the summer vacation he wanted to have contact with me and be close to me and identify with me. Then the important organizing memory of being left by his mother at age 2 to 3 years for a week was revived. When I interpreted his shame over his intense maternal longing, he thought of a giant baby bottle and his mother breast-feeding him. He arranged for a woman whom he hardly knew to share his apartment with him. He soon told two women he dated that he would not see them for 2 to 3 weeks, leaving them in order to defend against feeling abandoned by me. His castration anxiety was increased by his sexual success with different women on successive nights. A short time later, he had a frank primal scene dream after his mother made a date with him.

As noted, all during the early part of his analysis his reactions to any interruption were intense. He had a stronger desire to be fed when his castration anxiety was more prominent. Both were evident on one occasion (several months after the summer interruption) when I could not see him for his regular Friday hour. On Monday after the missed Friday hour he invited a young woman whom he did not know well to sleep with him, just as he had previously invited a woman to share his apartment with him after the summer interruption. He also thought of rejecting two women, just as he had actually done after the summer interruption. He was both afraid of and excited over seeing his mother on Wednesday, which was a holiday, when I again would not meet with him. His associations clearly expressed his castration anxiety.

He reported a dream from the preceding night in which he saw a man and woman have intercourse.

On Tuesday he imagined I would be with my family on Wednesday and disliked sharing me with anyone. He thought of telling a young woman he wanted to marry her. He wanted to be part of my family. He reported that he had forgotten one of his possessions in my waiting room after his Monday hour. He said that he wanted to travel all over when his analysis was completed. I interpreted this wish as a denial of the wish to hold on to me when he felt abandoned by me. He said he became dizzy just as I was saying he felt abandoned. He then said, "It's worse." He spoke of the couch moving, his moving, spinning, and rocking, and felt he was on an inclined plane sliding to the right. He wanted to be warm and to be held. When I noted his wanting to hold on to someone when I would not be here Wednesday, he felt slightly nauseated and also experienced an increased sense of disequilibrium.

In the Thursday hour he thought of my having a giant penis, his tearing it off and swallowing it. He had gone out with two women Tuesday night, seeing first one and then the other. He had seen his mother Wednesday, had been ambivalent about his father, and had felt he had to protect his penis. He felt my silence meant that I was asleep. He fantasied being fed, referring to the missed session. He alluded to a family romance fantasy, in which his father was a large provider of milk.

At no other time during his analysis did Mr. R. experience comparable symptoms of disequilibrium, nor did he report having had such symptoms of disequilibrium during his early or later childhood.

COMMENT

Mr. R.'s disappointment in his mother as the primary nurturing person in his early childhood as well as later was clear. It was evident from the two early memories and from his analysis that he attempted to cope with the absence of his mother by turning to his father. Often during his analysis when he was disappointed by me as his mother in the transference, he turned to me as father.

His attempts to seek his mother's care both historically (by getting lost and by making himself sick) and in the analysis were clear. When he was disappointed by me, his strong maternal transference became even stronger. When a teacher reminded him that they would soon finish working together, he experienced this as the loss of a substitute maternal object. His waking during the night with a "blocked ear" and fearing a loss of balance immediately after she reminded him of the anticipated loss fit with my hypothesis. That is, the anticipated loss of his main supervising teacher made him want to cling to her. His experiencing disequilibrium can then be understood as his remembering an earlier disequilibrium which occurred when clinging was interrupted by an abrupt movement. The summer interruption evoked extreme concern, which was heightened when he found his parents not only unavailable but needing him to care for them. The revival of the important organizing memory of being left by his mother for a week at age 2 to 3 years immediately after the summer interruption confirmed what was apparent, namely, that he reacted to the summer interruption as though his mother had left him. When his shame over the longing for his mother was interpreted, he wanted to be breast-fed and bottle-fed just as he had been in reality in early infancy. In the face of feeling abandoned, he first sought a substitute object and then turned passive into active and told two women he was dating that he would not see them for 2 to 3 weeks. He did to them what he felt had been done to him by his mother and by me.

On Monday after the missed Friday hour (and before the missed Wednesday hour) he repeated what had occurred just after the summer when he experienced my absence as he had experienced the loss of his mother in his third year. He frantically sought a substitute object; he then thought of rejecting two women. I interpreted to Mr. R. his wish to be with me and his use of defenses—to find a substitute object, turn passive into active (he rejected two women when he felt rejected), and his use of denial together with a counterphobic defense (he denied feeling abandoned and fantasied termination of his analysis and planned to travel all over). When I interpreted his denying his wish to hold on to me when feeling abandoned by me, he immediately became dizzy.

Thus an interpretation of the defense was followed by dizziness as an expression of the oral drive. His wanting to be warm and to be held can be understood as a wish to undo what had evoked the disequilibrium now and in infancy—the abrupt loss of the nuturing object. When I reinterpreted his wanting to hold on to someone when I would not see him on Wednesday, his increased sense of disequilibrium and nausea suggested that the current disequilibrium was a revival of an infantile disequilibrium evoked by having been moved abruptly to interrupt feeding/clinging. I want to emphasize that in anticipating the end of his analysis and planning to travel all over he denied the wish to cling to me and used a counterphobic defense. His wish to travel, *to be in motion,* can also be understood as an attempt to defend against an anticipated disequilibrium, psychic and potentially physical—he experienced this disequilibrium after missing his Friday hour and in anticipation of missing his Wednesday hour. His attempt to master the interruption in his analysis appeared to have revived the earliest experiences of mastery—interruptions of feeding/clinging. The dizziness that occurred in the earliest attempts of mastery was revived in the transference. His mother's seductive behavior and his increased castration anxiety gave an impetus to his longing for his mother regressively in the transference.

This patient's mother was aggressively controlling and depriving and disliked holding babies. It is therefore reasonable to assume that she would have moved him abruptly and rapidly to interrupt a feeding or his clinging to her in infancy. These circumstances laid the groundwork for Mr. R.'s intense maternal transference in his analysis and for his responding with dizziness when the defense against his wish to cling to me was interpreted. As Lewin (1952) noted, "For anxiety, though a signal, is not merely a signal. It has a content and it is a sort of 'memory'. That is, anxiety attacks not only serve as warnings; they also reproduce earlier life events" (p 311). Thus, Mr. R.'s dizziness can be understood as his remembering an earlier dizziness when clinging to his mother had been abruptly interrupted.

As is always the case with symptoms, the dizziness was multiply determined. When Mr. R. was 4 years old, a paternal figure played a game of throwing him in the air. This may have created a transient disequilibrium which also could have been revived and could have contributed to the dizziness he experienced on the couch. In view of Mr. R.'s background one can easily understand that he turned to his father as a substitute mother. He recalled that in his early years he held his father's hand when he was distressed. After the missed Wednesday, on Thursday he spoke of a family romance fantasy in which his father was a large provider of milk, making his father a "good mother" in order to be able to cope with the loss of his mother in the transference. Thus, his reaction to me can be viewed in another way: when he felt disappointed by me as mother in the transference, he wanted to cling to me as father. My interpretation of this wish was immediately followed by dizziness. It is also possible that my interpretation served to awaken him and the dizziness was part of a hypnopompic experience.

In a discussion of an earlier version of this paper, Parens (1974) noted that regression associated with an acute anxiety reaction may reactivate the type of vestibular mechanism I have described. Parens believes that if the abrupt interruption of feeding in a drowsy infant occurs during the latter part of the first year, after the ego has been structured into an agency, this event occurs during a hypnagogic state when the ego is in a state of regression and an altered state of consciousness prevails. Parens further suggested:

> When an infant's feeding is suddenly interrupted and he is abruptly moved, not only is there the vestibular event described by Dr. Friedman, but there is also an abrupt cessation of the most peaceful state humans may perceive: falling asleep, sucking at mother's breast. In this peaceful state drive gratification is insured and the ego is in a hypnagogic state. Because of this, it seems to me that the interruption in question is dramatic; it may, in fact, exaggerate the unpleasure induced by the vestibular event referred to by Dr. Friedman and thereby may give it the importance Dr. Friedman suggests. It may be gratuitous to note that in the economy of the psyche, the interruption of peacefulness in the state of the (pre)ego and of drive gratification might lead to the investment of a cathexis in the vestibular event of being moved.

Mr. R.'s libidinal regression occurred with such ease in the face of an increased castration threat and when the oral-aggressive wishes were not yet acceptable in the transference. Another factor contributed to his dizziness. The threat of being left on Wednesday was so great that there occurred a massive withdrawal of cathexis, inducing an altered ego state in which various kinds of disequilibrium were manifest (Stein, 1965). Mr. R.'s symptoms of disequilibrium may also have been due to modified sexual excitement or a defense against the loss, and an expression, of sexual excitement.

I want to stress that in my clinical opinion, the disequilibrium in Mr. R. largely represented a revival of disequilibrium from an early oral period when disequilibrium was not accompanied by fantasy. The symptom represents an altered state of consciousness which causes anxiety. There may be a secondarily elaborated fantasy in response to the symptom.

REVIEW OF THE LITERATURE

In 1905 Freud said, "I shall take thumb-sucking . . . as a sample of the sexual manifestations of childhood." He noted the relationship between grasping and sucking. "In this connection a grasping-instinct may appear and may manifest itself as a simultaneous rhythmic tugging at the lobes of the ears or a catching hold of some part of another person (as a rule the ear) for the same purpose" (p. 179f.).

Paul Schilder (1939) regarded clinging and the oral drive as closely linked genetically. In the clinical situation, disequilibrium occurs when there is a lack of support early in a patient's life; and furthermore, as a related phenomenon, dreams of flying and motion are common. Schilder's investigation of newborn infants showed that the act of sucking is always accompanied by a heightening of muscular tension, especially in respect to grasping. When grasping can be voluntarily initiated, it enables sucking to proceed more easily. Schilder confirmed that sucking reinforces the grasping reflex and vice versa. He suggested that these functions originally form a unit—the child sucks as he clings to his mother—but then undergo separate developments. Grasping becomes an independent function with a changed aim. In infancy, clinging secures the child's equilibrium, especially during feeding; and at a later stage, clinging serves the preservation of the upright posture.

Preservation of equilibrium is regulated by the vestibular apparatus.

In a study of patients who sustained a head injury with subsequent dizziness or vertigo, Friedman et al. (1945) found that the outstanding precipitating factor was a change in posture, whether sudden or otherwise. The authors concluded that both physical and psychological factors played an important role in the production of prolonged posttraumatic dizziness in the majority of cases. I would, of course, agree that physical factors are important. However, insofar as psychological factors may play a part, the finding that a change in posture was an outstanding precipitating factor in producing dizziness or vertigo would be consistent with my hypothesis. The traumatic injury to the head increased the patient's wishes to be cared for. On an unconscious level this injury revived the longings from the early mother-child nursing situation. Because of the increased force of the drive and the absence of a suitable object, i.e., a nursing mother, a change in posture revived the earlier disequilibrium that was experienced in the interruption of the infantile nursing/clinging.

Peiper (1961) observes that "Although infants vomit easily, they do not become seasick and are not disturbed by a rocking motion. The reflexes of position and movement must reach a certain stage of development for their coordination to be disturbed" (p. 149). These reflexes develop during the first year of life, so that the infant's first experiences of disequilibrium following an abrupt interruption of feeding/clinging would occur during the second half of the first year of life. I assume that at that time every infant would experience some transient disequilibrium when moved abruptly (especially in a half-awake half-asleep state).

In describing sensations associated with falling asleep, Isakower (1936) said that there are "distinct sensations of floating, sinking and giddiness" (p. 332). In some instances, the distinction between different regions of the body is blurred, and there is the visual impression of something shadowy, indefinite, and round. This shadowy round object swells to a gigantic size and comes nearer and nearer; or dry, sandy sensations in the mouth and skin occur on falling asleep as part of the wish for the breast in the face of unacceptable genital incestuous wishes. That is, when a strong incestuous genital wish is repudiated, regression to an oral wish takes place. I postulate that when the oral wish is unacceptable, the wish to cling occurs. If the wish to cling occurs in analysis when the object is not available, dizziness, floating, or other manifestations of disequilibrium can be seen. I view them as a revival of a primitive infantile dizziness, or as a revival of disequilibrium that occurred on falling asleep at an earlier age.

Lourie (1949) noted that motor phenomena of a repetitive nature occur when the infant is in a transitional stage of growth and development. Such motor phenomena also represent an attempt to experience kinesthetic sensations that play an important role in the infant's development. They serve ego growth and aid in obtaining balance; they may occur in the face of deprivation. In addition to their organizing and mobilizing effect, they may secondarily become associated with other needs and satisfactions. Some children only rock when they are pleased, as others engage in thumb sucking when they are satiated. The movements may occur to relieve tension and anxiety. Lourie further noted that when the secondary value of coping with tension and anxiety by rhythmic movements becomes prominent, it is the chief cause of their persistence after the first year. He noted the striking correlations between thumb sucking and rocking, which become interchangeable. Both are prominently used to relieve tensions as a prelude to sleep. This is not surprising since sleep would automatically evoke the wish to eat as a part of the oral triad described by Lewin (1950). A rhythmic motion would help to cope with and deny the disequilibrium that might result when no object is available and there is a wish to suck.

Greenacre (1941) cites Mrs. Blanton as observing that "walking with the baby quiets it even on the first day, and that in her experience, babies almost never cried when being carried through the hospital corridor. This too seems to support Ferenczi's and Freud's suggestion of the practical continuum of fetal and postnatal life; for the fetus has, in fact, been accustomed to being carried for nine months, subject to the rhythmical motion of the mother's walking" (p. 37). Since rhythmic motion and support are linked in the intrauterine state and almost always in the postnatal period, I would suggest that this may be an additional reason why the wish to cling and be supported is displaced onto rhythmic motion to express the drive.[1] This use of rhythmic motion may later be externalized in play with toys and serve the aim of mastery.

In 1914, Ferenczi described disequilibrium at the end of the psychoanalytic session:

> Many patients have a sensation of giddiness on rising from the recumbent position at the end of the psycho-analytic session. . . . [The patient] suddenly becomes conscious of the actual facts; he is not 'at home' here, but a patient like any other. . . . This sudden alteration of the psychic setting, *the disillusionment* (when one feels as *'though fallen from the clouds'*) may call up the same subjective feeling as is experienced in sudden and unexpected change of posture when one is unable to adapt oneself suitably by compensating movements and by means of the sense organs—that is to say, to preserve one's 'equilibrium'—which is the essence of giddiness [p. 239f.].

Peto (1970) noted that giddiness at the end of the analytic session is a special case of the regressive revival of being cast away by an archaic superego agency. I would add that ending an analytic hour may be seen as waking the patient; the giddiness which results may be understood as part of a hypnopompic experience. This giddiness may be the result of the regressive revival of an earlier actual giddiness that occurred when the infant's feeding or clinging was abruptly interrupted. The patient's associations to the giddiness itself as well as the dynamic context in which the giddiness occurs enable the analyst to determine its meaning.

FURTHER CLINICAL EXAMPLES

CASE 1

Miss S., in her 20s, sought analysis because of dissatisfaction with her life. What gradually emerged over several years of analysis was that her mother, though physically present, had never been available to her or responsive to her needs. Her father, a professional

---

1. Rocking during feeding is a pleasurable experience; other sensations of rapid movement, e.g., riding a roller coaster, may also be pleasurable.

man, was preoccupied with his work and himself and therefore was not available as a substitute object. In addition to having experienced a relative maternal deprivation, Miss S.'s home had been excessively stimulating sexually. She felt numb and foggy and had multiple Isakower phenomena during her analytic hours in the first three years of her analysis. After this analytic work during the initial three years, she began to feel like a whole person for the first time in many years.

In the fifth year of her analysis, she again fantasied intercourse as a fight and expressed her fear that the penis was a weapon that would give her vagina a jagged cut. Warding off the fantasied pain, she regressed and felt numb. She imagined I was giving a man extra time and a prescription for medication. What gradually unfolded was her anger at my not having helped her to plan a career, a wish to please me, and then a wish to identify with me. I interpreted her wanting to identify with me when she wanted to please me. She recalled trying to please her mother in the past; when her mother had been critical of her, she had felt "strange, disorganized, and disoriented" for several days. Next her wish to take her boyfriend's penis and be a man appeared. This suggested that she wanted to be a man both to ward off the danger of a penis cutting her vagina and to deal with the disappointment she experienced when she wanted to please me as she had wanted to please her mother in the past.

She then missed a Monday hour in order to have a long weekend. Following this she felt an increased hunger, thought she had seen me on the street, and wanted to be like me—be trained as an analyst. She attempted to ward off a wish to be like her mother. Then, after parking her car, she got out and "felt dizzy—lightheaded." Walking up the street, she thought of wanting to be like me and felt repelled by it. Her associations to falling led to not knowing what's happening and to childhood story characters. She said that Dorothy fell into a crack in the earth and fell and fell, like Alice in the rabbit hole. She thought of falling out of a tree and skidding in a car. I suggested that her wanting to be like me expressed a wish to hold on to me, an idea that also repelled her. She replied that she had felt that way as a child, when she wanted to hold on to someone and no one was there. She then expressed a wish to be outside herself in order to be able to observe herself. She wondered why she did not see herself as Cinderella at midnight turning into a pumpkin. "I always see myself as Alice falling through the rabbit hole with cards falling on her. She wakes up in a chair in front of a fireplace. The mother cat is washing two baby cats. It was time for tea." In my interpretation I suggested that she might have felt disequilibrium as an infant when feedings were interrupted and she was moved quickly. "Like being thrown over a shoulder to be burped," she said. She told of her mother physically supporting her as a child, holding her body in the air in a horizontal position so that she felt like she was flying. Further associations led to her feeling of falling off a slide when she falls asleep; thoughts of skating and skiing; and to her favorite nursery rhyme: "Rockaby baby in the tree top; when the wind blows the cradle will fall; down will come baby, cradle and all."

I have included this small fragment of a lengthy and complex analysis because it points to a specific and common occurrence: feedings are frequently interrupted for the purpose of burping the infant. Her associations led to the nursery rhyme "Rockaby baby," which suggests that the disequilibrium this patient felt as a baby when a feeding or clinging was interrupted made her feel that she was falling. I want to emphasize that this patient felt lightheaded without spinning. The clinical material suggests that the symptom of feeling lightheaded without spinning can be understood as having the same source as the symptom of dizziness which included spinning (as in the case of Mr. R.). Miss S.'s feeling "dizzy" at this time in her analysis also served the purpose of warding off what was about to emerge, namely, a wish to be orally impregnated by me. In connection with this wish, her feeling of dizziness can also be viewed as an expression of her sexual excitement. Some months later she felt dizzy when she felt sexually excited and fantasied holding me.

CASE 2

In the analysis of Mrs. G., a tall woman in her 30s, a major theme was her feeling of oral deprivation. She was breast-fed for several months, ate poorly as a child, and sucked her thumb. On my couch she tugged at the fringe of the pillow on which her head rested. She often ran her hand through her hair, sometimes twirling it and at other times tugging at a small lock of hair. In childhood she had held on to her hair while sucking her thumb. Associating to her play with her hair, she said that she had to have something "to cling to, to hold on to." Shortly thereafter I suggested that we might discover what her increased hair tugging expressed if she refrained from doing it. What then emerged more clearly was her fear of separation over the summer. Although she had spoken of her wish to have something in her mouth, she now spoke of this more clearly and vividly than in the past. She had an overpowering wish to have something in her mouth. A thinly disguised fellatio wish appeared in the transference. She wanted my penis as a breast substitute in the face of the approaching summer vacation.

Mrs. G. consciously inhibited clinging when she knew that I would soon be away. This inhibition intensified the wish to suck. Of course, the fellatio wish expressed not only a longing for the penis as a breast but also a wish for the penis as a penis. I would expect her to develop disequilibrium if clinging were inhibited and the wish to suck were not allowed expression. Later on in her analysis at a time when her oral longing was increased, she mentioned that her doctor wanted to prescribe a mild tranquilizer. I asked what her wanting to take this brought to mind. She responded to my question as a critical comment about her oral longing. After taking these tranquilizers over the weekend, she experienced acute sleepiness and disequilibrium while driving to her Monday hour. This sleepiness persisted during the hour and subsided only gradually in the course of several analytic hours. Thus, when she felt that her oral longing was not allowed, she experienced an altered state of consciousness with sleepiness and disequilibrium.

DISCUSSION

Over several years I have observed both children and adults who attempted to cope with a sense of imbalance, reacted with dizziness to the loss of an object, turned to drinking soda on my couch when frustrated in making a spinning toy, and slid down a hill in a baby-buggy contraption during the time of a missed hour. I considered that these various reactions might be explained by the type of early experience I have postulated. Subsequently I made the observations in the analytic cases reported in this paper. My experience with these patients and others confirms, I believe, what I initially considered as a tentative hypothesis. It led me to distinguish between two types of dizziness: (1) libidinized dizziness sought after by pleasurable rocking, occurring with masturbation accompanied by gratifying fantasies, or occurring as a derivative of the sensations experienced with satiation and going to sleep; (2) an anxious unpleasant dizziness associated with waking, falling asleep, or separation and loss of the object.

I want to emphasize that in two of my patients the partial regression to the early feeding/clinging situation with its accompanying dizziness occurred after a libidinal progression. In Mr. R.'s case, his oedipal conflict had become more prominent in the analysis. Another patient (not discussed here) expressed a desire to make a sexual overture to his wife, which represented a considerable libidinal progression for him. The ease of regression was undoubtedly enhanced by the threat of the libidinal progression.

These observations raise another question: is the symptom of dizziness an expression of a libidinal regression or a revival of an ego state. I believe it is both. The disequilibrium regressively expresses the oral drive, and at the same time a memory of an earlier ego state is revived and reexperienced. The full understanding of a symptom of disequilibrium requires the particular patient's associations. While one would expect variations in different patients' unconscious fantasies and therefore in the specific determinants of their disequilibrium, I see the genetic experience of an interrupted feeding/clinging by abrupt movements as a common determinant which may be significant or contributory in causing symptoms of disequilibrium.

BIBLIOGRAPHY

FERENCZI, S. (1914), Sensations of Giddiness at the End of the Psycho-Analytic Session. In: *Further Contributions to the Theory and Technique of Psycho-Analysis*. London: Hogarth Press, 1950, pp. 239–241.

FREUD, S. (1894), On the Grounds for Detaching a Particular Syndrome from Neurasthenia under the Description 'Anxiety Neurosis.' *S.E.,* 3:87–115.

————— (1905), Three Essays on the Theory of Sexuality. *S.E.,* 7:125–243.

FRIEDMAN, A. P., BRENNER, C., & DENNY-BROWN, D. E. (1945), Post-Traumatic Vertigo and Dizziness. *J. Neurosurg.,* 2:36–46.

GLENN, J. (1974), The Analysis of Masturbatory Conflicts of an Adolescent Boy with a Note on "Actual Neurosis." In: *The Analyst and the Adolescent at Work,* ed. M. Harley. New York: Quadrangle, pp. 164–189.

GREENACRE, P. (1941), The Predisposition to Anxiety. In: *Trauma, Growth, and Personality.* New York: Norton, 1952, pp. 27–82.

ISAKOWER, O. (1936), A Contribution to the Pathopsychology of Phenomena Associated with Falling Asleep. *Int. J. Psycho-Anal.,* 19:331–345, 1938.

LEWIN, B. D. (1950), *The Psychoanalysis of Elation.* New York: Norton.

————— (1952), Phobic Symptoms and Dream Interpretation. *Psychoanal. Quart.,* 21:295–322.

LOURIE, R. S. (1949), The Role of Rhythmic Patterns in Childhood. *Amer. J. Psychiat.,* 105:653–660.

PEIPER, A. (1961), *Cerebral Function in Infancy and Childhood.* New York: Consultants' Bureau, 1963.

PETO, A. (1970), To Cast Away. *This Annual,* 25:401–416.

SCHILDER, P. (1939), The Relations between Clinging and Equilibrium. *Int. J. Psycho-Anal.,* 20:58–63.

SPITZ, R. A. (1956), *No and Yes.* New York: Int. Univ. Press.

STEIN, M. H. (1965), States of Consciousness in the Analytic Situation. In: *Drives, Affects, Behavior,* ed. M. Schur. New York: Int. Univ. Press, 2:60–86.

EARLY NORMAL
DEVELOPMENT

Four Early Stages
in the Development of
Mother-Infant Interaction

T. BERRY BRAZELTON, M.D. AND
HEIDELISE ALS, Ph.D.

HAVING COME TO THE STUDY OF NEONATES BY WAY OF PEDIATRIC practice and psychoanalytic research on mother-infant interaction at the Putnam Children's Center, we became aware of the powerful influence of the individuality of the new infant in shaping his environment.[1] In the early 1950s, when most of our research was aimed at understanding the environmental forces which produced pathology in childhood, we were struck with the importance of seeing this pathology as the result of an interaction between the child and his environment. It appeared to be vitally important to understand why parents could function well with one kind of infant but not with another (Brazelton, 1976). This led us to try to

Dr. Brazelton is Associate Professor of Pediatrics, Harvard Medical School; Director, Child Development Unit, Children's Hospital Medical Center, Boston. Dr. Als is Assistant Professor of Pediatrics (Psychology), Harvard Medical School; Director of Research, Child Development Unit, Children's Hospital Medical Center, Boston.

This work was supported by grants from the Robert Wood Johnson Foundation, the Carnegie Foundation, and the William T. Grant Foundation.

Presented as the Helen Ross lecture, Chicago Psychoanalytic Society, Chicago, Illinois; April 13, 1978.

1. Because of the authors' close collaboration since 1972, the pronoun "we" has been used throughout, although only the senior author in fact worked at the Putnam Children's Center.

understand the kinds of equipment which each member of the mother-infant dyad brought to their interaction. We do not mean to exclude the father and siblings, nor the extended family, for all of these are of vital importance to the dyad of which we shall speak. But for simplicity's sake, we shall speak here of mothers and infants. In this process of interaction, we have become even more impressed with the power of such a dyadic interaction itself, and the importance of not analyzing each member as if he were an independent actor—independent of the effects of the interaction.

We felt that the earliest observable behavior of mothers and infants might be a clue to the influence each member of the dyad might have on the other. We found in our research at Putnam Children's Center that the prenatal interviews with normal primiparas, in a psychoanalytic interview setting, uncovered anxiety which seemed at first to be of almost pathological proportions. The unconscious material was so loaded and so distorted, so near the surface, that before delivery the interviewer felt inclined to make an ominous prediction about each woman's capacity to adjust to the role of mothering. Yet, when we saw each in action as a mother, this very anxiety and the distorted unconscious material seemed to become a force for reorganization, for readjustment to an important new role. We began to feel that much of the prenatal anxiety and distortion of fantasy was a healthy mechanism for bringing a woman out of the old homeostasis which she had achieved to be ready for a new level of adjustment. The "alarm reaction" we were tapping was serving as a kind of "shock treatment" for the reorganization required for her new role. We agree with Bowlby's (1969) concept of attachment and his emphasis on the "imprinting" of the mother on the new infant. We now see the shake-up in pregnancy as readying the circuits for new attachments; as preparation for the many choices which she must be ready to make in a very short, critical period; as a method of freeing her circuits for a kind of sensitivity to the infant and to his individual requirements which might not have been easily or otherwise available from her earlier adjustment. Thus, this very emotional turmoil of pregnancy and of the neonatal period can be seen as a positive force in the mother's healthy adjustment, enabling her to provide a more individualizing, flexible environment for the infant (Bibring et al., 1961).

Prospective fathers must be going through a very similar kind of turmoil and readjustment. In an ideal situation we might be offering both of them a lot more support and fuel for their new roles than we do. So far, we in medicine have not done well in substituting for the extended family in this earliest period, but we surely are just on the brink of exercising our potential as supports for young parents.

As we began in the early 1950s to attempt to document and understand neonatal behavior, very powerful mechanisms seemed to dominate the neonate's behavior (Brazelton, 1961). In the tremendous physiological realignment that the changeover from intrauterine to extrauterine existence demands, it has always amazed us that there is any room for individualized responses, for alerting and stimulus-seeking, or for behavior which indicates a kind of processing of information in the neonate; and yet, there is. Despite the fact that his major job is that of achieving homeostasis in the face of enormous onslaughts from his environment, we can see evidence of affective and cognitive responses in the immediate period after delivery.

This very capacity to reach out for, to respond to, and to organize toward a response to social or environmental cues seems so powerful at birth that one can see that even as a newborn the infant is "programmed" to strive, as he wakes from sleep and is on his way to a disorganized crying state, to turn his head to one side, to set off a tonic neck reflex, to adjust to this with a hand-to-mouth reflex and sucking on his fist. All of these can be called primitive reflex behaviors. But as soon as the newborn has completed this series, he sighs, looks around, and listens with real anticipation, as if to say, "This is what I'm really here for—to keep interfering motor activity under control so that I can look and listen and learn about my new world."

Our own model of infant behavior and early infant learning goes like this: The infant is equipped with reflex behavior responses which are established in rather primitive patterns at birth. He soon organizes them into more complex patterns of behavior which serve his goals for organization at a time when he is still prone to a costly disorganization of neuromotor and physiological systems, and then for attention to and interaction with his world (Als, 1979a). Thus, he is set up to learn about himself, for as he achieves each of these goals, his feedback systems say to him, "You've done it again! Now go on." In this way, each time he achieves a state of homeostatic control, he is fueled to go on to the next stage of disruption and reconstitution—a familiar model for energizing a developing system. We use Robert White's (1959) "sense of competence" as our idea for fueling the system from within. We also believe that the infant's quest for social stimuli is in response to his need for fueling from the world outside. As he achieves a homeostatic state, and as he reaches out for a disruptive stimulus, the reward for each of these states of homeostasis and disruption is reinforced by social or external cues. Hence, he starts out with the behaviorally identifiable mechanisms of a bimodal fueling system—(1) of attaining a state of homeostasis and a sense of achievement from within; and (2) the energy or drive to reach out for and incorporate cues and reinforcing signals from the world around him, fueling him from without. He is set up with behavioral pathways for providing both of these for himself—for adaptation to his new world, even in the neonatal period. Since very little fueling from within or without may be necessary to "set" these patterns and press him onward, they are quickly organized and reproduced over and over until they are efficient, incorporated, and can be utilized as the base for building later patterns. Greenacre's (1959) concept of early pathways for handling the stress and trauma of birth and delivery as precursors for stress patterns later on fits such a model. It is as if patterns or pathways which work were "greased up" for more efficient use later on. Our own concept is that others are available *too,* but these are just readied by successful experience.

With this model of available behavioral response systems which provide an increased availability to the outside world, one can then incorporate Sander's (1977) ideas of early entrainment of biobehavioral rhythms, Condon and Sander's (1974) propositions that the infant's movements match the rhythms of the adult's voice, Meltzoff and Moore's (1977) work on imitation of tongue protrusion in a 3-week-old, and Bower's (1966) observations on early reach behavior to an attractive object in the first weeks of life. As each of these responsive behaviors to external stimuli fuels a feedback system within the baby toward a realization that he has "done it"—controlled himself in order to reach out for and respond appropriately to an external stimulus or toward a whole adult behavioral set—he gets energized in such a powerful way that one can easily see the base for his entrainment. The matching of his responses to those in the external world must feel so rewarding that he quickly becomes available to whole sequential trains of behavioral displays in his environment and begins to entrain with them. He becomes energized to work toward inner controls and toward states of attention which maintain his availability to these external sequences. In this way, "entrainment" becomes a larger feedback system which adds a regulating and encompassing dimension to the two feedback systems of internalized control and externalized stimulus-response. Hence, entrainment becomes an envelope within which one can test out and learn about both of his fueling systems. Thus, he can learn most about himself by making himself available to entertainment by the world around him. This explains the observable drive on the part of the neonate to capture and interact with an adult interactant—and his "need" for social interaction. Figure 1 shows a schematic presentation of this mutual fueling process (Als and Brazelton, 1978).

But the infant is not alone in this process of learning about himself in the first few weeks and months. Because of the available energy, disrupted from old pathways in pregnancy—anxiety, if you will—the new parents are just as raw and ready for learning about themselves as the neonate. Just as they learn about each new stage in their development and find the appropriate control system, and experience the excitement of being fueled by the baby, the father and the mother are forced to learn about themselves. As each new stage in the infant's development presses them to adjust, they learn about the excitement *and pain* of disruption and the gratification of homeostasis as they hit a plateau. In this way, we see mothers and fathers learning about themselves as developing people while they learn about their new baby. This is also the way in which the fueling for both nurturance and learning comes about at each new stage in the baby's development. Otherwise, nurturing a new infant would be too costly and too painful. In a reciprocal feedback system, the rewards are built in for the parents as well as the infant.

We have adopted some of the concepts of a cybernetic feedback system as adaptable to our conceptual base (Tronick and Brazelton, 1979; Brazelton et al., 1979). This system allows for the feedback rewards of achieving homeostasis as well as the importance

PROCESS OF INTERACTIVE NEGOTIATION
BRINGING ABOUT EACH STAGE OF ORGANIZATION

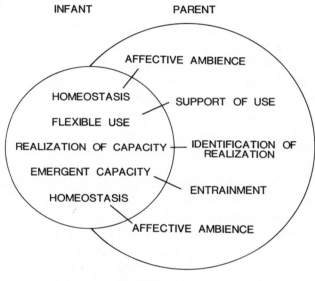

Figure 1

of forces for disruption and the subsequent learning to reorganize after each disruption. It represents a fueling model which fits with Erikson's (1968) stages of development, McGraw's (1945) spurts in development with periods of regression for reorganization and digestion of newly achieved skills, and Piaget's (1936) concepts of assimilation and accommodation.

The notion of a feedback system seems to fit our model particularly well, since it presents an adaptive model to stress and change, with a built-in self-regulatory goal. The immature organism with its vulnerability to being overloaded must be in constant homeostatic regulation—the physiological and the psychological. Handling input becomes a major goal for the infant, rather than a demanding or a destructive one. Such a system can handle disruption either by negative, stressful or by positive, attractive stimuli; but the organizing aspect of both is seen in the amount of growth of the system. Since positive stimuli permit growth and homeostasis with less cost, one can predict the value of a sensitive environmental feedback for the immature organism; just as one can predict with a more constantly stressful environment that there will be an attempt at precocious mastery; and finally, if the adult member or members are insensitive to the needs of the immature member of the dyad or triad, an expensive fixation or even breakdown in the system. If disruption or fixation does not occur, then stress can provide a learning paradigm for handling the stress and then recovery (Als et al., 1979a). Either way there is disruption of the old balance, but in one there is the energizing feedback of closing a successful homeostatic circle, with the infant thereby being readied and fueled for the next step in development.

We first began to see the value of such a conceptual base when we were developing the Brazelton (1973) *Neonatal Behavioral Assessment Scale.* The concept underlying the assessment is that the neonate can defend himself from negative stimuli, can control interfering autonomic and motoric responses in order to attend to important external stimuli, and can reach out for and utilize stimulation from his environment necessary for his species-specific motor, emotional, social, and cognitive development. Using the baby's own control over his states of consciousness, the examiner attempts to bring the baby from sleep to wakefulness and even to crying and back to sleep again as he assesses the neonate's capacity to respond to and elicit social responses from the environment. In a 20-minute assessment, an examiner can begin to feel a neonate's strengths in shaping those around him. The newborn responds clearly and differently to appealing and negative intrusive stimuli. Both kinds of stimulation provide some form of organization, but as one handles him and sees him achieve an alert state, using the examiner's cues, and as he then maintains a clearly alert state, one begins to realize how much a part of his organization the nurturing "other" can and must be. We work to achieve the infant's "best performance" on a series of responses to various stimuli—to voice, to face, to handling and cuddling, to the rattle, and to a red ball. As the infant becomes excited and responsive, one can see his increased and increasing sense of mastery and involvement with the adult examiner. His states of consciousness become the holding or cybernetic envelope for all his reactions; and as he responds individually to stimuli and as he moves from state to state, one can see and feel him respond to the stimulus, regain his balance, then move on to respond to the next stimulus. The process of responding—of realizing that he has responded by readjusting his state to incorporate that response, of realizing he has achieved a new but stable state—becomes the initial envelope for interaction with his world and for realizing his own control over his homeostatic systems. As one plays with a newborn, one realizes that the newborn is indeed displaying a marvelous capacity to regulate his internal physiological responses by the mechanisms of internal homeostatic control or "state" control. The newborn's "awareness" of this capacity becomes a first basis for internalizing his capacity to control himself and his environment as well as a base for the next steps. We believe that these observations might lend perspective to Hartmann's (1939) idea of precursors of ego development.

In following the system of organization through the infant's first 4 months of life, we were able to discern three more successive stages of disruption, progress, and the reachievement of homeostasis. Throughout the infant learns about himself, and the mother's self-awareness increases as she participates in helping him achieve the goals of each of these stages. These then become a rich base for the infant's affective and cognitive development as well as his awareness of himself—developmental accomplishments which might be equated with early ego development.

In order to delineate these stages, we would like to describe how we have been studying them in normal and abnormal mother-infant and father-infant pairs. We first became aware of the infant's capacity to respond clearly and differentially to an object and a person, as early as 3 weeks of age, in the course of our work at the Harvard Center for Cognitive Studies.[2]

2. This work was carried out by the senior author in direct collaboration with Barbara Koslowski and Mary Main, in the larger context of studies conducted in association with Jerome Bruner, Edward Tronick, Colwyn Trevarthen, and T. G. Bower.

By 3 weeks of age, the infant stared fixedly at the object with wide eyes, fixating on it for as much as 2 minutes without disruption of gaze or of attention. In this period, his face was fixed, the muscles of his face tense in a serious set, eyes staring, mouth and lips protruding toward the object. This static, fixed look of attention was interspersed with little jerks of facial muscles. Tongue jerked out toward the object and then withdrew rapidly. Occasional short bursts of vocalizing toward the object occurred. During these long periods of attention, the eyes blinked occasionally in single, isolated blinks. The body was set in a tense, immobilized sitting position, with the object at the infant's midline. If the object was moved to one side or the other, the infant tended to shift his body appropriately so that it was kept at his midline. His shoulders hunched as if he were about to "pounce." This complex behavior was observed long before a reach could be achieved, the infant utilizing an antigravity posturing of the shoulders (Bruner et al., 1972). Extremities were fixed, flexed at elbow and knee, fingers and toes aimed toward the object. Hands were semiflexed or tightly flexed, but fingers and toes repeatedly jerked out to point at the object. Jerky swipes of an arm or leg in the direction of the object occurred from time to time as the period of intense attention was maintained. In this period, the infant's attention seemed "hooked" on the object, and all his motor behavior alternated between the long, fixed periods of tense absorption and short bursts of jerky, excited movement in the direction of the object. He seemed to hold down any interfering behavior which might break into this prolonged state of attention.

As the object was gradually brought into "reach space" (a conceptual area 10 to 12 inches in front of the infant), his entire state of attention and behavior changed. His eyes softened and lidded briefly, but continued to scan the object with the same prolonged attention. His mouth opened as if in anticipation of mouthing it. The tongue came out toward the object and occasionally remained out for a period before it was withdrawn. His neck arched forward as his head strained toward the object. Shoulders hunched, and mouth protruded. Swipes of arms and extension of legs at the knee increased in number. Hands alternately fisted and opened in jerky movements toward the object, as early as 6 weeks of age.

The contrast of the infant's behavior and attention span when he was interacting with his mother, rather than an inanimate object, was striking as early as 4 weeks of age. We felt we could see brief episodes of these two contrasting modes of behavior as early as 2 to 3 weeks, but by 6 weeks we could predict correctly from watching parts of his body and observing his span and degree of attention whether he was responding to an object or to his mother.

Of course, the expectancy engendered in an interaction with a static object as opposed to a responsive person must be very different (B. L. White et al., 1964; Piaget, 1937). But what surprised us was how early this expectancy seemed to be reflected in the infant's behavior and use of attention. When the infant was interacting with his mother, there seemed to be a constant cycle of attention (A) followed by withdrawal of attention (W)—the cycle being used by each partner as he and she approached, then withdrew and waited for a response from the other participant. For the mothers and infants observed, this model of A-W of attention seemed to exist on several levels during an interaction sequence. If she responded in one way, their interactional energy built up; if another, the infant might turn away. The same was true of her response to his behavior. In order to predict and understand which behavioral cluster will produce an ongoing sequence of attention, one must understand the affective attention available in each member of the dyad. In other words, the strength of the dyadic interaction dominates the meaning of each member's behavior. The behavior of any one member becomes a part of a cluster of behaviors which are interacting with a cluster of behaviors from the other member of the dyad. No single behavior can be separated from the cluster for analysis without losing its meaning in the sequence. The effect of clustering and sequencing takes over if one assesses the value of particular behaviors, and in the same way the dyadic nature of interaction supersedes the importance of an individual member's clusters and sequences. The power of the interaction in shaping behavior can be seen at many levels. Using looking and not looking at the mother as measures of attention-nonattention, in a minute's interaction we observed an average of 4.4 cycles of such attention and apparent nonattention. Not only were the spans of attention and of looking away of shorter duration than they had been with objects, but they clearly were smoother as the attention built up, reached its peak, and then diminished gradually with the mother. Both the buildup and the decrease in attention were gradual. All of the infant's movements were smooth, cyclical, and one could indeed tell from looking at a toe or a finger whether the infant was in an interaction with an object or a parent—and by 4 weeks of age, even which parent it was.

When we analyzed the interaction by our techniques (Brazelton et al., 1973), using 18 mother and 19 infant variables (table 1), we began to see that there were clusters of behaviors on each side in a predictable rhythm. With newer analysis systems developed over the last 5 years (Brazelton et al., 1975; Tronick et al., 1977, 1979; Als et al., 1979b), we were able to document when the mother could be sensitive to the infant's homeostatic needs for interaction and recovery and when he became locked in a rhythmic interaction with her, as interaction I (fig. 2) shows. When she overloaded him or was not sensitive to him, he essentially turned her off or, as interaction II (fig. 2) shows, withdrew from the interaction with her (Als et al., 1979b).

We have been analyzing interactions between mothers and infants and fathers and infants in order to understand the limits of this reciprocal feedback system, and in order to test it as a diagnostic instrument for intervention. For when a mother watches her videotaped interaction with us, we find she can tell *us* when she and the baby are making it and when they are not. By the same token, she can begin to model herself toward the successful reciprocal periods. But, most striking, we have begun to discern the stages of development through which successful pairs proceed in order to achieve a firm reciprocal base for emotional development in the infant and the attachment process in the mother.

The provision of organization which takes place in continuous adaptation to and feedback from the environment potentiates the newborn's increasing differentiation. This differentiation comes from an internalized recognition of his capacity to reach out for and to shut off social stimuli. This same capacity, in turn, results in growing complexity of the interactional channels and structures and provides increasing opportunities for the individual system to become more differentiated. Given such a flexible system, the infant's individuality is continuously fitted to and shaped by that of the adult. Our model is that of a feedback system of increasing expansion and potentiation of the developing organism, a system embedded in and catalyzed by the interaction with his conspecifics (Als, 1979a; Als and Brazelton, 1978; Als et al., 1979c, 1979d).

Table 1

Infant and Mother Coded Behavioral Variables

Mother			Infant		
I	(1)	Vocalizing	I	(1)	Vocalizing
II	(2)	Smiling	II	(2)	Smiling
	(2A)	Laughing		(2A)	Laughing
III	(3)	Intent looking	III	(3)	Intent looking
	(4)	Dull looking		(4)	Dull looking
	(5)	Looking away		(5)	Looking away
				(6)	Eyes closed
IV	(6)	Reach	IV	(7)	Reach
	(7)	Touch		(8)	Touch
	(8)	Holding			
	(9)	Adjusting			
V	(10)	Moving into line of vision	V	(9)	Fussy, squirming
	(11)	Bobbing and nodding		(10)	Body cycling
	(12)	Leaning forward		(11)	Jerky, excited movements
	(13)	Leaning back		(12)	Leaning forward
				(13)	Leaning back
VI	(14)	Facial gestures	VI	(14)	Crying
	(15)	Hand gestures		(15)	Yawn
	(16)	Kiss		(16)	Spit up
	(17)	Wiping face		(17)	Bowel movement
	(18)	Miscellaneous		(18)	Tonguing
				(19)	Miscellaneous

The first item on a newborn's agenda is control over the physiological system, particularly breathing, heart rate, and temperature control. For preterm and at-risk newborns, this control is more difficult to achieve than it is for healthy full-term newborns. While control over these basic physiological demands is being achieved, the newborn begins to establish organization and differentiation of the motor system, affecting the range, smoothness, and complexity of movement. The next major agendum is the attainment of a stable organization of his states of consciousness. With this differentiation, the infant will have available all six states, from deep sleep to intense crying, and transitions between states will be carried out more smoothly. Achieving control over transitions be-

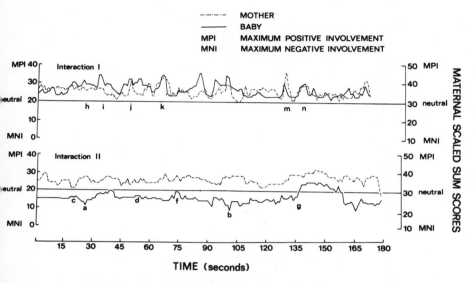

Figure 2. Well-Modulated Synchronous and Poorly Modulated Dissynchronous Interaction

tween states demands an integration of the control over the physiological and motoric systems and the states of consciousness. The adult caretaker can play the role of organizer (Sander, 1977) and can begin to expand certain states, e.g., the quiet, alert state, as well as the duration and quality of sleep states. In addition, the caregiver can help regulate the transitions between states for the infant.

As the state organization becomes differentiated and begins to be regulated, usually in the course of the first month, the next newly emerging expansion is that of the increasing differentiation of the alert state. The infant's social capacities begin to unfold. His ability to communicate becomes increasingly sophisticated. The repertoire of his facial expressions and their use, the range and use of vocalizations, cries, gestures, and postures in interaction with a social partner all begin to expand. On the basis of

well-modulated state organization he can negotiate his new range
and regulation of social interaction skills. Figure 3 is a schematic
presentation of the parent-infant mutual feedback system (Als et
al., 1979d).

Figure 4 shows the more detailed, second-by-second analysis of
the interactions of an infant boy and his mother at 25, 46, 68,

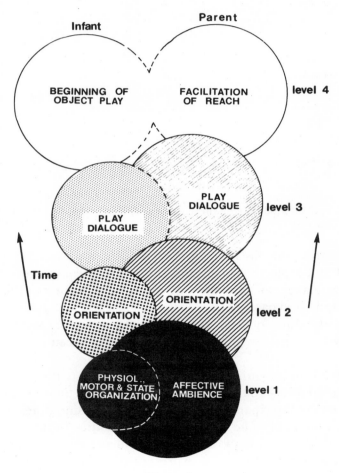

Figure 3

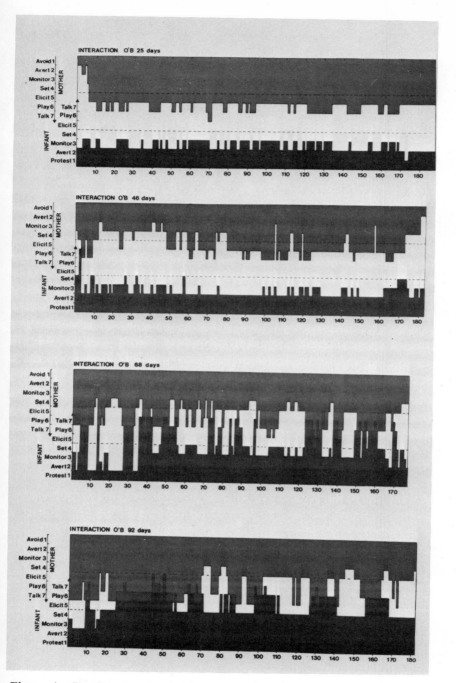

Figure 4. Developmental Changes of Infant-Mother Interaction over the First 3 Months

and 92 days (Als, 1979b; Als et al., 1979c). The infant's behavior is represented on the lower part of each subgraph, the mother's behavior on the top part of each subgraph. The partners' displays are graphed in mirror images of one another, presenting six states of interaction for each participant. The states are scaled to range from displays strongly directed away from the interaction, such as protest, avoid, and avert, through displays mildly directed toward the interaction, such as monitor and set, to displays strongly directed toward the interaction, such as play and talk. The closer the partners' respective positions to one another are on the graph, the more in heightened synchrony they are with one another; the farther away from one another on the graph their respective positions are, the more interactively distant they are from one another. More details of the analysis system and the scoring manual have been described by Als et al. (1979b).

At 25 days, the infant moves mainly from cautious monitoring back to averting, then attempts to monitor again.

By 46 days (about 6 weeks), the infant can repeatedly maintain a quiet, brightly alert, oriented state, labeled "set," toward the mother in this situation, and the newly emerging coo and play phase is beginning to be apparent in the initial sally. The mother's range has also widened by 6 weeks. She moves from intermittent averting, via monitoring, to eliciting and playing. The urgency of continuous prompting and organization exhibited in the tight cycling between eliciting and playing of the earlier interaction is no longer as intense. The infant has become more flexible, and the mother can leave some of the self-modulation up to him.

By 68 days (about 2 months), the infant's organization has become increasingly differentiated, moving initially between protest and play, and then, from 35 seconds on, between the phases monitor, set, play, and talk, until the very end, when he averts again. The repeated cycling through play and talk indicates the full emergence of the new differentiation of his alert state. He is now capable of engaging in interaction with a rich repertoire, integrating smiling and cooing, and he repeatedly achieves an amplitude of affective organization not previously attained. The mother simultaneously expands his peaks, and they achieve a high level of affective interlocking. She spends more time in set than before, indicating her expectant readiness for play and increasing ability to let him take the lead.

By 3 months (about 92 days), this new achievement of differentiation has become more solidified, as is indicated in the prolonged play episodes of the infant and the new baseline at set. The mother's new base is also at set with prolonged cycles through play and talk, indicating her confidence in the infant's self-regulation.

Figure 4 shows that the infant's homeostatic curve has literally moved up by two phases, from averting and monitoring at 25 days, with its peaks at set by 46 days, to its base at set and its peaks at play and talk by 3 months. The wave lengths of the homeostatic curve have also considerably increased, pointing to the smooth reintegration of the recent differentiation of both partners, now ready for new expansion of an increasingly solidifying base. This system thus gives us a way of documenting and quantifying the progress of early infant development within the matrix of social interaction, for the normal infant.

The model for the successful mutual negotiation of reciprocity and emergence of autonomy has previously been described by us (Als and Brazelton, 1978; Als et al., 1979d). First, the parent provides a specific and direct approach to the infant. Early on this may necessitate tactile and auditory and visual inputs of a very specific kind. Once the infant is oriented to the parent, the parent expands the affective and attentional ambience to maintain the infant's state. The infant begins to reciprocate with his ways of interaction. The parent maintains this interaction and gradually builds toward expanding it to include the next achievement, such as, early on, the mere maintenance of alertness, then the achievement of reaching out to sound. Once the new achievement has occurred—for instance, the infant has smiled or cooed—the parent acknowledges the achievement profusely, making time for it to become realized by the infant as an achievement and to become integrated into the current structure of competence. The expansion of current limits thus requires the sensitive gauging of the affective base necessary and the appropriate timing of the next step. It is a process of balancing the lending of support with reaching for the next level. It requires the parents' willingness to risk stressing the system when in balance and dealing with the resultant disorganization. When the limits are exceeded and disorganization results, the parent has to maintain perspective on the process and go back to that layer which currently ensures secure reorganization. Once back on base, the expansion process can begin again. The layers of interaction are thus passed through over and over again.

We think there are four clear stages of development implied in this interactive model (Als and Brazelton, 1978; Als et al., 1979d):

1. The infant achieves homeostatic control over input and output systems; i.e., he can both shut out and reach out for single stimuli, but then achieve control over his *physiological systems and states.*

2. Within this controlled system, he can begin to attend to and use the social cues to *prolong his states of attention* and to accept and incorporate more complex trains of messages.

3. Within such an entrained or mutual reciprocal feedback system, he and the parent begin to press the limits of (a) his capacity to take in and respond to information, and (b) to withdraw to recover in a homeostatic system. The sensitive adult presses him to the limits of both of these and allows him time and opportunity for the *realization of his having incorporated them as part of his own repertoire.* The mother-infant "games" described by Stern (1974) are elegant examples of the real value of this phase as a system for affective and cognitive experience at 3 and 4 months.

4. (This phase is perhaps the real test of attachment.) Within the dyad or triad, the baby is allowed to demonstrate and incorporate a sense of his own autonomy. At the point where the mother or nurturing parent can indeed permit the *baby* to be the *leader or signal-giver,* when the adult can recognize and encourage the baby's independent search for and response to environmental or social cues and games—to initiate them, to reach for and play with objects, etc.—the small infant's own feeling of competence and of voluntary control over his environment is strengthened. This goal of competence harks back to the first stage and completes at a more complex level of awareness the full circle of feedback to self-competence in dealing with inner and outer feedback systems. We see this at 4 to 5 months in normal infants during a feeding— when they stop to look around and process the environment.

When a mother can allow for this and even foster it, she and the infant become aware of his burgeoning autonomy. In psychoanalytic terms, his ego development is well on its way!

In summary, this model of development is a powerful one for understanding the reciprocal bonds that are set up between parent and infant. The feedback model allows for flexibility, disruption, and reorganization. Within its envelope of reciprocal interaction, one can conceive of a rich matrix of different modalities for communication, individualized for each pair and critically dependent on the contribution of each member of the dyad or triad. There is no reason that each system cannot be shaped in different ways by the preferred modalities for interaction of each of its participants, but each *must* be sensitive and ready to adjust to the other member in the envelope. And at each stage of development, the envelope will be different—richer, we would hope.

We regard these observations as evidence for the first stages of emotional and cognitive awareness in the infant and in the nurturing "other." A baby is learning about himself, developing an ego base. The mother and the father who are attached to and intimately involved with this infant are both consciously and unconsciously aware of parallel stages of their own development as nurturers. We, as professionals interested in fostering this early development, must begin to look for and to see these ingredients in the first few months and recognize the power of real reciprocity as we set up an intervention. For we feel that we have been stuck for too long in a nonreciprocal "therapeutic" model of judgments, of criticism, of looking for pathology and ignoring strengths in a mother-father-infant triad. If we can visualize the interaction as flexible and our role as supportive to the envelope, perhaps we can begin to utilize the available energy and the strengths at a time when we can help the dyad or triad right the interaction. Within this model of looking for and having expectation for recovery, we feel we can more often create a self-fulfilling prophecy, or Rosenthal (1966) effect, with mother-infant and father-infant pairs, and we will support them toward a rewarding and internalized system of success.

BIBLIOGRAPHY

ALS, H. (1979), Assessing an Assessment. In: *Organization and Stability of Newborn Behavior,* ed. A. Sameroff [Monograph of the Society for Research in Child Development]. Chicago: Univ. Chicago Press, in press.

———— (1979b), Social Interaction. In: *Social Interaction and Communications in Infancy,* ed. I. C. Ugiris. San Francisco: Jossey-Bass, in press.

———— & BRAZELTON, T. B. (1978), Stages of Early Infant Organization Accomplished in the Interaction with the Caregiver. Read at the meeting of the American Cleft Palate Association, Atlanta, Georgia.

———— LESTER, B. M., & BRAZELTON, T. B. (1979a), Dynamics of the Behavioral Organization of the Premature Infant. In: *Infants Born at Risk,* ed. T. M. Field, A. M. Sostek, S. Goldberg, & H. H. Shuman. New York: Spectrum Publications, in press.

———— TRONICK, E., & BRAZELTON, T. B. (1979b), Analysis of Face-to-Face Interaction in Infant-Adult Dyads. In: *The Study of Social Interaction,* ed. M. E. Lamb, S. J. Suomi, & G. R. Stephenson. Madison: Univ. Wisconsin Press, pp. 33–76.

———— ———— ———— (1979c), Stages of Early Behavioral Organization. In: *Interactions of High-Risk Infants and Children,* ed. T. M. Field. New York: Grune & Stratton, in press.

———— ———— ———— (1979d), Affective Reciprocity and the Development of Autonomy. *J. Amer. Acad. Child Psychiat.,* in press.

BIBRING, G. L., DWYER, T. F., & VALENSTEIN, A. F. (1961), A Study of the Psychological Processes in Pregnancy and of the Earliest Mother-Child Relationship. *This Annual,* 16:9–72.

BOWER, T. G. (1966), The Visual World of Infants. *Sci. American,* 215:80–92.

BOWLBY, J. (1969), *Attachment and Loss,* vol. I. New York: Basic Books.

BRAZELTON, T. B. (1961), Psychophysiological Reactions in the Neonate I. *J. Ped.,* 58:508–513.

———— (1973), *Neonatal Behavioral Assessment Scale* [Clinics in Developmental Medicine, 50]. London: William Heinemann; Philadelphia: J. B. Lippincott.

———— (1976), Assessment of the Infant at Risk. *Clin. Obst. Gyn.,* 16:361–375.

———— KOSLOWSKI, B., & MAIN, M. (1973), Origins of Reciprocity. In: *Origins of Behavior,* ed. M. Lewis & L. Rosenblum. New York: Wiley, 1:49–76.

———— TRONICK, E., ADAMSON, L., ALS, H., & WISE, S. (1975), Early Mother-Infant Reciprocity. In: *Parent-Infant Interaction* [Ciba Foundation Symposium 33]. Amsterdam: Elsevier, pp. 137–154.

———— YOGMAN, M. W., ALS, H., & TRONICK, E. (1979), The Infant As a Focus for Family Reciprocity. In: *Social Network of the Developing Child,* ed. M. Lewis & L. Rosenblum. New York: Wiley, pp. 29–43.

BRUNER, J. S., MAY, A., & KOSLOWSKI, B. (1972), *The Intention to Take*. A film distributed by Media Guild (Solana Beach, Calif.).

CONDON, W. S. & SANDER, L. W. (1974), Neonate Movement Is Synchronized with Adult Speech. *Science*, 183:99–101.

ERIKSON, E. H. (1968), *Identity: Youth and Crisis*. New York: Norton.

GREENACRE, P. (1959), On Focal Symbiosis. In: *Dynamic Psychopathology in Childhood*, ed. L. Jessner & E. Pavenstedt. New York: Grune & Stratton, pp. 243–256.

HARTMANN, H. (1939), *Ego Psychology and the Problem of Adaptation*. New York: Int. Univ. Press, 1958.

McGRAW, M. B. (1945), *The Neuromuscular Maturation of the Human Infant*. New York: Hafner Press.

MELTZOFF, A. N. & MOORE, M. K. (1977), Imitation of Facial and Manual Gestures by Human Neonates. *Science*, 198:75–78.

PIAGET, J. (1936), *The Origins of Intelligence in the Child*. New York: Int. Univ. Press, 1954.

———— (1937), *The Construction of Reality in the Child*. New York: Basic Books, 1954.

ROSENTHAL, R. (1966), *Experimenter Effects in Behavioral Research*. New York: Appleton-Century-Crofts.

SANDER, L. W. (1977), The Regulation of Exchange in the Infant-Caregiver System and Some Aspects of the Context-Contest Relationship. In: *Interaction, Conversation, and the Development of Language*, ed. M. Lewis & L. Rosenblum. New York: Wiley, pp. 133–157.

STERN, D. N. (1974), The Goal and Structure of Mother-Infant Play. *J. Amer. Acad. Child Psychiat.*, 13:402–421.

TRONICK, E., ALS, H., & ADAMSON, L. (1979), Structure of Early Face-to-Face Communicative Interactions. In: *Before Speech*, ed. M. Bullowa. Cambridge: Cambridge Univ. Press, in press.

———— ———— & BRAZELTON, T. B. (1977), The Infant's Capacity to Regulate Mutuality in Face-to-Face Interaction. *J. Communic.*, 27:74–80.

———— & BRAZELTON, T. B. (1979), The Joint Regulation of Infant-Adult Interaction. *J. Cyber. Inform. Proc.*, in press.

WHITE, B. L., CASTLE, P., & HELD, A. (1964), Observations on the Development of Visually Guided Directed Reaching. *Child Develpm.*, 35:349–364.

WHITE, R. W. (1959), Motivation Reconsidered. *Psychol. Rev.*, 66:297–333.

The Role of Hearing in
Early Ego Organization

CHARLES B. TERHUNE, M.D.

MY INTEREST IN THE TOPIC OF THIS PAPER REPRESENTS A SYNTHESIS
of my experience in the practice of pediatrics over many years
and my more recent interest in developmental ego psychology.
What I propose to do might be described as an attempt to excavate
the deepest layer of the tell that represents human ego development. I have long been intrigued with the individuality of infants
only a day or two old, their differing responsiveness to stimuli, and
the rapidity with which bonding takes place between the infant
and his mother. I have also been impressed with the paucity of
material in the literature describing evidence of ego function in
the first 3 months of life. Doubtless, this is because such function,
if it exists at all, is on a very crude, primal level. However, if significant bonding takes place early in life—and some say it does as
early as 2 weeks—is it not possible that this is built on some
archaic form of ego function? Surely, it must indicate in some degree a memory function because there is a consistent, repetitious,
expectant quality in the infantile response to cues given by his
mother and a quality of concern, aversion, and then withdrawal
in his behavior when the expected cues are not forthcoming
(Brazelton et al., 1975). This, then, would suggest that in addition
to memory, there is affect, and in a limited way intentionality and
delay.

The author would like to express sincere appreciation to Dr. Malcolm
Marks for his many helpful and creative suggestions during the preparation
of this paper.

I have also been impressed that sensory deprivation in the newborn may have grave effects upon personality development both immediately and in later life. Much work has been done with infants blind from birth to indicate the difficulties they have in ego development (Burlingham, 1961, 1964, 1965, 1967; Fraiberg, 1968, 1971); and, indeed, infants deaf from birth are frequently suspected of being autistic. It is also relevant that sensory deprivation in adults (particularly in regard to verbal dialogue with other humans) may lead to psychoticlike states. For specific details one may read the writings of Capt. Joshua Slocum (1900), Robert Manry (1966), Charles A. Lindbergh (1953), and others who have taken long solo voyages and experienced delusional or hallucinatory states while out of contact with other humans.

Freud, in his early writings on childhood (1905) and later on anxiety (1916–17), tells the following brief anecdote:

> While I was in the next room, I heard a child who was afraid of the dark call out: 'Do speak to me Auntie, I'm frightened.' 'Why, what good would that do? You can't see me.' To this the child replied: 'If someone speaks, it gets lighter' [p. 407].

I feel that it gets lighter for all of us in many senses of the word when we have someone with whom to converse, and that an elemental form of conversing begins in infants at birth and develops rapidly in intensity and subtlety during the ensuing weeks.

A brief philosophical consideration seems appropriate. The spoken word is transitory in time; the visual image, however, frequently may be recovered, if desired, again and again. Does it then not stand to reason that the infant would capture sounds instantly and attempt to reproduce them as a means of furthering his communication with his mother, and that this ability (to capture the sounds) may be a necessary, innate power possibly more essential than the retention of a visual image?

It is rather remarkable that although the ear is the organ of the sensory modality that is singularly essential for the psychoanalyst in his daily work, to date, little attention has been given in the psychoanalytic literature or in the development of psychoanalytic theory to the ear and hearing. A recently published index of the *Journal of the American Psychoanalytic Association* (1976) has

5 references to the ear and hearing, whereas there are 27 references to the eye and vision. A similar disparity exists in the index of *The Psychoanalytic Study of the Child* (1975), in which there are only 2 references to the ear and hearing and 22 to the eye and vision. A brief review of dictionaries of synonyms, phrases, and quotations reveals that optical references exceed auditory ones in approximately a four to one ratio.

Common phraseology, however, is rich in idioms related to the ear and hearing. We speak of "getting an earful," "lending an ear," "pricking up our ears," "eating till it comes out of our ears," "getting our ears pinned back," "turning a deaf ear," "having an ear to the ground," "putting a bug in someone's ear," "having an ear for music," and "playing by ear"; a "hearing" is a review before an investigating body or an opportunity to be heard; we say that one will "hear from us" to describe a reprimand; or we "hear out" someone if we listen to the end; and, finally, we say "hear! hear!" to show approval or agreement.[1] The importance of the ear and hearing can best be summarized by quoting from Knapp's paper, "The Ear, Listening and Hearing" (1953) (one of the two papers relating to the ear and hearing in the *Journal of the American Psychoanalytic Association*):

> . . . the ear, often an inobtrusive part of our body scheme, plays a definite role in psychic life. . . . Its symbolic role is in turn influenced by its special functions—reception of sound and perception of words. It may serve passively as a funnel through which we are fed important instinctual stimuli, often strongly and deeply repressed, particularly during sleep. *It may function actively as a probe,* a weapon, or a sensitive antenna, with *which we extend the boundaries of the visible world and grasp important data for the formation of ego and superego* [p. 688; my italics].

In this paper I shall attempt to establish the primacy of hearing as an agency of early ego organization at a time when the "boundaries of the visible world" are, at best, poorly defined; thereby I hope to expand in some small measure our understanding of the role hearing plays as a "funnel through which we are fed impor-

1. Isakower (1939) emphasizes the exceptional position of the auditory sphere, though he relates it to the superego.

tant instinctual stimuli." Finally, I shall submit a theory that hearing the mother's voice may indeed be an earlier organizer of the psyche than the smiling response described by Spitz.

Anatomically the ear is a functionally complete structure with a myelinated nerve supply long before birth (Streeter, 1901), and responsiveness to sound has been observed as early as the 31st intrauterine week (Peiper, 1924). Sonntag and Wallace (1935) report a marked increase in fetal movement in response to the noise of a doorbell buzzer; this movement was especially strong and consistent when the buzzer was placed over the fetal head. Similarly, it has long been known that the fetal heart rate increases if sharp, loud noises occur near the mother, and that infants will respond even on the first day of life by being either soothed, alerted, or distressed, depending on the tone, duration, and intensity of ambient sounds. Certain types of stimuli such as low frequency tones and continuous or rhythmic sounds are soothing to the infant, whereas high frequency tones (over 4000 CPS) and loud or sudden sounds are distressing. Thus, as might be expected, tape-recorded heart beats, a metronome and lullabies are soothing, and indeed more soothing than silence. Brody and Axelrad (1970) quote the work of Birns who, "after exciting infants ranging from 36 to 96 hours old, found that the infants could be soothed by auditory stimulation . . . [and] that neonates can differentiate among [high and low] tones of varying intensity" (p. 15). They further quote Fantz who showed that perception occurs in very young infants, demonstrating that the young infant is capable of cortical activity. There is indeed evidence that the maturational crisis that Benjamin places at approximately 1 month of age (see Rubinfine, 1959) coincides with the emergence of cortical activity as evidenced by changes in EEG tracings which occur at that age.[2]

Thus, it is certain that the infant hears, but what he *does* with what he hears is a little less certain, though numerous authors have addressed themselves to this issue. Brazelton (1975) reports, "Even premature babies have a wonderful capacity for choosing a female voice rather than a male's. . . . As soon as he is captured with an auditory stimulus the baby quiets down, has a studied look on his

2. A more comprehensive and detailed description of the neonate's auditory competency can be found in Appleton et al. (1975).

face even when his eyes are closed, and turns towards his mother's voice" (p. 98).

Gesell and Amatruda (1941) state: "It is quite possible that ontogenetically the infant is at first most susceptible to the sound of a voice, particularly to the fundamental laryngeal tones with a vibration frequency of 100 to 400 cycles per second, the vibration frequency of his own vocal cords" (p. 270). Could this be why we coo at babies? Settlage (1964) writes: "Infants a few weeks of age have been observed to respond to the mother's voice with a lessening of tension even though the mother was not in contact with them and in spite of simultaneous exposure to the sounds of other voices" (p. 64), and Barr (1972) states that "by the age of one month, the infant smiles to the sound of his mother's voice and begins vocalization with cooing, gurgling and grunting sounds" (p. 9). Lewis (1971) asserts that "the child can be soothed specifically by the voice of his mother as early as the first few weeks" (p. 15). Culp (1973), Turnure (1967), and Self (1971), using a variety of experimental methods, have demonstrated that an infant as young as 4 weeks of age can discriminate his mother's voice from that of strangers in the absence of visual contact with the mother.

Mills and Melhuish (1974), working with babies 20 to 30 days old, demonstrated that these babies expended a greater effort in sucking (a pacifier) in order to hear the mother's voice. In the experiment, a transducer was placed in the pacifier which, when the baby began to suck, lighted a panel behind a screen where either the mother or an unfamiliar voice would begin to read to the infant. There was a strikingly significant statistical difference in the time spent sucking in response to the maternal voice and that of the stranger. Bell and Ainsworth (1972) report what all mothers know—that by the quality of his vocal productions an infant can elicit a variety of caretaker responses; and that these caretaker responses, including those using the auditory mode, in turn elicit specific behavior from the infant. Brazelton and his co-workers (1975) have shown that the infant responds differently to the voice of the mother and that of a stranger; moreover, they found a remarkable degree of mutual cuing in infants only a few weeks old.

Thus, in addition to being able to hear, it would appear that the infant at approximately 1 month of age is beginning to use the auditory apparatus in part, at least, as a "funnel through which [he is] fed instinctual stimuli." It is my belief that many of these instinctual stimuli are used by the infant as building blocks—foundation stones—in the very earliest development of his ego functions. In order to integrate the above material with our knowledge of developmental ego psychology, I shall briefly review those aspects of developmental ego psychology that are pertinent to my assumption.

Not long after Freud (1923) published *The Ego and the Id,* where he states: "We might add, perhaps, that the ego wears a 'cap of hearing' " (p. 25), Glover (1930) offered the theory that early ego formation amounts to a coalescence of ego nuclei, the latter being formed as a by-product of the infant's interactions with the objects of his instincts. He posits: "In the sense of organized reactive function, *we are entitled to say that a 'real' ego system exists from shortly after birth*" (p. 116; my italics).

Hartmann (1939) considered adaptation as a primary function of the ego and suggested that the ego evolves out of an undifferentiated matrix containing those apparatus which will serve the drives and that these functions exist from the beginning of life (p. 15). He states, "The newborn infant is not wholly a creature of drives; he has inborn apparatuses (perceptual and protective mechanisms) which appropriately perform a part of those functions which, after differentiation of ego and id, we attribute to the ego" (p. 49). Among the ego apparatus present early in life are those underlying the ego functions of perception, intention, object comprehension, thinking, recall phenomena, and others. Hartmann also proposed the term "average expectable environment" to describe the mothering person and her abilities to provide nurture and protection for the infant. Hartmann (1955) further delineates the concept of neutralization of aggressive and libidinal drives which makes instinctual energies available for ego building. Another theory of Hartmann's that has bearing on my thesis is that of the development of object relations. He proposed that a normal infant proceeds from an objectless stage of primary narcissism to a stage in which the object is viewed as need-gratifying, to the stage of object constancy—a line of development also outlined by Anna Freud (1965).

In his many contributions to the theories of early ego formation Spitz (1965) underscored, as does Mahler (1968), the importance of the mother, citing the "circular exchange" between mother and infant as *the* necessary essential for psychological development, and even for physical survival. In this paper, I shall primarily consider the smiling response—the "first organizer of the psyche."

Describing the infant's discovery of the object world and the growing distinction between it and his own physical and mental self, Jacobson (1964) states, "we do not know precisely at what time the psychic apparatus becomes capable of retaining memory traces of pleasure-unpleasure experiences; but there is no doubt that long before the infant becomes aware of the mother as a person and of his own self, engrams are laid down of experiences which reflect his responses to maternal care in the realm of his entire mental and body self" (p. 34f.). It is one of these very engrams that I believe represents an earlier first organizer of the psyche than the smiling response described by Spitz.

I propose that the infant's percept of the mother's voice is the earliest manifestation of ego function, and not the gestalt of the human face. Kris (1956) said, "The earliest memory function arises in the refinding of the needed and later beloved object" (p. 677). Kris does not specify the perceptual modality by which the "beloved object" is "refound." It is my belief that the infant refinds by hearing before he does by vision. I submit this proposal as an expansion of Spitz's theory rather than as a refutation of it because Spitz's concept of nodal points in the development of the psyche seems most valid to me. It is my contention that the infant's response to the mother's voice is such a nodal point. Spitz (1959) states that the smiling response, which occurs approximately in the third month of life in response to the gestalt of the human face, is the first organizer of the psyche. Yet, he quotes John Benjamin (see Rubinfine, 1959) as postulating that:

> . . . by the end of the first four weeks, a measure of organization and integration of muscular behavior has taken place which justifies differentiating this period from the subsequent two months in which an increasing measure of psychological development becomes discernible. The observation is indisputably correct.

> However, one of the essential criteria which . . . defines the in-
> ception of a new stage is missing. . . . That criterion is the spe-
> cific affective behavior, which I consider the indicator of the in-
> ception of each successive stage. Until such an indicator . . . can
> be isolated, I would be inclined to consider this as a subdivision
> of the first stage described by me [Spitz, 1959, p. 15f.].

Personal observation over more than 25 years of pediatric practice suggests to me that infants become aware of their mother's
voice as early as 1 month of age, and that they manifest this awareness of the mother's voice by stopping their cry in anticipation of
her arrival and of a feeding experience. It is my contention that
this quieting of the baby's cry represents just such an affective behavior. Moore and Fine (1968) define affects as "Subjectively experienced feeling states, usually perceived as pleasurable or unpleasurable in relation to the gratification or frustration of instinctual drives" (p. 18). Cannot one then say that the quieting of
the baby's cry in anticipation of the feeding experience is evidence
of a "feeling state" perceived as pleasurable in relation to the
gratification of an instinctual drive?

Although the work of Brazelton, Gesell, Birns, Lipsitt, Fantz,
and others demonstrates that auditory perception is present in the
neonate and to a limited extent has a diacritic property, it does
not suggest that this represents an ego function. However, the infant's ability to perceive the mother's voice above other voices and
to be quieted by it would seem to me to be an early manifestation
of a variety of ego functions. In addition to a more refined form
of diacritic perception, it would also represent a beginning of frustration tolerance, of drive deferment, of awareness of an object,
and of awareness of an "outside" as opposed to a purely coenesthetic self. If one defines ego as that agency of the mental apparatus which acts as a modifier between drive and environment,
this early awareness of the mother's presence and diacritic perception of the mother as a separate individual (i.e., a part of the
environment) would indicate that it is indeed an early manifestation of ego function. This behavior on the part of the very young
infant in response to his mother's voice further suggests that his
mental apparatus has acquired the capacity for anticipation, a

capacity for delay, a capacity for intentional movement (or in this case, cessation of movement—indeed, perhaps an inhibition of movement implying some voluntary control), and a capacity to control the pressure of an unpleasurable stimulus. It also suggests a very beginning of awareness of the mother as a separate object, possibly endowed with object cathexis, and therefore a beginning differentiation of self and object. As Lichtenberg (1975) put it: "The child . . . begins to 'live' a bit less in his own body and a bit [more in] . . . his outer world" (p. 461).

As mentioned above, attention to the mother's voice also represents an awareness of an outside, a beginning of reality testing, a beginning of memory traces, a beginning of secondary process thinking, and a beginning of a capacity for neutralization. It may also represent a separation of conscious and unconscious thinking and, in a limited sense, a beginning of communication between self and object. The capacity for early acoustic discrimination would thus meet the criteria of Hartmann's concept of adaptation as a primary function of the ego, as well as the other ego functions he mentions—perception, intention, object comprehension, thinking, and recall phenomena. Mahler (1968) feels that at about the second month of life the infant becomes dimly aware of a need-gratifying object, and by the third month of life is aware that his needs are gratified by the object. I believe that in the case of an average expectable baby born into the average expectable environment, these events may occur as early as 4 weeks of age and are manifested in the manner noted above. Semantic communication is a skill confined only to humans (and possibly cetaceans). It therefore seems reasonable that the human infant would learn early in life to rely upon this unusual and exclusively human skill in recognizing his mother's voice. Furthermore, semantic communication is the major mode of human interchange throughout life and, as noted, is the mode used almost exclusively in psychoanalysis.

Doubtless, every psychotherapist and analyst has had the experience of dealing with patients who seemed more attuned to the tone and inflection of the therapist's voice than to the verbal content of his interventions. My experience has been that such patients are often low-level borderline personalities, prone to rapid regression and fusion of self-object images, with little capacity for drive delay, intentionality, or anticipation. These people's object relations are largely on a need-gratifying level, and they frequently exhibit a childlike, almost infantile clinging quality in their relationships with the therapist or their peers. One such patient of mine has made a number of statements such as: "I feel 'alone' if your voice doesn't sound the way I want it to" and "I can tell by the tone of your voice that you've 'gone away' from me" (we were both still sitting in the same chairs). On one occasion she telephoned and, when I answered, said, "Thank you, I just wanted to hear your voice and know that you still existed." She then said good-bye and hung up the phone. A colleague who uses a recording device on his telephone has told me of a similar patient who would call his recording device several times a day just to hear his voice. I believe that patients of this type present a regressive or arrested type of behavior dating back to a preverbal developmental level and possibly to a developmental level as early as that outlined above.

SUMMARY

A brief review of the anatomic, physiological, and psychological aspects of the development of the auditory apparatus has been presented and an attempt has been made to integrate these data with certain aspects of developmental ego psychology. An expansion of a portion of existing theory has been submitted. That expansion consists of the concept that the first indication of ego function is the capacity for delay observed in the restless infant upon hearing the sound of his mother's voice, an event observable several weeks before the onset of the smiling response. I would like to suggest that this thesis be further tested by experimental methods such as those worked out by Brazelton and his co-workers. Such studies should use observers trained in ego psychology and psychoanalysis, as Mahler and her associates did at the Master's Children Center, or as Ernst Kris did at the Yale Child Study Center (see Ritvo et al., 1963).

Finally, I hope that by advancing this revision of theory, our skills in preverbal reconstruction may be furthered and our understanding of the role our own voice may play in therapeutic success (or failure!) may be enriched.

BIBLIOGRAPHY

APPLETON, T., CLIFTON, R., & GOLDBERG, S. (1975), The Development of Behavioral Competence in Infancy. *Rev. Child Develpm. Res.,* 4:106–117.

BARR, D. F. (1972), *Auditory Perceptual Disorders.* Springfield, Ill.: Thomas.

BELL, S. & AINSWORTH, M. D. S. (1972), Infant Crying and Maternal Responsiveness. *Child Develpm.,* 43:1171–1190.

BRACKBILL, Y., ADAMS, G., CROWELL, D., & GRAY, M. (1966), Arousal Levels in Neonates and Pre-School Children under Continuous Auditory Stimulation. *Child Psychol.,* 4:178–188.

BRAZELTON, T. B. (1975), Discussion of J. H. Kennell, M. A. Trause, & M. H. Klaus, Evidence for a Sensitive Period in the Human Mother. In: *Parent-Infant Interaction* [Ciba Foundation Symposium 33]. Amsterdam: Elsevier, pp. 95–102.

———— (1977), Personal communication.

———— TRONICK, E., ADAMSON, L., ALS, H., & WISE, S. (1975), Early Mother-Infant Reciprocity. In: *Parent-Infant Interaction* [Ciba Foundation Symposium 33]. Amsterdam: Elsevier, pp. 137–154.

BRODY, S. & AXELRAD, S. (1970), *Anxiety and Ego Formation in Infancy.* New York: Int. Univ. Press.

BURLINGHAM, D. (1961), Some Notes on the Development of the Blind. *This Annual,* 16:121–145.

———— (1964), Hearing and Its Role in the Development of the Blind. *This Annual,* 19:95–112.

———— (1965), Some Problems of Ego Development in Blind Children. *This Annual,* 20:194–208.

———— (1967), Developmental Considerations in the Occupation of the Blind. *This Annual,* 22:187–198.

CULP, P. (1973), Effect of Mother's Voice on Infant Looking Behavior. *Proc. 81st Ann. Convention Amer. Psychol. Assn.,* pp. 55–56.

FRAIBERG, S. (1968), Parallel and Divergent Patterns in Blind and Sighted Infants. *This Annual,* 23:264–300.

———— (1971), Separation Crisis in Two Blind Children. *This Annual,* 26:355–371.

FREUD, A. (1965), Normality and Pathology in Childhood. *W.,* 6.

FREUD, S. (1905), Three Essays on the Theory of Sexuality. *S.E.,* 7:125–243.

———— (1916–17), Introductory Lectures on Psycho-Analysis. *S.E.,* 15 & 16.

———— (1923), The Ego and the Id. *S.E.,* 19:3–66.

GESELL, A. & AMATRUDA, C. (1941), *Developmental Diagnosis.* New York: Hoeber, 2nd ed.

GLOVER, E. (1924), The Significance of the Mouth in Psycho-Analysis. *Brit. J. Med. Psychol.,* 4:134–155.

———— (1930), Grades of Ego-Differentiation. In: *On the Early Development of Mind.* New York: Int. Univ. Press, 1956, pp. 112–122.

Hartmann, H. (1939), *Ego Psychology and the Problem of Adaptation.* New York: Int. Univ. Press, 1958.

———— (1952), The Mutual Influences in the Development of Ego and Id. *This Annual,* 7:9–30.

———— (1955), Notes on the Theory of Sublimation. *This Annual,* 10:9–29.

ISAKOWER, O. (1939), On the Exceptional Position of the Auditory Sphere. *Int. J. Psycho-Anal.,* 20:340–348.

JACOBSON, E. (1964), *The Self and Object World.* New York: Int. Univ. Press.

Journal of the American Psychoanalytic Association: Cumulative Index, vols. 1–22/1953–1974. New York: Int. Univ. Press, 1976.

KNAPP, P. H. (1953), The Ear, Listening and Hearing. *J. Amer. Psychoanal. Assn.,* 1:672–689.

KRIS, E. (1956), The Personal Myth. *J. Amer. Psychoanal. Assn.,* 4:653–681.

LEWIS, M. (1971), *Clinical Aspects of Child Development.* Philadelphia: Lee & Febiger.

———— (1975), Personal communication.

LICHTENBERG, J. (1975), The Development of the Sense of Self. *J. Amer. Psychoanal. Assn.,* 23:453–484.

LINDBERGH, C. A. (1953), *The Spirit of St. Louis.* New York: Scribners.

MAHLER, M. S. (1968), *On Human Symbiosis and the Vicissitudes of Individuation.* New York: Int. Univ. Press.

MANRY, R. (1966), *Tinkerbelle.* New York: Harper & Row.

MILLS, M. & MELHUISH, E. (1974), Recognition of the Mother's Voice in Infancy. *Nature,* 252:123–124.

Moore, B. E. & Fine, B. D. (1968), *A Glossary of Psychoanalytic Terms and Concepts.* New York: Amer. Psychoanal. Assn., 2nd ed.

PEIPER, A. (1924), Beitrag zur Sinnesphysiologie der Frühgeburt. *Jb. Kinderheilk.,* 104:195–201.

The Psychoanalytic Study of the Child: Abstracts and Index to Volumes 1–25. New Haven: Yale Univ. Press, 1975.

RITVO, S., McCOLLUM, A. T., OMWAKE, E., PROVENCE, S. A., & SOLNIT, A. J. (1963), Some Relations of Constitution, Environment, and Personality As Observed in a Longitudinal Study of Child Development. In: *Modern Perspectives in Child Development,* ed. A. J. Solnit & S. A. Provence. New York: Int. Univ. Press, pp. 107–143.

RUBINFINE, D. L. (1959), Report of Panel: Some Theoretical Aspects of Early Psychic Functioning. *J. Amer. Psychoanal. Assn.,* 7:561–576.

SELF, P. (1971), Individual Differences in Auditory and Visual Responsiveness in Infants 8 Days to 6 Weeks. Doctoral Dissertation, University of Kansas.

SETTLAGE, C. F. (1964), In: Nelson's *Textbook of Pediatrics.* Philadelphia: Saunders, 8th ed.

——— (1974), Personal communication.

SLOCUM, J. (1900), *Sailing Alone Around the World.* New York: Century Company.

SONNTAG, L. W. & WALLACE, R. F. (1935), The Response of the Human Fetus to Sound Stimuli. *Child Develpm.,* 6:235–258.

SPITZ, R. A. (1959), *A Genetic Field Theory of Ego Formation.* New York: Int. Univ. Press.

——— (1965), *The First Year of Life.* New York: Int. Univ. Press.

STREETER, G. (1901), On the Development of the Membranous Labyrinth and the Acoustic and Facial Nerves in the Human Embryo. *Amer. J. Anat.,* 1:139–166.

TURNURE, C. (1967), Infant Response to the Mother's Voice As a Function of Age and Voice. Doctoral Dissertation, Yale University.

Developmental Considerations
of Ambivalence

Part 2 of An Exploration of the Relations of Instinctual Drives and the Symbiosis-Separation-Individuation Process

HENRI PARENS, M.D.

LIKE A NUMBER OF PSYCHOANALYTIC TERMS, "AMBIVALENCE" HAS been used with a variety of meanings. Moore and Fine (1968) define ambivalence in its broad sense as describing "the simultaneous existence of opposite feelings, attitudes, and tendencies directed toward another person, thing, or situation" (p. 19). Without assuming that the narrower definition is more valid or gives rise to the broader one, I shall restrict ambivalence to mean that the self experiences coexisting feelings of love and hate (hostility or rage) toward the same libidinal object.[1] Two conditions, therefore, must be met for ambivalence to exist in the psyche. First, it requires the development of a sufficiently intrapsychically structured libidinal object (Spitz, 1965). In my opinion, it does not require that

Director and Principal Investigator, Early Child Development Program and Project, Eastern Pennsylvania Psychiatric Institute and Medical College of Pennsylvania; Faculty and Supervisor in Child Analysis, Philadelphia Psychoanalytic Institute; Associate Clinical Professor of Child Psychiatry, Medical College of Pennsylvania.

1. According to Holder (1975), ambivalence was generally used by Freud in this sense.

the object have attained stable *libidinal* object constancy (which, in the sense of Mahler et al. [1975] and McDevitt [1975], occurs during the third year of life).² From the beginning of the separation-individuation phase (Mahler, 1965; Mahler and Furer, 1968), during the third quarter of the first year of life, the libidinal object is sufficiently structured to be remembered as specific and distinguishable from others. We may assume that the object then begins to be experienced as an object, albeit still as a component of the primitive, symbiotic and narcissistic, self representation (Parens, 1971).

Second, both love and hate feelings emerge out of the self's relation to the object. They probably cannot exist prior to the time when the libidinal object is sufficiently structured, at about 6 months. In the course of longitudinal direct observations, I gained the impression that the earliest precursor of hate is the rage reaction of infancy. I believe that rage is the earliest manifestation of the trend hostile destructiveness, and is its simplest paradigm (Parens, 1979a). In my use of these terms, hate is a later development of hostile destructiveness. Although hate does not exist in the first months or even the first year, there is much evidence that during the latter part of the first year the child experiences *negatively valenced feelings*. I regard these as precursor affects in the spectrum to which hate belongs (see also Greenacre, 1979). Similarly, although object love does not seem to exist prior to about 18 months, the child rather consistently manifests *positively valenced feelings*—affects precursor to object love—in interaction with the libidinal object during the second half of the first year of life.

On the other hand, there is general agreement that by the time of the phallic-oedipal phase—or the first genital phase, as I now prefer to call it (Parens et al., 1976)—ambivalence plays a large

2. The concept *object constancy* continues to be defined variably, Fraiberg's (1969) clarifying efforts notwithstanding. Spitz (1966), Anna Freud (1968), and Erna Furman (1974) believe that object constancy—in contrast to the way Mahler, McDevitt, and others define *libidinal object constancy*— begins during the second half of the first year of life. This view resonates well with my formulations of the child's early ego and drive development, object relatedness, and capability to experience affects during the latter part of the first year of life.

part in psychic life (Freud, 1909, 1913, 1926; Holder, 1975; Mc-Devitt, 1977). For example, Freud made numerous references to the part ambivalence plays in the development of the infantile neurosis. In 1913, he emphasized that the boy's oedipus complex is a "conflict arising out of [his] . . . ambivalent attitude towards his father" (p. 129). So too, in 1926, Freud noted that Little Hans was "in the jealous and hostile Oedipus attitude towards his father, whom nevertheless . . . he dearly loved. Here, then, we have a *conflict due to ambivalence*" (p. 101f.; my italics). I shall use "conflicts of ambivalence" in this sense.

There also exists much evidence supporting the view that ambivalence already makes its appearance during the rapprochement subphase (see also McDevitt, 1977; Mahler et al., 1975) and during the classical anal conflict, both of which tend to begin about the middle of the second year of life. Additional support for this view can be inferred from the assumption that the object is further established as libidinal object during rapprochement, and that true object love—object libido (Parens, 1979b)—and object-directed hate seem to emerge.

Some of our observational data [3] suggest that ambivalence may emerge even earlier than the middle of the second year of life. There appears to be a gray area extending from about 6 months of age, when the normal infant seems to structure a recognitive *representation* of the libidinal object (manifest in convincing evidence that the mother has become the libidinal object), to about 18 months of age when (with rapprochement-subphase developments) we infer strong evidence of object permanence, object libido (true object love), and hate. I shall present some of our findings which may shed light on this gray area of ambivalence.

From a developmental point of view, two factors recommend the proposition that ambivalence evolves through two basic conflicts in early childhood. The two conflicts of ambivalence show (1) significant differences which are determined by their different levels of structural (ego and id) and object-related developments; (2) there is an important difference in the path taken by girls and

3. In our project 15 primary research subjects have been observed with their mothers from birth for 2-hour sessions twice weekly. For further methodological details see Parens (1979a, chap. 4).

boys in the formation of their ambivalent cathexes. The *first conflict of ambivalence,* the coexistence of love and hate feelings toward the libidinal object, progressively emerges during the preoedipal period of development. This conflict has a source and gathers contributions in its course toward the *second conflict of ambivalence,* which arises out of the oedipus complex. (See table 1 for an overview of the development of ambivalence.)

Table 1

Development of Ambivalence (Abraham, 1924)

Phasic Development	Ambivalence in Object Relations
1. Normal autistic	1. Preambivalent, absolute primary narcissism
2. Symbiotic	2. Preambivalent, not so absolute primary narcissism
3. First part separation-individuation phase	3. First conflict of ambivalence; *dyadic*
4. Second part separation-individuation phase	4. Further elaboration of first conflict of ambivalence; ± resolution of dyadic ambivalence
5. Oedipus complex	5. Second conflict of ambivalence; *triadic*
6. Latency	6. Relative postambivalence
7. Adolescence	7. Reactivation and resolution of residual dyadic and triadic conflicts leading to postambivalence

THE FIRST CONFLICT OF AMBIVALENCE

Hypothesis: The *first conflict of ambivalence* occurs in the context of *dyadic* object relatedness. Some of its determinants and precursors may be set down in the psyche during the symbiosis. It seems to originate at the end of the first year during the differentiation-practicing subphases; and it gains large tributary during the rapprochement subphase when it becomes focused, organized, and the preexisting ambivalence may be intensified or ameliorated.

NORMAL AUTISTIC PHASE

During this phase, the immaturity of ego apparatus and functions as well as the primary narcissistic state of the drives and their degree of undifferentiation preclude the existence of love or hate feelings toward an object. At this time experiences of excessive unpleasure can be inferred from the infant's rage reactions which are manifest a few hours after birth. The neonate cannot perceive or (cognitively) assign the source or even the nature of such excessive unpleasure, nor can he cognitively direct the discharge of the rage induced in him. Nonetheless, from some of the manifest reflex behavior we can infer a tendency to discharge unpleasure-induced destructiveness—however primitive in form and function this tendency may be—toward the outside rind of the archaic self, mechanisms which Freud (1914) ascribed to primary narcissism and the pleasure-ego. On the basis that it is possible to condition human infants 4 to 6 weeks old (Scott, 1963), we may assume that at this age the infant has the capability for some primitive form of learning, of memory-trace formation. Similarly, we assume that the undoing of excessive unpleasure by maternal intervention is also recorded in the psyche from soon after birth.

It is of interest that we readily see expressions of unpleasure (rage) from birth, while there are few clear manifestations of pleasure until the emergence of the social smiling response at about the second month of life (Spitz, 1965; Wolff, 1963). We may assume that the pleasure-ego functions at a most archaic level and that it is secured to function by such automatisms (Hartmann, 1939) as physiological ridding mechanisms, innate releasing mechanisms, and by primary narcissism. Although I assume that the infant under 6 weeks has archaic learning capabilities, it would not be warranted to presume more than the most primitive degrees of structural differentiation. Even though conditioning is possible within 30 to 45 days after birth, there is no satisfactory evidence that memory traces of rage experience coalesce into nuclei of hostile destructive impulses attached to a patterned unpleasure experience during these early weeks of life.

NORMAL SYMBIOTIC PHASE

The emergence of the nonspecific social smiling response gives one the impression that the child, at a most primitive level, experiences and becomes aware of an object. During this phase of not so absolute primary narcissism (Mahler and Furer, 1968, p. 10), the symbiotic dyad becomes represented intrapsychically in a manner yet to be formulated. We know from Spitz's (1965) work that one task of the symbiotic phase (3 to about 10 months) is to evolve and attach a libidinal cathexis to a specific person who thereby becomes a libidinal object.

Through observations, one can follow the progressive differentiation of the 3- to 6-month-old child's smiling response. From nonspecificity it evolves into a hierarchy of *specific* smiling responses, elicited most easily and broadly on seeing mother, somewhat less so on seeing father and siblings, and even less to persons seen irregularly. With unfamiliar persons, the child manifests, rather than a smiling response, a more or less intense stranger response. At about 5 to 6 months, many children show evidence not only of recognizing mother, but also of being preferentially and more easily comforted by her, of missing her when she is not present, and of expecting her to undo experiences of excessive unpleasure.

From these behaviors we infer that from about 6 months of age, the child registers pleasure and unpleasure experiences in the context of a somewhat reliably structured primitive libidinal relationship. We assume that small amounts of narcissistic libido and aggression are transiently invested in the mother, who is still experienced as a part of the self. To the extent that the 6-month-old child's recognition of the mother achieves a degree of stability, to that extent we may assume not only that cathectic attachments are beginning to hold, but also that the child is becoming capable of recognitive memory (Fraiberg, 1969) and of elaborating out of engrams, it seems to me, at least some *recognitive form of psychic representation*.

The fact that the mother can become a relatively stable libidinal object permits us to draw some cautious inferences regarding primitive object cathexes and representations. Although Piaget's (1954) formulations of *object permanence* and *evocative memory* have contributed much to our understanding of the child's developing psyche (Bell, 1969; Décarie, 1965; Fraiberg, 1969; Mahler et al., 1975), some colleagues have on occasion taken these formulations to mean that the child is incapable of any form of memory or psychic representation prior to about 16 months of age. My findings concur with those of Spitz, especially on anaclitic depression (1946, 1965), and with the findings of those who assume that some form of object constancy—in contrast to *libidinal* object constancy—begins near the end of the first year of life (A. Freud, 1968; Fraiberg, 1969; E. Furman, 1974), as well as with the considerations of Frank (1969) regarding the setting down in the psyche of what eventually become "unrememberable" and "unforgettable" affective experiences.

The findings of these investigators and direct observations reveal that relatively much development occurs during the second half of the first year of life. The assumption of recognitive psychic representations, paralleling recognitive memory, provides us with a tool that can help clarify the child's experiences and intrapsychic recording prior to the advent of evocative memory and object permanence. I found it helpful in understanding 6-month-old Louise, whose reaction to the temporary loss of her mother illustrates a well-known clinical phenomenon.

Louise. When well-developing Louise S. was just under 6 months old, her mother entered the hospital for gall bladder surgery. Since Louise's birth, Mrs. S. had ably cared for her several children. There was clear evidence of a good attachment between Louise and her mother, with specificity for mother, as well as libidinal attachment to father and siblings.

When Mrs. S. returned home from the hospital 5 days later, Louise "did not recognize" her and pulled away when Mrs. S. reached for Louise. Mrs. S. was shocked and distressed but did not force herself on the child. Two hours later, after a number of refusals, Louise accepted her mother's offer to hold her and now clutched Mrs. S. tightly. For the next 48 hours Louise clung to her mother, showing acute separation anxiety when her mother moved away. Subsequently, Louise experienced increased separation reactions and showed a high alertness to visual and auditory stimuli.

In exploring this often encountered reaction in young children of "not recognizing" the mother or the parents after separations of several days or weeks, we first considered that Louise's attachment to her mother was just lost in mother's absence. But Louise's initial refusals were contradicted by her subsequent clinging to her mother and her acute separation anxiety for the next 48 hours. We concluded, therefore, that her infantile ego actively caused this failure to recognize the newly structured libidinal object. Louise's clinging and separation anxiety just 2 hours after she had not recognized her mother indicated, we felt, that Mrs. S. was indeed a more or less established libidinal object for Louise. Since such libidinal object structuring cannot be assumed to occur in a 2-hour period, Louise's experiencing Mrs. S. as libidinal object, we hypothesized, was the result of an object attachment established prior to Mrs. S.'s going to the hospital. We had, in fact, already recorded the unique importance of Mrs. S. to Louise from their interactions before the separation imposed by the mother's surgery.

Why did Louise not recognize her mother who 2 hours later, and for many months to come, proved more valuable to her than all other objects? I suggest that Louise experienced her mother's absence as painful when she found her mother did not appear as expected to undo the numerous daily experiences of accumulating unpleasure associated with cyclical need constellations (Freud, 1926). I wonder if the pain of missing the specific libidinal object led to a primitive form of repression of the recognitive representation of that object as well as the denial of its libidinal cathexis. Then, when the actual object was seen again, the infantile ego did not immediately register the recognitive memory of the libidinal object because of the work done by that very young ego to protect the child against excessive pain.

With this explanatory inference in mind, I now turn to the question of the beginning of ambivalence: what do repeated, patterned experiences of object-associated gratification (pleasure) and of rage (excessive unpleasure) create in the 6-month-old child's psyche and how do they become represented?

A nursing infant held by his mother, during this period of evolving libidinization of the object, stares at her face, especially her eyes and forehead, for many minutes during each feeding. One gains the impression that while oral gratification takes place, the face of the mother as well as her smell, body tone, and affective ambience are taken into the psyche through receptive sensory apparatus, and over several months become elements of the specific libidinal symbiotic partner (Spitz, 1965). Observation justifies the inference that a positively valenced, narcissistic, libidinal cathexis is attached to that part-object which gratifies well. So too, under conditions of repeated rage experiences associated with mother, this primitive part-object is invested with a negatively valenced, rage-associated, destructive cathexis. In the infantile psyche, the economic aspect of drive activity already prevails, and primitive feelings that are precursors to love (good, positive affective valence) and rage (bad, negative affective valence) exist. Which of the two gains dominance is determined by affective life experience (Kernberg, 1974).

We are, of course, on highly speculative grounds when we attempt to conceptualize the status of the self-object representation at this time in ontogeny. But let me assume that at about 6 months a recognitive form of psychic representation of that self-object begins to hold. Even while that libidinal object is experienced as an object, the boundaries between self and object are not delineated and that between inside and outside is vague.

In describing the pleasure-ego, Freud (1915) postulated that the infant assimilates to the self what is pleasurable, experienced as "good," and ejects from the archaic self to the outside what is painful, experienced as "bad." I find it difficult to assume, however, that at this point in development primitive representations of the self-object are split according to gratification (good) and excessive frustration (bad). While the pleasure-ego operates on the basis of primary narcissism and tends to polarize what is to be retained within and what ejected from the archaic self, certain infantile experiences suggest that other factors operate, quite early, alongside this tendency. For instance, much undoing of pain, which the child experiences as good, is registered as coming from outside the coenesthetically experienced self, i.e., from the partner of the symbiosis. For instance, the primitive but crucial coenesthetic experience that "help comes from the outside" (Mahler, 1952) can readily be inferred, as the infant waits for gratification while the mother prepares to feed. Furthermore, at this age, during the feeding process, the specific libidinal object that cannot coenesthetically be felt as part of self is invested with precursor love feelings. We cannot assume that frustration affects (bad) are always assigned to the outside. More specifically, sufficient recognitive memory probably exists when the libidinal object becomes structured, and it may be more in keeping with direct observations to assume that this object is to some degree recognized as the source of gratification *as well as* frustration.

The question of when and how splitting into good and bad self and object representations originates is pertinent to this problem. Do these early precursors of love and rage cathexes attach themselves to separate nuclei of primitive self-object representations? Following Erikson (1959) we assume that basic trust is an experiential phenomenon that precipitates out of the daily events of the first year of life. During the second and by the third trimester of life, under average conditions, the symbiotic partner seems to be narcissistically and omnipotently expected to gratify.

Observation shows that many infants less than 6 months make loud demands when gratification is delayed, rage often preceding gratification by only seconds. Does a "bad object" representation (or engram) here quickly give way to a "good object" representation? When the infant is in a state of need and begins to expect gratification, we assume that he "hallucinates" a "good" part-object representation. At what point in the course of this need event does he hallucinate a "bad, frustrating" part-object representation? When the 6-month-old experiences pain, does he hallucinate the rage-associated, frustrating part-object or the gratifying part-object?

When Louise did not "recognize" her mother, she seemed to have repressed all recognitive representation of her mother, good and bad. If that object was represented in split form, why did she let slip from her memory the representation of the "good" part-object, which, I believe, she missed so painfully? Because of the painful feeling of loss it induced in the ego? But is that object representation, then, not the "bad" representation?

I cannot answer these questions. At times, it seems to me there are too many obstacles to assuming that object representations in their earliest forms are only split or fragmented (Kernberg, 1966, 1975). Rather, it seems to me that two processes may occur simultaneously, proceeding ontogenetically from opposite poles: (1) parts, functions, particular object-related experiences become invested emotionally, as nuclei of the psychic apparatus (Glover, 1956), or as units of self-object-affect (Kernberg, 1966), which progressively become structured as "whole" organizations and organisms; (2) an overall amorphous, undifferentiated self-object, inside-outside, experienced *en masse,* gradually becomes sorted out, progressively better focused, and organized into its component parts, much as Spitz (1965) suggests for the structuring of the libidinal object.

Although both precursors of love and rage feelings become attached to the evolving libidinal object, are there any conditions in the child's psyche that would make him experience ambivalence? The most likely answer is: no. First, the immaturity of the id and ego limits the 6-month-old's experiences of affects to *precursors* of love and hate. Second, recognitive memory requires the object-related affective experience to be in the present. Generally one affective experience predominates in the present and is the experience that the child will cathect. But at the interface between frustration and gratification, a mix, alternation of, or transition in, affective experience prevails, and I cannot even suggest what may then happen in the infantile psyche. I can only make certain assumptions. It would seem that for ambivalence to be experienced the ego must begin to function at the level of evocative memory of which the 6-month-old is not yet capable. Evocative memory functioning would allow the affective cathexis not activated by the present experience to be perceived (even if only preconsciously or unconsciously) when the polar cathexis is activated. Thus, hate could be consciously felt toward the object, while the ego would at the same time preconsciously or unconsciously experience the object-love cathexis. This, I conclude, the 6-month-old does not achieve. However, although ambivalence per se may not exist during the symbiosis, precursor love and hate feelings *do* become embedded in the psyche by virtue of their connection with the object and the drives and will most likely eventually contribute to ambivalence (see also Greenacre, 1979).

DIFFERENTIATION AND PRACTICING SUBPHASES

From about 5 to 6 months, under average expectable conditions, forces within the child initiate the separation-individuation process (Mahler et al., 1975). This is a critical crossroad in development: when the symbiosis is at its height, a maturational disposition within the child begins the process of separation and individuation.

Dynamics operative in the child quickly become complex. Spitz (1946, 1965) found that in the second 6 months of life the child who has sufficiently invested his mother emotionally will, on actually being separated from her for a protracted period of time, become progressively depressed; and if the mother does not return (or there is no substitute for her) within about 3 months, the *anaclitic depression* which has resulted will become irreversible.

Coleman and Provence (1957) as well as Mahler and Furer (1968) have added a critical finding to that of Spitz, namely, that anaclitic depressions are also found when the mothering person, though physically present, is emotionally unavailable to the child less than 1 year old. While the child may sufficiently invest emotionally in the mother, such a mother, due to her own too constant and too deep depression, chronically impoverished object relatedness, or more serious disturbance, can only poorly invest emotionally in her child.

Vicki. From the time she was about 7 months old we began to note in Vicki a progressively intensifying and pervasive depression (Parens et al., 1974). Her overburdened mother cared for her with irritability, resentment, and at times harshness. During her ninth month Vicki's depression became so severe that we began psychotherapy with her and her mother.

In Vicki, we made an observation that is pertinent to the vicissitudes of hostile destructiveness and libido in object relations, in the context of the child's overall development: we were impressed with the marked absence of typical practicing-subphase explorations and locomotor mastery activities. This led us to infer that the pain of Vicki's depression not only turned the libido (Freud, 1914) but also nondestructive aggression and the ego's efforts at adaptation inwardly, thus preempting practicing-subphase activity (Parens, 1979a, 1979b). This finding and postulate support Spitz's (1946) view that the discharge toward the outside and the expression of aggression, including destructiveness, in these children are obtunded and that the hostile destructiveness mobilized is turned inwardly against the self (Solnit, 1966, 1970). It would seem, then, that the internal representation of the object, which is still amalgamated with the symbiotic self representation—"I-not I" (Mahler et al., 1975; Parens, 1971)—also receives a large component of the hostile destructive cathexis, even though in actuality destructiveness appears to not be discharged against the object.

During the course of psychotherapy, Vicki ably extracted the libidinal supplies she needed (Mahler, 1963). Her seemingly well-regulated, small-dosed motoric and verbal expression of hostility toward her mother was impressive. At present Vicki is almost 8 years old. Her remarkable recovery compels me to conclude that the hostility which turned upon the self to cause Vicki's anaclitic depression was slowly and gradually neutralized as libidinal objects could make up for the libidinal deprivation and hostility (her own and mother's) that Vicki had suffered during the symbiotic phase.

The findings of Spitz and Mahler, showing the infant's reaction to object loss at this age, have been corroborated by a number of clinical observations and studies in humans (Bowlby, 1958, 1960; Provence and Lipton, 1962; Solnit, 1966, 1970) and also in other primates (Goodall, 1971; Harlow et al., 1959, 1960, 1962; Kaufman and Rosenblum, 1967). Again we confront the question: what can we infer from these studies about the status of ego, drives, and object-related developments at this age, and particularly for this study, of object cathexes, object representations, and affective experience. Erna Furman (1974) raises a similar point. Discussing the reactions of a less than 1-year-old to the loss of the mother, she says, "something must happen to the object representation of the mother" (p. 42). Further, in a 1-year-old's search for his deceased brother, she believed that one could observe "the object constancy of the representation of the dead brother" (p. 42). Speaking of the child in the second half of the first year of life, she too finds it necessary to assume some form of intrapsychic representation of the object even before the child has evolved the capability for object permanence. Furman "felt that at this stage the total loss of the love object would be conceived as such, setting the stage for intrapsychic reactions affecting object cathexis and object representations" (p. 42). I have the same impression. Another troublesome but striking finding and inference seemed to add weight to this impression.

Richie. We first saw Richie when he was 1-2-11.[4] He was depressed, hyperalert, his eyes sad and distrustful. At 14½ months, he appeared subdued and younger than 8½-month-old Eddie, one of our normal infants. Richie just sat, barely stretching to reach toys around him, his movements sluggish.

Pictures of Richie at 4 and 5 months show him bright-eyed and smiling widely; his very expressive face and posturings revealed the richness of his very early emotional life. When the photos were taken, he and his parents were living with a middle-aged paternal aunt. When Richie was 6½ months old, his father insisted that they move away from this aunt. Two weeks later the father left. Being alone with the baby, this very young mother could not tolerate his complaining and not eating, and would put him in the hall "to cry out his whining." Richie changed profoundly, seeming to withdraw. His mother reported that when Richie was 10 months old, she had a fight with her husband during which a pot of boiling water fell on Richie's back and burned him. On the basis of assumed battering and incompetence, the mother was not allowed to continue caring for her child. Richie remained in the hospital until 14 months of age when his middle-aged paternal aunt took him into custody. When his mother visited him at the aunt's, Richie avoided contact with her and for days thereafter was upset and difficult to care for. Here are a few details of his ontogeny, as recorded in observation.

At 1-2-25 of age, depression continues, so do affective and motor retardation with notable dampening of sensorimotor exploratory activity. Hyperalertness to objects continues. Occasionally now he smiles, bounces on his knees; several times, seemingly spontaneously, he threw

4. Age expressed in years-months-days.

toys vigorously and was quickly reprimanded by Mrs. V. Despite the sympathetic response of our Project mothers and staff, object relatedness was sharply restricted, except that he turned to Mrs. V. and, depressed, would lean against her.

At 1-3-8, depression still dominating but lifting; he was less morose, smiling more at objects. Motor activity was much expanded; he scurried, crawled across the Infant Area, reached out to several adults. Using a number of toys, he was much more involved in exploring things and objects. He threw toys down vigorously from the toy cart and had to be contained. He seemed to have moved in object relatedness from: "people can't be trusted, they only hurt you," to: "OK, I'll take a chance; I'll try again." He was especially attentive to Mrs. V., engaging her with toys, leaning against her chest, suddenly depressed. Due to nightmares, during this period he wakened during the night, screaming; he could be comforted by his great-aunt in a few minutes.

At 1-8-23 in assessing his accelerating developmental strides, we felt that ego functioning was at a more advanced level and objects were more positively invested emotionally. While there was still more than usual affect fluidity with quick swings from pleasure to depression, his smile now was warmer, less of a grimace. Aggression seemed better controlled; there was no manifest explosiveness. He now folded his hands on his chest to prevent them from grabbing or reaching for things he felt he should not have; he also shook his head "No" at such moments. We felt that the load of hostile destructiveness mobilized and automatized in him was larger than that of our primary research subjects, including those who manifested a large share of hostile destructiveness. He again had nightmares every night. He now smilingly entertained his great-aunt and Mrs. V. by repeating things at which they laughed.

From this time we began to see a striking phenomenon. On this day, at age 1-8-23, he approached 4-month-old Karen, sat by her on the blanket spread on the floor, stayed there several minutes, immobile, head down, low-keyed. He reached for her pacifier on the blanket, toyed with it gently, slowly. The great-aunt, uneasy, distracted him, as did Mrs. I., Karen's mother. After about 3 minutes he devised a game of bringing blocks to his great-aunt, while he glanced low-keyedly at Mrs. I., who was playfully interacting with Karen. He cleared up affectively, and brought a block to Karen, ending up sitting on her blanket. He then brought dolls to his aunt, wanting her to hold them. While we were explaining to the great-aunt that these were proxies standing for him (Parens, 1973; with Pollock and Prall, 1974), he brought to her Karen's rattle which, he conveyed, he wanted her to shake for the doll-proxy. He smiled when she did so. Several times he then climbed into his great-aunt's arms and just lay there looking painfully depressed for several minutes. We inferred, and then could gradually confirm, that seeing Karen and her mother interact warmly may have roused Richie's memories of yearning for such mothering, yearnings dating back to 7 to 14 months when he was in the deepest phase of anaclitic depression.

From 1-8-23 on, we repeatedly saw the following reaction in Richie. While cheerful, playful, or otherwise engaged in some affectively positive activity, he would suddenly stop, become immobile, head down, acutely depressed, and remain so for a few minutes. We found that at these times he would be staring at Mrs. I., when the latter was engaged with Karen in some intimate mother-child interaction such as breast feeding, just holding, comforting, or playing. He then looked as if he were waking from a dissociative state and resumed an activity away from the mother-child scene which he seemed to have so cathected.

One day, inching closer and closer, Richie ended up on Mrs. I.'s lap, and was for a while held by her side by side with Karen. Mrs. I. responded to Richie's yearning state, as did several of the mothers and observers, by wanting to nurture and comfort him. The dissociative staring at the Mrs. I. and Karen dyad evolved into a special, mutual, much-felt interest between Mrs. I., Karen, and Richie.

Summary: In the period of 14 to 20 months of age, we saw Richie move out of his anaclitic depression, showing great improvements in his affective state, drive disposition, and ego functions. In terms of aggression, he moved from massive turning of hostile destructiveness inwardly, to muted explosiveness, discharging rage to the outside onto inanimate objects, and then to significant control of outer-directed explosiveness, by a variety of defenses including inhibition and beginning neutralization. At 20 months, in order to control destructive discharges, Richie began to use mechanisms which our primary research children employed from about 10 to 12 months of age on. With respect to libidinal object relatedness, the shift from "needing but not trusting objects" to "beginning to trust and turn to them again" turned him back from a borderline adaptation (Kernberg, 1966, 1975), or worse, antisocial object-need disavowal (Parens and Saul, 1971), or autistic withdrawal.

Yet, what we can learn about ambivalence, especially its precursors during the period from 6 to 16 months, from traumatized children like Vicki and Richie is very limited. A major obstacle for us is that their symptomatic depression masked or did not allow unequivocal evidence of affectionate reactions to the symbiotic partner; nor did we then see object-directed rage reactions in Vicki. However, our observations support two relevant hypotheses: (1) Memories of experience from the second 6 months of life are stored in the psyche and may be recovered. As has long been hypothesized in psychoanalysis, these may leave an enduring imprint on that psyche, self, and object relatedness (see Freud's [1940] note on the indelibility of the earliest cathexes). The infantile ego will actively attempt to master the marked ache that such traumatic cathexes continue to inflict on the self (as was true in Richie's case). (2) Profoundly negative affective states, on the spectrum of rage and hate, deriving from and attached to object relatedness, are set down in the psyche during this developmental period and can in due time have their impact on ambivalence.

The child in an "average expectable environment" does not undergo traumatizations of the sort experienced by Vicki and Richie. From the fortunate child we learned something quite different about the emergence of ambivalence during the first part of the separation-individuation phase. Especially during the practicing subphase, some of our well-endowed and well-developing children were thrust into rage reactions toward their beloved mothers. The emerging conflict between self and mother, its character, sharpness, and intrapsychic reverberations, raised the question whether ambivalence could be inferred in the 10- to 16-month-old child. In addition, we were compelled to ask whether this observable behavior is a manifestation of a special conflict of ambivalence, which emerges especially during the practicing subphase.

PRACTICING-SUBPHASE CONFLICT

Some of our children showed a large upsurge in the aggressive drive accompanied by sharply mounting strivings for autonomy—assertiveness, efforts to do things oneself or control (at times omnipotently) and master the self and the environment (Parens, 1979a, 1979b). At times of pleasure these strivings give the impression so aptly described by Greenacre's (1957) "love affair with the world" and by Mahler's concept of "elated practicing." In my view, these strivings for autonomy (Erikson, 1959) serve both differentiation and practicing, which, in accord with Mahler's theory, are evidence of the child's thrust to become psychologically an individual. *Differentiation* is that aspect of the separation-individuation process which is manifested in the behavior of the less than 1-year-old who is physically close to mother and pushing away from her against mother's greater or lesser resistance. *Practicing* reflects the child's exercising of newly emerging sensori-motor capabilities and skills and his primordial efforts to master himself and his rapidly expanding universe.

When difficulties arise in the child's earliest efforts at differentiation—as a result of carrying over a prior troubled symbiosis or of mother's strong opposition to her child's first attempts to individuate—negatively valenced feelings toward her will be manifest in behavior. In our quite healthy children, we found that a struggle with mother arises especially out of their practicing activities. When these strivings for autonomy are thwarted by environmental resistance, the children experience mounting unpleasure and, when that resistance is protracted, they often show evidence of a large upsurge of hostile destructiveness. Since the mother, in the service of protecting the toddler or breakable things, is the most frequent obstacle to the gratification of these autonomy strivings, the destructiveness mobilized in the child is naturally directed toward her. The commonly found *interpersonal* conflict which now results takes on the character of a battle of wills between child and mother. When the pressure of aggression is especially sharp, it may create an acutely difficult situation for the self and the object, as Mary and Jane illustrate.

Mary.[5] When Mary W. was 1-0-13 of age, we saw the mounting pressure of Mary's strivings for autonomy lead her mother to repeated prohibitions and limit-setting because Mrs. W. felt that Mary's behavior presented some hazard, was inconvenient, or unsocial. Mrs. W. did not want Mary to go into the hall, or reach for cups of coffee or ashtrays or other children's toys, and she often was brought to her feet to contain her daughter who, at this time, seemed pressured from within and propelled exactly in the direction of these forbidden objects.

5. Some of the material on Mary and Jane is presented in film (Parens and Pollock, 1977).

Mary reacted to her mother's restrictions with mounting hostile feelings toward her. She complained angrily, her face flushed, muscles tense; shaking and yelling, she eventually reacted with rage. We saw Mary visibly work to control the actual discharge of hostile destructiveness toward her mother. We saw evidence of the development of defenses and the beginnings of a sharp conflict between Mary and her mother.

At age 1-1-3, Mary's hitherto moderate objections, verbal complaints and inhibited motor discharge of hostility gave way to the actual discharge of destructiveness toward mother. When Mrs. W. brought Mary back from the hall, the first few times Mary smiled and permitted herself to be passively returned to the Infant Area. But then progressively she complained more vigorously, vocally, bodily contorting to extricate herself, and eventually she cried angrily, waved her left arm in a striking movement against her mother several times and kicked her, at first from a distance but twice actually struck her mother with her arm. Once she also struck herself.

As a result of this encounter, Mary showed evidence of intrapsychic distress; and for the first time while crying, she could not be comforted by the good efforts of her mother. The following observation was recorded: Mary is crying angrily in mother's arms, she seems to want to get out of those arms; mother puts her down gently, without observable rejection, and Mary cries even more loudly and angrily. Mother cannot hold her and cannot put her down. Mother picks Mary up and holds her while sitting in a chair, and Mary calms some. As she sits on mother's lap, she does not mold into her mother's body, which she has always done easily, but rather sits upright, separated from mother's torso. Mrs. W., wanting to comfort her more actively, reaches to touch Mary's arm; Mary pushes her hand away, in unequivocal rejection. A moment later this is repeated. Mary's affect is sober and serious.

I interrupt the narrative to draw attention to the inferences we drew from these data. We assumed that the conflict between child and mother, an *interpersonal* conflict, led to the emergence of an *intrapsychic* conflict in the child. When Mary's strivings for autonomy were thwarted by her mother, she experienced progressively mounting hostile feelings toward her frustrating mother. This state of unpleasure, however, led the child to need comforting from the gratifying good mother, and Mary, crying and angry, turned for comforting to this same mother toward whom her hostile feelings were directed. The infantile ego is now presented with antagonistic feelings toward the love object: when Mary was angry

with her mother, we inferred that she invested the infantile representation of her mother with hostile destructiveness; and while she
wanted to be comforted, she experienced her as the good mother;
in addition, she gave evidence of attempts to protect her mother
against this hostile destructive discharge (cathexis) by its inhibition. The dominance of good and hostile feelings toward the
mother seemed to alternate and led to a transient immobilization
of the ego.

Now, Mary sat on mother's lap, and as mother tried to comfort her,
Mary remained tense and did not permit mother to put her down.
She gradually poised herself on her mother's lap, sitting on it but separated from mother's torso. She rejected her mother's comforting hand
twice, and mother stopped actively trying to comfort her. After 30–60
seconds so poised, Mrs. W. got up carrying her daughter, hoping to
distract her by engaging her interest in a toy. But as Mrs. W. bent
down, Mary suddenly began to cry as if she had been struck a blow!
When mother returned to her chair, Mary calmed quickly and continued to sit upright on her mother's lap. Gradually, her body tone
softened and she relaxed passively into her mother's body, thumb in
mouth, where she remained, awake, for 20 to 30 minutes.

This segment of behavior seemed to indicate that sharp feelings
of anger toward the beloved mother caused Mary's immobility. I
wondered if the budding ego was paralyzed in its very early efforts
to integrate precursor love and hostile feelings toward the object,
in its work of splitting and integrating the good and bad component representations of the libidinal object. Gradually, assisted
by the mother's good efforts, the cathexis of the good mother
representation seemed to gain the upper hand and Mary accepted
the comforting offered to her.

That demands on the ego were made by an *intrapsychic* crisis
seemed supported by Mrs. W.'s report, which we confirmed, that
this same evening, 13-month-old Mary began to communicate with
her mother vocally, using preverbal inflection and rhythms that
sounded like words. It was a distinct new step toward verbal communication. The significance of this newly acquired ego skill is
aptly reflected in Freud's insight (1893) that the first man who
threw an invective at his enemy instead of a spear was the founder
of civilization. We hypothesized that the new skill arose out of the

demands made this day on the ego by the child's hostile destructive feelings toward her libidinal object, an object already highly invested with precursor love feelings. In this, of course, I am only illustrating one detail of Ernst Kris's concept that to a degree "frustration promotes development" (Solnit, 1978), that the "favorable development of . . . ego functions is closely related not to the absence but to an optimal distance from conflict" (Kris, 1950, p. 28), a derivative of Hartmann et al.'s view (1946) that development occurs in the context of an optimal gradient of gratification and frustration.

Three days later, at age 1-1-6, the struggle between Mary and her mother continued at the same intensity, but Mary was more quickly responsive to mother's prohibition, giving evidence of anticipating it. She went a step further in dealing with mother's verbal "no" by complaining in vocal argumentative tones, all the while complying with mother's dictate without requiring physical assistance.

Visit after visit, this struggle was evident. About one month after its onset, the conflict in Mary slowly began to resolve, waxing and waning as it did so. At age 1-2-25, the conflict again peaked; frustration mounted to a point where she stopped accepting mother's limits and began to give in to the anger mother's prohibitions aroused. At first she expressed her anger by vocal sounds that had the quality of cursing and scolding. One observer thought she said, "Damn." At one point Mary hit out toward her mother in the air, as she walked away from her.

In the next 2 weeks further resolution of this crisis was apparent. About 2 months after its onset, Mary conveyed the wish that mother relent in her prohibition against Mary's going down the hall to the Toddler Area. Another week later, Mary's 12-year-old brother who was visiting took her to the Toddler Area for snacks. One month later she went there with her mother's permission.

Jane. At age 0-10-3, Jane's reaction to her mother's prohibition of some of her exploratory activity heralded and forewarned the onset of a struggle for control. At age 0-10-17, Jane and mother were at an impasse. Jane wanted to go out the double door, which Mrs. K. prohibited. Jane went to the door about 15 times, challenging mother's dictate not to go out. The first 3 times mother pulled her back, and Jane had a tantrum. Mrs. K. was an experienced and talented mother who seemed to have a good grasp of the difficult situation that confronted her.

Gradually, Jane's reaction to mother's repeated prohibition on that day became less and less angry as she seemed to be coping, dose by dose, with the repeated frustration of her wish. In the Project, this impasse remained at the forefront of Jane's relation to her mother for 6 weeks.

The harshness of this protracted experience led to dramatic adaptive attempts on Jane's part. At 0-10-20, Jane again wanted to go out the double door. When her mother fetched her, Jane became angry, but the tone of that anger was not as harsh as it had been 3 days earlier. On this day, Jane came upon turning the 5th or 6th conflictual inter-action into a playful situation. From that point on, she progressively mastered this nagging, recurrent striving to do as she wished. At age 0-11-1, Jane made some 20 attempts to go out the double door. The pressure of drive derivatives that called for gratification was evident not only in the repeated appearance of this behavior during each visit, but also in the efforts made by the ego to adapt to the push of her wish which came into conflict with the love object. From her behavior we inferred efforts that included the defenses of making-a-game of the conflict, inhibition, splitting the representations of mother, and the internalization of limit-setting dictates of the love object, which repre-sents the earliest developments of superego precursors (Parens, 1979a).

At age 0-11-18 Jane continued to show evidence of this conflict with mother and her efforts to cope with it. After I month's vacation, when she returned to the Project, Jane just went out through that door. It would not satisfy us simply to assume that mother no longer pro-hibited Jane's going out. Nor did Jane's self-assertiveness or her striv-ings for autonomy and separateness lessen. The struggle seemed to have evaporated like one of Winnicott's (1953) transitional phenomena.

An Intrapsychic Conflict Due to Ambivalence

Observations in the practicing subphase compel us to assume that the pressure of emerging strivings for autonomy, when exces-sively frustrated, often leads to the emergence of hostile destruc-tiveness toward the libidinal object. If the child encounters environmental opposition, he has a notable automatic response: the pressure from within often seems to propel the child in exactly the direction prohibited by mother. There the child usually en-counters persisting opposition from mother, which in turn en-genders further hostile feelings toward her.

Again and again, our observations of these 10- to 14-month-old toddlers led to the inference that such encounters between child and mother created an *intrapsychic conflict* within the child. That an interpersonal conflict can create the conditions for the development of an intrapsychic conflict is due, I believe, to the child's *valuation of the object* (libidinal object cathexis). "It is by these unavoidable unpleasure experiences that, attaching to the powerfully positive cathexis of that symbiotic partner, *the libidinal object also becomes the first object qua object of the infant's destructive impulses*" (Parens, 1979a).

The specific question I am attempting to study is: does the fact that the libidinal object becomes the object of the child's hostile destructiveness create a conflict of ambivalence in his psyche? We do not have tools to help us reach assured conclusions, but we proceed cautiously by examining the issue from two complementary positions: (1) from our clinical experience in assessing children's behaviors and inferring the underlying dynamics (see Anna Freud, 1966, especially pp. 14–15, 21); and (2) by assessing, as best we can, the developmental status of self-object relatedness, cathectic stability and representation, affects, and the ego's memory function.

1. What do Mary's transient immobility on mother's lap and subsequent more differentiated skill in vocal communication, or Jane's making a game of the struggle with mother look and feel like to the observing, empathic, analyst? Having known these children from birth and having observed them twice weekly for 2-hour periods, I have the impression that these children were coping with feelings of rage toward their beloved mother. I do not believe that their behavior indicated either fear of the object's anger or fear of loss of mother's love. To me, it seemed to be mostly fear of destroying the most valued of all libidinal objects. Over a period of 8 years of observing these children and their mothers, we have, like other child analytic observers, on numerous occasions felt frustrated by the preverbal child's inability to tell us what he or she is experiencing and have had to rely on our clinical judgment.

2. In order to try to answer the question: is fear of destroying the most valued libidinal object synonymous with ambivalence? I find it useful to look at these data from the second position. With regard to the developmental status of self-object relatedness, the object is still experienced as a part of the self, as the symbiotic

partner. But it is neither just a part-object nor only a need-fulfilling object. The mother is now warmly smiled at even when the child is not in a state of need; an adventitious meeting of eyes with mother will often bring a warm smile to the child's face. Furthermore, mother's status as libidinal object is significantly more stable and established than it had been several months earlier at the height of the normal symbiotic phase. That is, the libidinal and aggressive cathexis invested in the object, as inferred from the child's motoric and affective interactions with mother, expectation of mother's availability and nurturance, seems much more cemented and steadfast than it was 3 to 6 months earlier. One also gains the impression from these affective and motoric interactions that although the mother and self are not yet diacritically experienced as separate, a number of factors begin to delineate the self as different from "other than self." The progressively more strongly libidinized sensorimotor organization of the self, the enriching discovery of so many new things during the child's explorations which are coenesthetically felt (transiently cathected) as other than self, and the growing awareness of distancing from mother, especially registered at moments of "emotional refueling" (Mahler)—all these lead me to assume that the self-object representation probably is more and more experienced coenesthetically and diacritically as consisting of two psychic organizations that are becoming more and more cohesive and organized into self and object. During the rapprochement subphase, which follows this developmental period, the child will turn her or his attention especially to the then strongly experienced awareness of being separate from mother.

With regard to the status of affects, occasionally one can observe in the emotional expressions of the child a quality of love attachment to mother which comes near to being affection, love. Such a moment is illustrated in Jane's bringing her cheek to mother's in a moment of tenderness between them. Similarly, in Mary's struggle with her mother, we saw moments of rage that came near to an expression of hostility or hate. Since such moments may be brief and not stably manifest, I would still catalogue these affects as precursors of object love and hate. They are, nonetheless, much closer to love and hate than the positively and negatively valenced affects expressed 3 to 6 months earlier.

With regard to the developmental status of the ego's memory function, here too the child has advanced from the beginnings of recognitive memory functioning. *Recognitive memory* is the capability of the infantile ego to recognize an object previously seen. It implies some memory trace and cathexis of that object, though these are unstable, are not experienced in the object's absence, but can be reactivated when the object is again visualized. The object, thus, is not seen *de novo*. *Evocative memory,* on the other hand, is the capability to remember the representation of an object when the object is no longer in the child's field of vision. When that is achieved, Piaget taught us, the child is capable of *object permanence.*

Piaget's (1954) proposition that person permanence occurs prior to object permanence is especially pertinent. When as psychoanalysts we employ the term object permanence, it is not always clear whether we are using the word "object" to mean thing or person, a point discussed by W. G. Cobliner (in Spitz, 1965). Those of us who use the term object permanence assume that it emerges between 14 to 18 months, according to Piaget's findings. Bell (1969) tested Piaget's hypothesis and confirmed it, but introduced an important qualification. Piaget proposed that person permanence occurs earlier than object permanence "because persons stimulate many of the baby's schemata simultaneously and thus foster the process of assimilation." Bell found, however, and underscored that "a baby will be able to develop the concept of the permanence of persons earlier than that of things only when a certain harmonious interaction with his mother prevails." Bell "places greater emphasis on the notion that the development of person-permanence is sensitive to the quality of the interpersonal stimulation" (p. 52). I think most analysts would support Bell's position.

The evolving of recognitive memory into evocative memory is pertinent to this study of ambivalence. The development of memory, like that of all other adaptive functions of the ego, is progressive, so that the ratio between recognitive memory and evocative memory functioning shifts. In other words, during its development, evocative memory and the capacity for person permanence and object permanence do not operate on an all-or-none basis. Memory will at times function at a more advanced level (evocative) or at a less advanced level (recognitive), a phenomenon well known to child analysts. Testing 33 middle-class children, Bell found not only that person permanence is a progressive development, but also that evidence of person permanence occurred in 43% of these subjects at *11 months* of age. At this age, early elements of person permanence were also present in about 70% of all her subjects (p. 57). Bell's study supports the possibility that at about 11 months affective object-related experiences may have achieved sufficiently stable cathexis and sufficiently stable intrapsychic representation to be remembered in the absence of their activation in the present.

The clinical impression that the child fears destroying his most valued libidinal object is further strengthened by the finding that the beginnings of superego precursors and of the ego's neutralization function emerge during the last quarter of the first year of life (Parens, 1979a; Spitz, 1965). Both of these emerge in the context of the child's encountering the mother's prohibitions, to which the child tends to react with much unpleasure and hostile destructiveness.

Although some uncertainty remains, especially from the side of the insufficient maturation of affects and the instability of evocative memory vis-à-vis person permanence, it seems to me that the child's ego first registers the condition of ambivalence in a conflict between his hostile destructiveness to and his strong libidinal cathexis of the mother. The young ego, rendered anxious by the attitude of the self and the object, sets itself the great task of mediating between the drives and reality, begins to internalize dictates from the libidinal object, and begins to neutralize destructiveness toward it.

RAPPROCHEMENT SUBPHASE

In the course of healthy development during this subphase ambivalence to the beloved symbiotic partner inevitably is further elaborated, as we know from two sources: (1) the observations made in our Early Child Development Project; (2) from the work of Mahler and her co-workers (1968, 1972, 1975) we know that the rapprochement crisis—an intrapsychic crisis engendered by ambitendent wishes to remain fused with the symbiotic partner versus to separate and individuate—unavoidably leads to coexisting conflicting feelings of love and hate toward the same love object.

Since at this time of life we have much evidence from which we can infer object love and hate toward the libidinal object, we can more assuredly say that the child experiences ambivalence during the rapprochement subphase (see also McDevitt, 1977). Two factors play a special part in the mobilization of hostile destructive feelings in the child: (1) the continuation, at a more advanced developmental level, of the differentiation and practicing-subphase conflict of autonomy; and (2) the rapprochement crisis itself. Both factors further elaborate and enlarge or, in fact, may lessen whatever ambivalence has already been activated.

During the rapprochement subphase, strivings for autonomy tend to lessen to some degree. They are robbed of the elation they induced during the practicing subphase by several factors: (1) the lessening of the excitement and heightened narcissism associated with the upsurge of aggression and the developmental spurt of the sensorimotor organization of the ego; (2) the greater ego development leads to better cognition, reality perception, and lessening of omnipotence; and (3) the newly aroused libidinal need for the object's love induced by maturation and development of both ego and libido (Parens, 1979b). Whatever its antecedents, however, the rapprochement task creates its own large component of ambivalence in the child.

Candy. During the symbiotic and the first part of her separation-individuation phases, Candy's relationship with her mother was warm, close, and notably free of stress and strain. Her development progressed gratifyingly. Rapprochement followed the lines drawn by Mahler (1965, 1968) with renewed closeness to and constant sharing of current interests and activities with mother. Then we saw evidence of a sharply delineated rapprochement crisis.

When she was 1-7-21, Candy stayed close to her mother, busily playing near her from the beginning of the session. Several children took off their shoes and went to the matted playroom. Candy, too, took off her shoes, excitedly getting ready to join the others. However, once her shoes were off, she sobered and went back to the sofa, onto mother's lap. After 5 seconds on mother's lap, Candy began to cry and

twisted her body away from mother as though she were suddenly experiencing acute pain. Mrs. G. reacted sensitively by letting her daughter get down. Candy dropped to the floor, crying, twisting, kicking her
legs in a mild temper tantrum, an unusual reaction for her. Surprised,
Mrs. G. tried to comfort Candy by talking and touching; and finally,
by mutual accord, picked her up. But once in mother's arms, Candy
again started to cry and twisted herself away. Again mother complied
and let Candy down. Three times mother and daughter reenacted this
same sequence, Candy's ambitendent behavior winding down with the
6th "hold me close!" communication. Candy's pain and distress, arising
out of her conflicting wishes, were strikingly mirrored in the mother's
feelings.

Four days later aggressive discharges poured out of Candy. At one
point, Candy again became irritable, cried, twisted herself in and out
of her mother's arms. The sum of her current behavior suggested that
hostile destructiveness was aroused by and directed toward her mother.

At 1-7-28 Candy stayed close to her mother, on "their sofa," the entire session. With much pleasure, she engaged first her mother, then
one of the observers, in a game of throwing a doll off the sofa. We inferred from this activity that Candy was ridding herself of and aggressively separating from the object. During this enacted separation, her
face and actions seemed harsh. But when she brought the doll close to
herself, taking possession of and caring for her, she appeared gentle and
well satisfied. (At other times, separation was pleasurable and being
close caused distress.) Her discharge of hostile destructiveness was at-
tenuated by the defense of making-a-game of it and was discharged
with pleasurable affect, the anger being dissimulated.

During the next 2 weeks the sharpening of the rapprochement crisis
mobilized much hostile feelings in Candy. At that time the mother began to leave her children with a caretaker on Fridays for several hours.
Upon her return Candy greeted her unsmilingly and occasionally struck
her. Peers now often became the target of her blows, due largely to
the displacement of destructiveness from the object of rapprochement.
Three weeks later, Candy took a further step toward working through
her current developmental dilemma when she selectively engaged one
of the observers pleasantly while her mother stood by readily available
to her.

At 1-9-13, the radius of Candy's movement away from her mother
widened significantly. For the first time since 1-7-21 she went into the
hall leading from the Infant Area to the Toddler Area without her
mother, separating for a distance of about 20 feet. She used other people well, asking one adult to pick her up when she became anxious

about separation and to bring her back to the Infant Area. She took a pull toy she had recently invested emotionally, separated from her mother, warded off Mary's efforts to take the pull toy from her, went to a table behind "her sofa," took the pull toy apart, and made its parts disappear into the drawer of that table. She opened and closed that drawer, pushing the pieces out of sight when they became visible—all creating the impression that she was working through the separation from the emotionally invested toy. After a 10-minute separation from mother, Candy returned to her and both enjoyed the reunion.

A distinct quieting of hostile destructiveness toward her mother occurred with the quieting of Candy's rapprochement crisis, the relation between child and mother remaining predominantly affectionate and quite easygoing. But, as we soon found, this was only the calm before the rough seas of her castration and oedipus complexes, which soon began to emerge.

As we saw in Candy, the ambitendent wishes in the child lead to a state of helplessness of the ego, which creates an intrapsychic crisis, as McDevitt, Bergman, and Mahler have reported. Where sufficient anxiety mounts, by virtue of its unpleasure experience, further hostile destructiveness is mobilized and directed toward the self and the love object. Observation reveals that the libidinal object (as auxiliary ego), by her reactions, plays a significant collaborative part in allaying or intensifying rapprochement-derived anxiety in the child, thereby reducing or increasing the mobilization of hate feelings and the experience of ambivalence. Another important factor is the pattern of the rapprochement crisis in a particular child, that is, the quality, intensity, and frequency of intrapsychic tension created by the ambitendent wishes. In children like Candy, one large, protracted rapprochement crisis, if we may think of it that way, creates a state of continued heightened tension, as a result of which mobilization of anxiety, hate, and ambivalence is sustained. A more gradual working through of the rapprochement task is less likely to produce periods of equally intense anxiety, hate, and ambivalence.

THE SECOND CONFLICT OF AMBIVALENCE

Hypothesis: The second conflict of ambivalence occurs in the context of first genital(phallic)-phase triadic object relatedness. It both arises within the classical oedipus complex and gives rise to its core conflict. It is largely determined by the then-current status of ambivalence in dyadic object relations and may in turn retrogressively reactivate and/or intensify dyadic object-related ambivalence.

The marked hostile destructiveness toward the rival love object, characteristic of this developmental period, reflects both an upsurge of aggression and a further gender-related distinction between boys and girls. After several months of increasingly more troublesome interactions between Jane and her mother, a relationship that until then had been significantly positive and affectionate, Jane's experienced mother complained that her daughter (2 ½ years) was becoming very difficult to handle. One morning Jane's mother asked with a half-smile: "Anyone want her for a year?" We had observed the upsurge of hostile, rivalrous behavior toward her mother and had already recorded (3 months earlier) that Jane was beginning to experience her oedipus complex.

Observations of mother-child dyads made us strongly aware of the fact that normal girls like Jane, Mary, and Candy experience their practicing subphase conflict and rapprochement crises with their mothers, and due to their oedipus complex experience a further intense conflict of ambivalence, again with their mothers. The normal boy, on the other hand, who also experiences his practicing-subphase conflict and rapprochement crises with his mother, experiences his basic oedipal conflict of ambivalence with his father, not his mother. The thesis of a "first conflict of ambivalence," which develops in dyadic object relatedness during the preoedipal period of life, and a "second conflict of ambivalence," which emerges in triadic object relatedness during the first part of the oedipus complex, highlights the fact that girls have both of these conflicts with their mothers, while boys have the first with their mothers and the second with their fathers. While the resulting ambivalence varies widely—depending on the qualities of intrapsychic developments and pressures as well as object relations—many a girl's ambivalence toward other females tends to be more intense than her ambivalence toward males. In the boy, ambivalence toward male and female tends to be distributed between them. I should emphasize, however, that ambivalence is not predetermined; rather, it is the result of experience, being determined by the vicissitudes of instinctual drives and ego functioning in the child in reciprocal interaction with his objects. In other words, the schema of conflicts of ambivalence proposed here and the resultant distribution of ambivalence in object relations suggested by it is a simplification. Nonetheless, it is often encountered clinically even when it is embedded in a maze of dynamic complexity.

In attempting to delineate these two conflicts of ambivalence, I have noted that the second conflict is far more complex than the first. Upon entering the phase of the oedipus complex, the little girl loves and hates her mother, who is now more or less acutely experienced as the rival for the father. The complement is experienced by the 3-year-old boy. The heterosexual oedipal relation in each child is highly invested with a powerful cathectic valence. Further developments in the ego also add significantly to the greater complexity of the oedipal conflict of ambivalence. They do so especially through the production of intense feelings of guilt vis-à-vis the hated love object and the structuring of the superego (Freud, 1923).

While the findings from our Project and from clinical analyses show these triadic dynamics of ambivalence, a further complication sets in during the latter part of the oedipal phase. Both the girl and the boy repeatedly have the experience that the heterosexual oedipal love object does not gratify oedipal wishes and thereby frustrates the oedipal child intensely. In the course of clinical psychoanalyses one invariably encounters feelings of rage toward that frustrating love object, feelings which go back to the latter part of the oedipal phase and even later. From then on one encounters some degree of ambivalence toward the heterosexual love object. Therefore, a second factor contributes an opposing pull within the second conflict of ambivalence. Clinical findings suggest that while ambivalent feelings are experienced toward both love objects during the course of the oedipus complex, those which emerge toward the rival for the heterosexual love object remain by far the most powerful and conflict-inducing.

From Freud's formulations (1913, 1923) and the analyses of

adults and children, we know that the hostile destructiveness mobilized by the child's oedipal wishes is largely responsible for the development of the superego. Freud (1913) observed that the threat of consummating destructiveness toward the oedipal rival in the face of the love feelings toward that rival arouses an intense feeling of remorse. At this time, the superego becomes structured. All this requires no elaboration here. Both love and hate play a central role in the structuring and the character of the superego as well as the ego's defenses.

SUMMARY

This study of the development of ambivalence is an outgrowth of an effort to examine the interrelations of the symbiosis—separation-individuation process and instinctual drives. Ambivalence is evident during the rapprochement subphase of separation-individuation, when the child gives evidence of experiencing coexisting feelings of object love and hate toward the sufficiently structured libidinal object. However, longitudinal observation of children from birth reveals evidence suggestive of early intrapsychic conflict arising out of coexisting positively and negatively valenced feelings toward the libidinal object, feelings which already play a significant part in the child's psychic life from the end of the first year of life. This is readily observable in healthy children in reaction to limit-setting during the practicing subphase. Strong negatively valenced feelings often encountered during practicing essentially result from frustration of strivings for autonomy (individuation) by the libidinal object who is also the symbiotic partner. Although we cannot speak with certainty, during this period the positively and negatively valenced feelings experienced toward the libidinal object are impressive precursors of love and hate and create at least a significant, perhaps precursor, form of ambivalence.

Viewed developmentally, ambivalence seems to evolve ontogenetically through two basic conflicts: the first conflict of ambivalence has its beginnings during the first part of the separation-individuation phase, especially during the practicing subphase, and consolidates during the rapprochement subphase, especially in the arena of rapprochement crises. This first conflict occurs in the context of dyadic object relations. The second conflict arises out of rivalry with the loved parent of the same sex, an unavoidable component of the oedipus complex. This second conflict occurs in the context of oedipal triadic object relations.

This simplified formulation suggests the generalization that the boy usually has his first conflict of ambivalence in the relation to his mother, and the second in the relation to his father. In the girl, on the other hand, both conflicts occur principally in her relation to her mother, a factor that sharply multiplies her difficulties in that most central of all human relationships.

BIBLIOGRAPHY

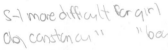

ABRAHAM, K. (1924), A Short Study of the Development of the Libido. In: *Selected Papers of Karl Abraham.* New York: Basic Books, 1953, pp. 418–501.

BELL, S. M. V. (1969), *The Relationship of Infant-Mother Attachment to the Development of the Concept of Object-Permanence.* Ann Arbor, Mich.: University Microfilms.

BOWLBY, J. (1958), The Nature of the Child's Tie to His Mother. *Int. J. Psycho-Anal.,* 39:350–373.

———— (1960), Grief and Mourning in Infancy and Early Childhood. *This Annual,* 15:9–52.

COLEMAN, R. W. & PROVENCE, S. (1957), Environmental Retardation (Hospitalism) in Infants Living in Families. *Pediatrics,* 11:285–292.

DÉCARIE, T. G. (1965), *Intelligence and Affectivity in Early Childhood.* New York: Int. Univ. Press.

ERIKSON, E. H. (1959), *Identity and the Life Cycle* [*Psychol. Issues,* Monogr. 1]. New York: Int. Univ. Press.

FRAIBERG, S. (1969), Libidinal Object Constancy and Mental Representation. *This Annual,* 24:9–47.

FRANK, A. (1969), The Unrememberable and the Unforgettable. *This Annual,* 24:48–77.

FREUD, A. (1965), Normality and Pathology in Childhood. *W.,* 6.

———— (1968), In: Panel Discussion. *Int. J. Psycho-Anal.,* 49:506–512.

FREUD, S. (1893), On the Psychical Mechanism of Hysterical Phenomena. *S.E.,* 3:25–39.

———— (1909), Notes upon a Case of Obsessional Neurosis. *S.E.,* 10:153–320.

———— (1913), Totem and Taboo. *S.E.,* 13:1–161.

———— (1914), On Narcissism. *S.E.,* 14:67–102.

———— (1915), Instincts and Their Vicissitudes. *S.E.,* 14:109–140.

———— (1923), The Ego and the Id. *S.E.,* 19:3–66.

—— (1926), Inhibitions, Symptoms and Anxiety. *S.E.*, 20:77–174.

—— (1940), An Outline of Psycho-Analysis. *S.E.*, 23:141–207.

FURMAN, E. (1974), *A Child's Parent Dies*. New Haven & London: Yale Univ. Press.

GLOVER, E. (1956), *On the Early Development of Mind*. New York: Int. Univ. Press.

GOODALL, J. VAN L. (1971), *In the Shadow of Man*. Boston: Houghton Mifflin.

GREENACRE, P. (1957), The Childhood of the Artist. *This Annual*, 12:47–72.

—— (1979), Reconstruction of the Process of Individuation. *This Annual*, 34:121–144.

HARLOW, H. F. (1960), Primary Affectional Patterns in Primates. *Amer J. Orthopsychiat.*, 30:676–684.

—— & HARLOW, M. K. (1962), Social Deprivation in Monkeys. *Sci. American*, 207:136–146.

—— & ZIMMERMAN, R. R. (1959), Affectional Responses in the Infant Monkey. *Science*, 130:421–432.

HARTMANN, H. (1939), *Ego Psychology and the Problem of Adaptation*. New York: Int. Univ. Press, 1958.

—— KRIS, E., & LOEWENSTEIN, R. M. (1946), Comments on the Formation of Psychic Structure. *This Annual*, 2:11–38.

HOLDER, A. (1975), Theoretical and Clinical Aspects of Ambivalence. *This Annual*, 30:197–220.

KAUFMAN, I. C. & ROSENBLUM, L. A. (1967), The Reaction to Separation of Infant Monkey. *Psychosom. Med.*, 29:648–675.

KERNBERG, O. F. (1966), Structural Derivatives of Object Relationships. *Int. J. Psycho-Anal.*, 47:236–253.

—— (1974), Instincts, Affects and Object Relations. Read at the Fall Meeting of the American Psychoanalytic Association.

—— (1975), *Borderline Conditions and Pathological Narcissism*. New York: Jason Aronson.

KRIS, E. (1950), Notes on the Development and on Some Current Problems of Psychoanalytic Child Psychology. *This Annual*, 5:24–46.

MAHLER, M. S. (1952), On Child Psychosis and Schizophrenia. *This Annual*, 7:286–305.

—— (1963), Thoughts about Development and Individuation. *This Annual*, 18:307–324.

—— (1965), On the Significance of the Normal Separation-Individuation Phase. In: *Drives, Affects, Behavior*, ed. M. Schur. New York: Int. Univ. Press, 21:161–169.

—— (1972), Rapprochement Subphase of the Separation-Individuation Process. *Psychoanal. Quart.*, 41:487–506.

—— & FURER, M. (1968), *On Human Symbiosis and the Vicissitudes of Individuation*. New York: Int. Univ. Press.

———— & McDevitt, J. B. (1968), Observations on Adaptation and Defense *in Statu Nascendi. Psychoanal. Quart.*, 37:1–21.

———— Pine F., & Bergman, A. (1975), *The Psychological Birth of the Human Infant.* New York: Basic Books.

McDevitt, J. B. (1975), Separation-Individuation and Object Constancy. *J. Amer. Psychoanal. Assn.*, 23:713–742.

———— (1977), Separation-Individuation and Aggression. Read at the Association of Freudian Psychologists, New York.

Moore, B. E. & Fine, B. D. (1968), *A Glossary of Psychoanalytic Terms and Concepts.* New York: Amer. Psychoanal. Assn.

Parens, H. (1971), A Contribution of Separation-Individuation to the Development of Psychic Structure. In: *Separation-Individuation,* ed. J. B. McDevitt & C. F. Settlage. New York: Int. Univ. Press, pp. 100–112.

———— (1973), Discussion of Film Presentation "Developmental Conflicts in a 2½-Year-Old Child" by H. Nagera. In: *Summaries of Scientific Papers and Workshops.* Association for Child Psychoanalysis, 1974.

———— (1976), Vicissitudes of Hostile Destructiveness in the Child at Risk. Read at the Meeting of the American Psychoanalytic Association, New York.

———— (1979a), *The Development of Aggression in Early Childhood.* New York: Jason Aronson.

———— (1979b), An Exploration of the Relations of Instinctual Drives and Symbiosis—Separation-Individuation Process: Part 1. *J. Amer. Psychoanal. Assn.* (in press).

———— & Pollock, L. (1977), Film #5: *Toward an Epigenesis of Aggression in Early Childhood.* #2: *Aggression and Beginning Separation-Individuation.* Audio Visual Media Section, Eastern Pennsylvania Psychiatric Institute, Philadelphia, Pa.

———— & Prall, R. C. (1974), Film #3: *Prevention: Early Intervention Mother-Child Groups. Ibid.*

———— Stern, J., & Kramer, S. (1976), On the Girl's Entry into the Oedipus Complex. *J. Amer. Psychoanal. Assn.*, 24:79–107.

———— & Saul, L. J. (1971), *Dependence in Man.* New York: Int. Univ. Press.

Piaget, J. (1954), *Les relations entre l'affectivité et l'intelligence dans le developpement mental de l'enfant.* Paris: Centre de Documentation Universitaire.

Provence, S. & Lipton, R. C. (1962), *Infants in Institutions.* New York: Int. Univ. Press.

Scott, J. P. (1963), The Process of Primary Socialization in Canine and Human Infants. *Monog. Soc. Res. Child Develpm.*, 28, No. 1.

Solnit, A. J. (1966), Some Adaptive Functions of Aggressive Behavior. In: *Psychoanalysis,* ed. R. M. Loewenstein, L. M. Newman, M. Schur, & A. J. Solnit. New York: Int. Univ. Press, pp. 169–189.

———— (1970), A Study of Object Loss in Infancy. *This Annual,* 25:257–272.

———— (1978), Personal communication.

SPITZ, R. A. (1946), Anaclitic Depression. *This Annual*, 2:313–342.

———— (1965), *The First Year of Life.* New York: Int. Univ. Press.

———— (1966), Metapsychology and Infant Observation. In: *Psychoanalysis,* ed. R. M. Loewenstein, L. M. Newman, M. Schur, & A. J. Solnit. New York: Int. Univ. Press, p. 123–151.

WINNICOTT, D. W. (1953), Transitional Objects and Transitional Phenomena. *Int. J. Psycho-Anal.*, 34:89–97.

WOLFF, P. H. (1963), Observations on the Early Development of Smiling. In: *Determinants of Infant Behavior,* ed. B. M. Foss. New York: John Wiley, 2:113–138.

Hatching in the Human Infant
As the Beginning
of Separation-Individuation

What It Is and What It Looks Like

RUTH CODIER RESCH, Ph.D.

THE WORK OF MAHLER AND HER CO-WORKERS (1975) HAS ADDED A
new dimension to our thinking about the dynamics of growth in
infancy and toddlerhood. They have used a direct observational
framework through which they have extended psychoanalytic and
developmental theories into infancy. With this method they have
defined and described a number of phases in the separation-
individuation process in the first 3 years of life. Among these is
"hatching," which they identify as a change point, principally in
alertness, occurring in the early months of the first year:

Dr. Resch is Clinical Assistant Professor and Director of the Infant-Toddler
Observation Nursery in the Division of Child and Adolescent Psychiatry,
Downstate Medical Center, Brooklyn, N.Y.

I am deeply indebted to Dr. Adolph Christ for his belief both in me and
in rigorous natural observational research and for his unflagging generosity
and support of the entire project of which this study has been one part. My
appreciation also to two research assistants, Dierdre Coltrera and Shirley
Gatano.

This paper, together with videotape material, was presented at the Annual
Meeting of the American Psychoanalytic Association, May 1977. This work
was supported in part by NIMH—Psychiatry Education Branch, Grant No.
5-T01-MH05816-25.

> The "hatching process" is, we believe, a gradual ontogenetic evolution of the sensorium—the perceptual-conscious system—which enables the infant to have a more *permanently alert sensorium* whenever he is awake. . . . In other words, the infant's attention, which during the first months of symbiosis was in large part *inwardly* directed, or focused in a coenesthetic vague way *within the symbiotic orbit,* gradually expands through the coming into being of outwardly directed perceptual activity during the child's increasing periods of wakefulness . . . we came to recognize at some point during the differentiation subphase a certain new look of alertness, persistence and goal-directedness. . . . This new gestalt was unmistakable to the members of our staff, but it is difficult to define with specific criteria [p. 53f.].

Indeed it *is* unmistakable—in addition, it has a quiet momentousness to it. Like infantile sexuality, once our attention is drawn to the phenomenon, our vision is changed by what we have seen. In this paper I will expand upon the concept of hatching and present, from a videotape observational study, what hatching seems to be, how it comes about, and what it might mean. In brief, I have come to see hatching as a bio-perceptual-affective integration. At that time growth achievements in a number of separate functions—perception, motor skills, perceptual-sensorimotor coordinations, and affects—come together.

When these separate maturational and developmental achievements are integrated at a particular level in early infancy, a new psychological organization is created. This organization provides the basis for a new emerging sense of self, of effectance. It is a beginning of pleasure in the world beyond the self and beyond the normal symbiotic situation. Specifically, hatching appears to be an integration that is a marker between symbiosis and beginning differentiation.

METHOD

The observations to be described were made in the Infant Toddler Observation Nursery in the Division of Child and Adolescent Psychiatry at Downstate Medical Center. The setting is quite similar to the Masters Center of the Mahler group, the Galenson-

Roiphe nursery formerly at Einstein Medical Center, and Louise Kaplan's at New York University. Our nursery is a comfortable living room, with a sleeping and eating area attached, where small groups of normal babies and their mothers come together for a morning, as they would in one of their homes. They come for two mornings a week, having committed themselves to a year's participation.

The main thrust of the current research in this nursery has to do with the most basic situation of separation: how the baby, and later the toddler, becomes aware of and deals with the mother's ordinary movements to and away from him and with her disappearances. That is, I am studying the cognitive-affective matrix from which defense and adaptation in the normal separating process develop.

The critical difference between this nursery and the others is the manner of the data collection and therefore of data analysis. With television we have a faithful recording of primary behavior, behavior sequences, in a natural setting. This record affords us the opportunity, and responsibility, to follow up on our clinical-observational hunches by going back over the moving pictures *many* times to submit our formulations to critical scrutiny—what I have elsewhere (1976a) described as solidly data-based hypothesis generation, a propaedeutic model of research. I believe that videotaping offers us a detailed moment-by-moment infant behavioral analogue to the intrapsychic free association process that has been the hallmark of psychoanalytic study. While the analogy is a metaphor, the two techniques share important and useful characteristics—the potential for noticing and linking *un*obvious details and relationships, for recognition of unexpected, unsought-for patterns.

Systematic techniques on the one hand and *rigorous natural* behavioral records on the other hand can together illuminate many previously unnoticed relationships. I did not in fact set out to study hatching. One morning in the nursery I saw a baby do what I *thought might* be hatching before my eyes. Following this "Ah-ha" experience of recognition, I began to look at tapes of other babies to see whether the behavioral changes I observed were particular to this baby or occurred in others as well.

This study, which is based on 25 hours of tapes of seven babies in a 3-month period, is an effort to delineate further the phenomena of hatching toward more fully descriptive, and thence to more operational, definitions. I would like to emphasize that critical attention at these formative stages will make hypothesis-testing studies in the complex phenomena of psychoanalysis both more realistically possible and potentially more successful.

The video data (see Appendix) illuminated the participation of four major areas in the baby's development toward hatching. There are perceptual, motor, sensorimotor coordinations and affects. I have found it fruitful to use Anna Freud's concept of developmental lines (1965). It is a model which permits one to trace separate ego functions as they coordinate into larger syntheses with object relations directed toward adaptations to and gratifications in the outer world.

PERCEPTUAL DEVELOPMENTS

Developments in the perceptual system are, first of all, influenced by the state of consciousness. Wolff (1963) has traced an early shift toward a more brightened state of consciousness at about 3 months. Both his work and that of Tennes et al. (1972) suggest that this change corresponds to the development of the social smile.

Prior to hatching, the quiet alert state in our babies has a rather vague quality. While the babies are clearly attentive, the eyes are veiled. The ordinary alert state lacks the sharpness and clarity that are regularly seen later.

Secondly, there is a progression in the general use of perceptual functions and of vision especially. Prior to hatching, the baby in the everyday nursery situation is most dominantly a perceptually receptive organism. The infant primarily takes in the world around. For a time before hatching, hearing and vision in the alert state often appear to have a "mesmerized" quality. The babies are relatively glued to single stimuli, i.e., they are rather stimulus-bound.

At hatching, it is the shift in alertness that the Mahler group noticed as so striking. The videotape study demonstrates that there is a more stable change in duration of quiet alert states. More important is a fairly dramatic shift to a clear and sharp state. Using the Mahler data, Willey (1978) tried to specify further the facial characteristics of this qualitative state change.

In terms of use of perception, there is a relative shift to a more active and baby-determined perceptual organization. As the "mesmerized" quality lessens, gaze becomes more flexible; the baby can more easily and actively shift gaze back and forth among different interesting sights and sounds. The baby now is not so glued to one stimulus or object of perception.

MOTOR DEVELOPMENTS

Prior to hatching the baby's skills and investment are largely in the fine motor sphere, that is, the achievement and use of a fairly smooth grasp. The area of mobility is near prehension.

At hatching, the motor development has moved to the impressively complex achievement of a stable autonomous sit posture. The area of mobility is now a self-determined reach-grasp. Both of these developments combined extend the infant's directed mobility outward in space in a highly significant manner.

SENSORIMOTOR COORDINATIONS

Prior to hatching, the eye-hand-mouth coordination is the dominant achievement (Hoffer, 1949). Spitz's films on grasping beautifully show this coordination. What the eye sees the hand can grasp; and what the hand grasps, the eye can see (Piaget, 1936). Our tapes also show what a difficult and delicate undertaking this achievement is.

In Piaget's formulations of sensorimotor cognition, primary circular reactions in behavior predominate prior to hatching. These are primarily actions *on* the body or actions *on* the body with objects—eye-hand-mouth-suck. Primary circular reactions, being essentially autoplastic (on the body), are symbiotic phase cognition par excellence.

At hatching, the eye-hand-mouth coordination expands into what I call the eye-hand-mouth-sit coordination. The latter, I believe, is a pivotal development in the hatching process. It seems to function rather as a keystone that finally brings the others into an integration. When the eye-hand-mouth coordination comes together with the autonomous capacity to sit, the baby becomes capable of a far wider and more stable range of mobility, a more effective area of reach-grasp. I emphasize *autonomous* sit, because babies are sat up with help well before this time (in laps, in infant seats, carriers, high chairs, and the like). Not until the autonomous sit is achieved, however, does the baby acquire the full mobility and perceptual versatility that the stable spine in the sit position affords. Gesell (1934) very early in his work recognized the organizing character of changes in postural skills. In the sit position, the arms and hands are freed from support duties. The visual field is no longer limited by the prone and supine postures or by the deterioration of an unsteady sit. The Gesell developmental scales, as well as those that followed (Cattell, Bayley) are structurally organized around changes in posture and in mobility.

Secondary circular reactions appeared in the video data at hatching. They are the next stage in cognition. They employ actions of the body to produce and reproduce attractive external events and to make interesting sights last. Secondary circular reactions represent a shift to the alloplastic domain, that is, interest in and active action upon external objects and events. With this also comes the beginning of the cognitive progression toward object permanence—knowledge of existence and whereabouts of moving and disappearing objects. As such, secondary circular reactions are really the cognitive beginning of psychological differentiation in Mahler's sense of a primary shift from the body-self-mother orbit to an emerging sense of self-in-the-world.

INTEGRATION

When a baby appears *hatched* in Mahler's alertness sense in our videotapes, all of these developments—perceptual, motor, and sensorimotor—have taken place. Each of them is a major and fairly complex development. Most of them have been documented more or less extensively in the literature. Obviously they are not new. What is new is the observation that all of these become integrated at this time. This integration, I believe, is more fully represented in the process that the Mahler group so aptly termed hatching.

It also should be said that the implicit background for the full integration is one of optimum facilitating parenting—the essential dimension of object relations as the bridge to the outer world.

These separate developments came together in nearly the same way in all of the seven babies I observed. In one baby early crawling performed the same function of broadened access to mobility as the autonomous sit posture did for the others, i.e., the coordination of the reach-grasp in a widened circle of activity. This particular baby was fitted with an orthopedic brace between his shoes. He solved the motor impediment by using the brace as a base from which to push off into crawling, rather than effecting the more difficult twist into a sit position. The important achievement, however, is the same for this baby as for the others: the widened circle of effective activity.

Mahler et al. place hatching "at the peak of symbiosis," which leaves somewhat unclear its relation to the process of differentiation they chart for the first 3 years. The video-observational study clearly shows hatching as an *integration* of *several* sets of developments. This integration is the stage setting that marks the major shift from symbiosis to emerging individuation. It is the beginning of differentiation; it is the shift from autoplastic to alloplastic. Thus it represents a major functional and psychological shift in the way the baby views the world.

The baby can now sit independently of anyone's help, is now free to utilize reach-grasp from a very stable posture that allows a much wider circle of effective activity. The baby now has the cognitive and motor coordinations that enable him to get hold of what is becoming an intensely interesting world, a world made more vivid by increased alertness and more flexible use of the perceptual systems.

This description brings me to what hatching is all about: the affective shift. The world is now energized with interest and with increasing pleasure in function. The baby can now get hold of the world and do things with it—and that is exciting, from the

baby's view. The shift in state of consciousness is also an *affective*
brightening. It is an affective infusion of interest in the outer
world, an emerging pleasure in what the baby instrumentally can
now *do* with objects and people. Having hatched, these infants
rapidly progress to the early practicing subphase, the first phase of
differentiation.

Hatching, then, is the coming together of eye-hand and reach-
grasp coordinations with the autonomous mobility in the sit position and changes in cognition. This idea accords well with Spitz's
concept of "organizers" (1959) and Werner's hierarchic integration
(1957). I want to underscore the recognition that it is a momentous shift—albeit a relatively quiet one.

On the one hand, this perceptual-sensorimotor integration is the
means by which the cognitive shift from primary circular reactions
(autoplastic, directed to the body) takes place to secondary circular
reactions (alloplastic, directed to outer objects and people across
larger spaces). On the other hand, this "new look" not only represents a shift in the sensorium, it is an affective and cognitive shift
of interest to the outer world.

I mentioned earlier my own "Ah-ha" experience after watching
one baby hatch in the nursery. That was not totally an offhand remark, for I would like to suggest that, developmentally, hatching
is perhaps the first cognitive-affective "Ah-ha" experience.

We are all familiar with the "Ah-ha" character of the achievement when an infant first walks. The world looks different and is
accessible in an entirely new way. The normal infant responds to
that achievement with a huge shift in interest and affect. Indeed,
for the Mahler group, walking is the induction into the later practicing subphase. The world, they say, is the second year toddler's
"oyster." That phrase is surely evocative of the zest, pleasure in
function, and enlarged exploration that one almost palpably sees
in infants in the second year. In addition, this change reverberates
in everyone around a new toddler.

I would like to suggest that the "Ah-ha" of the first walker is a
later, more dramatic version of the earlier hatching process. Here
it is apt to use Piaget's term (1936) "décalàge" from cognition in
the way that Louise Kaplan (1972) applied to to emotional development. A "vertical décalàge" is a repetition of an early behavior

pattern at a later, more complex stage of development. The induction of the new toddler into the later practicing subphase, with its accompanying elation, is a vertical décalàge. In psychological terms, it is a more complex repetition of the hatching transition into the early practicing subphase, with its emotional brightening and muted delight with the world (though at hatching the infant's world is a much smaller one). Hatching has a similar, albeit quieter, affective momentousness to it because it truly is the induction into beginning differentiation—the *very first* "Ah-ha" experience with the world!

Among the group of "vital pleasures" that George Klein (1976) outlined with considerable sensitivity to developmental issues is an elaboration of White's idea of "effectance pleasure" (1959, 1963). Without observational data, Klein wrote as follows:

> When the baby starts to grasp articles, sits up, crawls, tries to walk, he begins a process that eventually yields the sense that the locus and origin of these achievements is in himself. When the child thus feels the change as originating with himself, he begins to have a sense of *being* himself, a psychologically, not simply physically, autonomous unit [p. 225].

Thus, in the late 1960s when he was actually formulating these ideas, Klein also was struggling with the terms of individuation. With regard to the affective situation, he said that effectance pleasure "differs from pleasure in functioning in that, in effectance, the focus is not simply upon the exercise of skill or function per se, but on pleasure derived from the instrumental power of skill as a tool of one's intention" (p. 225).

These are the critical early links between the perceptual-motor-cognitive developments and the development of affect. After smiling, hatching becomes observable as a microcosm; it is the next of the crucial organizers. The baby's first social smile lights up everyone around. The infant's world is warmed emotionally by that smile, and ordinary adults respond powerfully to it. As Spitz has shown, this smile reorganizes the infant's symbiotic world.

In hatching, I think that we see a similar affective warming, this time for the infant—an infusion of pleasure into the link between the infant's new sense of instrumental functioning and the world about him. The infant for the first time actually gets hold of the world and goes after it—and that not only produces "interesting new sights" (to borrow Piaget's phrase), but is joyously satisfying to the infant.

Summary

Intensive longitudinal video observations of infants and mothers in the natural context of a morning nursery make possible detailed study of many early psychological developments. This paper expands on the observations of Mahler et al. on hatching and discusses it as a time of bio-perceptual-affective integration. I have traced the development of state of consciousness, perception, motor skills, perceptual-motor coordinations, cognition, and affect as they progress toward this integration. Hatching is discussed as a new psychological organization which marks the boundary between symbiosis and early practicing in the separation-individuation progression. This paper proposes hatching as a critical organizer in the early months. These observations enable us to begin a practical synthesis of observational data of perceptual-motor-cognitive developments and the psychoanalytic theory of the development of affects and object relations.

Appendix

Given the setting, frequency, and regularity of our video observations, the behaviors discussed in this paper are by no means fleeting or unique. The following samples illustrate the developmental progression in two children and are representative of many other observations that constitute the video-recorded data base for this study.

These samples are continuous behavior narratives, transcribed from the videotapes. The study itself, however, was done directly from the tapes. Self-explanatory baby behaviors relating to the developments discussed in the paper are italicized; comments and formulations about behavior are placed in brackets immediately following the salient observed behavior.

TAD

Prior to Hatching

Segment 1 (5 months, 2 weeks). At the beginning of the observation, Tad is seated on the floor. His mother is also seated on the floor, alongside Tad. Although Tad is supported by his mother's holding his left hand, he is *wobbly and teetery in his sitting.* Tad occupies himself with sucking and chewing on his right hand [primary circular reaction]. He has a neutral expression on his face. He does not appear to take notice, nor does he respond to his mother's shaking his hand. Tad gazes around himself a number of times, *without seeming to focus* upon anything in particular. His *gaze is vague and ill defined.* Tad momentarily focuses on a rag doll that is at his feet. A second or two later, he reaches for it. He pushes the doll's hand into his mouth and continues to suck and chew it as he had previously done with his own hand [primary circular reaction; Tad's actions are not too coordinated: rather rough and not well controlled].

Tad appears to be only *vaguely aware* of what he has in his mouth. He loses interest in the doll just as unpredictably as he gained interest in it [brief attention]. He focuses visually on the doll and then a second or more later feels for it [awkward momentary delay between perceptual and motor coordination].

Tad *begins to fall over* and he looks around himself. He now falls toward the other side, toward his mother. She lifts him and places him directly in front of her, sitting, and *supports him.* During this process, Tad has dropped the rag doll. He does not in any way register its loss or search for it [primary circular reaction; object permanence: stage of no special reactions]. Tad seems to have no reaction or response to the change in his position, vis-à-vis mother or the room. Tad now focuses upon a person crossing the room in front of him. He then turns and almost accidentally finds and plays with his feet [primary circular reaction].

Tad now *reaches beyond his feet, loses balance, and falls* onto his stomach. He makes a half-smile with his eyes and mouth. He lifts his head and looks around the room. His mother lifts him off the blanket he had fallen onto. She holds him in a standing position on her lap while Tad *unsteadily scans* the room.

Segment 2 (5 days later; close-up of face). Tad is again seated on the floor and is engaged in a great deal of visual scanning. He seems to be *mesmerized* by the sights around him (or as though he is simultaneously lost in deep thought). He is suddenly startled by a loud noise, blinks, jumps a little, and looks about himself and his surroundings. Tad smiles and visually follows the movement of a baby that is being placed at his side. He begins kicking a little and then again seems to become *mesmerized* watching another baby across the room [gaze dominates motor activity].

Segment 3 (same day). Tad is now sitting between his mother's feet, which are tucked close to his body and provide him support for sitting. His mother reaches around in front of him to give him a toy, which he takes from her. He looks at it and becomes interested in a sound across the room. His hands together with the toy drop between his thighs. Tad does not play with the toy. Instead he is engaged in looking at what the other children are doing across the room. Tad looks *transfixed*. He is suddenly startled, blinks several times, and then becomes alert to other things going on around him. Tad is considerably *less wobbly* in his sitting than he had been 5 days ago. [On the whole, Tad appears to be passively related to his surroundings in this observation. He uses relatively little motor activity in comparison with the amount of visual activity he engages in.]

Hatching

Segment 4 (6 months, less 1 day). Tad is sitting on the floor, a neutral expression on his face. He is being handed a piece of zwieback from behind by his mother. Tad takes the biscuit from her, and she seats herself in a chair close behind Tad. He curiously looks at the zwieback in his hands and then places it in his mouth. He sucks on it for a few seconds while looking around the room. The zwieback falls from Tad's mouth onto the upper part of his chest [rough eye-hand-mouth coordination: improving]. He inadvertently catches it and returns it to his mouth [object permanence: stage of no special reactions]. He sucks on it again for a few seconds, and then it falls from his mouth again.

Tad then seems to engage in a not very fully attentive search for the zwieback. He looks on his stomach and then down between his legs. He sees the biscuit lying between his legs, feels for it, and believes he is lifting it off the floor. When Tad looks at his hands, clearly expecting to find the biscuit there, he is disappointed to discover that there is nothing there [object permanence: stage of accommodation, kinesthetic tactile]. His eyes seem to sadden for an instant, and then he looks about himself in what seems to be a general but aimless expectancy for the zwieback.

Tad's hands are between his legs. His hands happen onto the zwieback and, as he touches it, he looks down [accidental tactile discovery]. Having found it by feel, he lifts it from the floor and passes it to his other hand [midline coordination]. Placing the zwieback in his mouth, Tad begins to suck and chew on it once again for a while.

Having securely placed the biscuit in his mouth, he now looks away from it. [His sitting position is balanced and more stable. His retrieval of the zwieback shows improving eye-hand coordination. Although his coordination and perception of the location of objects are still quite rough, Tad's movements are not nearly as aimless and without modulation as they had been.]

While Tad is busily sucking on the zwieback, his eyes alternate from watching a person cross the room to taking the zwieback out of his mouth and watching it in his hands [motor coordination now easily coexists with gaze shifts]. The segment ends as Tad is engaged in laboriously changing the zwieback over from one hand to the other. Unintentionally it drops to the floor. This time he looks around aimlessly, appears to have no notion whatever of where it went. It is lost altogether to him and there is no further search [object permanence: no special reactions].

Segment 5 (6 months, 4 days). Tad, sitting on the floor, is being offered a cookie by his mother who is standing on his right side. Tad eagerly takes the cookie and places it in his mouth. While sucking on the cookie, he *visually scans* the room. He pauses to watch another mother in the room who is sitting on a couch across the room. His *attention now seems to shift* to this woman's baby, seated on the floor in front of him. His *gaze then shifts again* to another activity going on behind the baby. Tad attentively follows the movements of the baby's mother as she plays with her baby, rattling and then handing the baby a toy, and then resuming her seat on the couch [more fluid gaze].

Once the mother has been seated, Tad continues *visually scanning the room in a continuous and purposeful manner.* Tad returns to watching the other baby and curiously stares at the baby for several moments (the baby is about two feet from Tad). Tad now shifts his attention to his hands that are still holding the cookie in his mouth. The cookie has been softened by Tad's continuous sucking of it, and it now falls to the floor. Tad looks very mildly surprised [object permanence, stage 3: acts of interrupted prehension].

Tad first looks to the hand that had been holding the cookie and keeps looking straight at this hand [object permanence: looking where the object was last seen]. He does not track the fall of the cookie to the floor. He repeatedly opens and closes his hand, watching it intently

[object permanence: repetitive grasp, where it was last felt]. It seems
to be an effort to recapture the tactile feel of the cookie in his hand.
He brings his hand toward his mouth, pulls it away looking at it. He
brings it toward himself again and then seems to realize that the cookie
isn't there. He drops his hand to his leg. Seeming to continue a search,
Tad looks down at his hand, then between his legs, and turns inquisi-
tively to the other baby in the room [object permanence: visual accom-
modation]. After a moment, he looks down again at his hand and then
feels for the cookie in his hand. Still not finding it in his hand, he looks
between his legs, beyond and to the side. His mother comes into view
and Tad reaches his hand out to his mother [secondary circular reaction; object permanence: repetition of prior acts, looking and feeling].

Hatched

Segment 6 (6 months, 2 weeks). Tad is *sitting stably and erectly* on
the floor. There is an open-shelved toy cabinet to his back on one side
and a large wooden toy cart to his other side. Tad is *carefully and intently watching* the movements made by a little girl (about 3 years old)
just beyond the toy cart. He looks away and down as the little girl
moves from behind the cart to sit and read a book, about a foot or so
in front of him.

Tad now looks up and focuses on the girl reading the book. He
studies her intently, rather *transfixed* by her, as she flips the pages of
the book. *Suddenly and abruptly he looks away* [intentional shift of
gaze]. Tad reaches forward for the soft fabric-covered blocks a few
inches beyond his feet. Unsuccessful in his reach for the blocks, Tad
lifts his arms, looks vaguely about, and finds a cloth book with his
hands at about the same time his eyes do [closer coordination of eye
and reach].

Turning to see more clearly what he has found, Tad attempts to lift
the book off the ground. He succeeds on his second try and, holding the
book in both hands, Tad brings the book to his mouth, holding it there
for a split second. Lifting the hand that is in possession of the book
away from his mouth, Tad plays a new game of raising and lowering
the book at different heights [primary circular reaction gives way to
secondary circular reaction: experiments with dropping objects from
different heights]. As part of the game, Tad moves the book away from
himself and toward the side. He accidentally bangs his hand on a board
in the cart. Puzzled, Tad turns to see what has made the noise and in
doing so unintentionally drops the cloth book as he reaches for the
board [multiple actions].

Tad, seeming to realize he has dropped the book, looks down at the floor. He sees the book, and raises it to his mouth [object permanence, stage 3, interrupted acts: drops cloth, reaches board, looks for cloth]. Tad now sucks and chews the book while watching the little girl bring cloth blocks from behind the cart to about a half a foot in front of Tad. Several times Tad takes the book out of his mouth [resumption of primary circular reaction: suck, chew, look]. While doing this with one hand, Tad is reaching for the blocks the girl is bringing over with his other hand. Tad lowers his hand whenever the girl places the blocks on the floor before him, as though he might be imitating her actions.

Tad is so *engrossed in studying* the girl's actions that he keeps his hand suspended momentarily in mid-air while he follows her visually across the room [very alert, intent interest in external activity]. Tad now concerns himself with watching his hands and the book as he takes the cloth book in and out of his mouth. He brings his other hand to the book and continues to play the game while holding the book in both hands [primary circular reactions]. Tad's attention is turned away from the book to the conversation the adults are having across the room. Tad spots the little girl across the room and follows her visually as she gets up and walks behind the cart [multiple actions].

While paying close attention to the actions of the girl, Tad removes the book from his mouth, places it on his lap almost without having to notice, and continues watching the girl [smooth and automatic visual-motor coordination]. Tad's attention drifts from the little girl to one of the women on the couch [bright alert gaze; flexible use of gaze]. For a few seconds he studies the women and pays close attention to the conversation the adults are having. After a few moments, Tad looks down at the book on his lap, raises it with both arms, lets it drop and then retrieves it again [secondary circular reaction]. This game of dropping and finding the book is done intentionally by Tad. [This demonstrates not only the improvement in his coordination since the last observation, but also that he is now capable of doing two things at one time. For example, Tad attempted during this observation to reach for the cloth blocks while playing and sucking his book with his other hand.]

MAG

Prior to Hatching

Segment 1 (4 months, 7 days). Mag is lying on her side on a blanket on the floor. She is bright-eyed, though *staring vaguely* out into the room. Not paying direct attention to what she is doing, Mag is pulling

at the legs of her pants and at the same time she is forming her mouth
into a cooing shape and making sounds. Mag suddenly lets go of her
pants legs and rolls back onto her back, in a loss of balance [primary
circular reaction, autoplastic activity]. She begins to kick, raise, and
lower her arms once she has found herself on her back. One of her
hands *happens to find* one of her feet. She holds onto her foot for a second or two and then lets go [limited grasp range]. In the meantime,
she turns her head around and attentively looks in the direction of
voices of other mothers across the room. It is almost perchance that
while her head is turned, Mag *happens to notice* a baby across the
room and *weakly stares* at the baby for several seconds. Losing interest
just as unexplainably as she had gained interest, Mag turns her eyes
and body away from the other baby.

With a sudden burst of energy, Mag catches her feet with both hands
as she turns. Mag *looks aimlessly* around herself and the room and
smiles. Lying on her back, Mag sees her mother, kicks, and smiles at
her. Mag catches her feet again and continues looking at her mother
for several seconds, smiles again, and unintentionally turns onto her
side again while continuing to play with her feet. Mag gazes in the
direction of the other mothers across the room as they are talking [gaze
shifts more stimulus-dominated than self-motivated]. She remains staring in that general direction for several moments. Her *gaze* seems to
have direction but still has a *nonspecific* quality to it.

Hatching

Segment 2 (4 months, 29 days). Lying on her right side on the floor,
Mag is busy handling a wooden jack-in-the-box with her free left hand.
Mag is surrounded by toys: a plastic daisy mirror is by her head; a
rag doll is by her stomach and legs; a ball and several small toys are
by her feet. Mag *studies* the box with her eyes and hands, exploring
the different planes and pushing the box on edge and back with her
hand. Occasionally Mag looks up and gazes about the room.

She pauses and focuses a moment on the adults' conversation across
the room. Mag turns her head to follow the person crossing the room
and then turns in the opposite direction toward another baby's voice
[only one action at a time, looking or handling]. Mag attentively
watches the baby and then smiles as she watches someone cross directly
in front of her. Mag resumes handling the box and manages to turn it
onto its side [primary circular reaction]. Her attention now drifts to
the baby who is sitting and playing about a foot away.

While Mag is watching the baby, a visiting child about 4 years old
comes over to Mag and removes a small toy from in front of Mag. She

then turns over the jack-in-the-box as though to help Mag. Mag watches the child's actions but keeps her eyes on the box. She reaches out for the child's hand. The child abruptly takes hold of Mag's hand and places it on the box again. The child leaves; Mag watches the child as the latter goes, looks at the box, and pushes it [primary circular reaction].

While Mag pushes the box away, her hands thrust downward. In her movements she touches the doll by her side but *does not grasp or search.* There is a plastic rattle on the floor immediately in front of her eyes, but she does not reach for it. As her hands continue in motion downward, they touch another rattle which makes a noise, and she grasps it [primary circular reaction]. She looks down at her hands to see what she has found, brings it up nearer her face to see it. She raises and puts the rattle down several times. She studies it intensely for a moment and then brings it to her mouth. She is fairly *deft in handling* the rattle with both hands, despite the fact that she is lying on her side with one elbow pinned under her body. She *occasionally looks up from the rattle and then around the room, then turns her attention to* the rattle again.

Segment 3 (5 months, 13 days). Mag is *sitting for the very first time* in her life on her own. Her back happens to be to her mother, and she is *smiling radiantly* at another mother who is sitting on the couch. She is leaning far forward, which does not give her good balance, but she nonetheless seems *rather steady for a first-time sitter.* She suddenly looks away in response to a noise from across the room. Then she looks down at the floor immediately before her. She sees a plastic cup, reaches to grasp it, lifts it, and puts it to her mouth [primary circular reaction, autoplastic]. Mag is sagging further forward, but has not lost balance. Her mother lifts her from behind, while Mag continues to hold the cup. The camera loses track of Mag for some moments as the video shifts from one camera perspective in search of a better one.

Mag is on her mother's lap gazing about herself and nonspecifically toward the camera for several seconds. Sometime during the move from the floor to mother's lap, Mag has acquired tissues and is holding one in each hand. Mag is touching her mother with the tissues, turns and *smiles radiantly* at her mother while Mrs. M. chats with another mother across the room.

Hatched

Segment 4 (5 months, 20 days). Mag is sitting on the floor grasping a wooden block in one hand while *alertly watching* another baby in the room who is sitting and playing with a toy a few inches away from

Mag. She is again surrounded by toys. A plastic bin filled with all sorts of colorful, small and medium-sized toys is before her; several toys are scattered by her legs and by her side. There is another toy bin by her side.

Mag looks away from the baby as the baby crawls away from Mag. Mag spots the daisy mirror before her, drops the block she had been holding, and picks up the mirror. She eagerly presses it to her mouth and then puts it down [primary circular reaction]. Mag now turns to the block she had dropped, studies it for a moment with her hands and eyes. She picks it up, studies it again, and brings it to her mouth. Mag now transfers the block to her other hand and rests it gently on her legs for a while. She *visually scans the area* around her, perhaps for a new toy. Not seeming to find anything, Mag returns to the block she is holding in her hand. She lifts it and puts it down again [more flexible use of gaze].

Hearing the voice of a baby, Mag looks up to see where it is coming from and smiles when she spots the baby. Mag looks about the room, returning to look at the block in her hand. Playing with the block, Mag *transfers* it from one hand over to the other, *watching her hands carefully* as she does so. She brings the block to her mouth and once again *briefly looks around* the room, rests the toy on her legs, brings the block to her mouth, and repeats the process again.

Mag now lifts the block with one hand above her head and slams it onto the ground. She picks the block up again, studies it for a moment, brings it to her mouth, and then puts it down again [beginning secondary circular reaction]. Mag repeats the entire process, although this time she energetically throws the block down and away from herself. Unconcerned with the whereabouts of the block, Mag does not even look around to see where it has fallen; instead she becomes interested in the daisy mirror that is resting in her lap. Studying it with her eyes and hands, Mag brings it to her mouth [object permanence, stage 2: no special reaction]. Then while sucking on the daisy, Mag focuses her attention on another baby crawling across the room directly in front of Mag.

Segment 5 (same day). Mag is lying on her stomach on the floor. She studies the plastic teether she is moving in her hand. Mag looks up from the teether, turns away facing in the direction of the camera for a moment, and returns her gaze to her play. Mag puts the teether in her mouth, takes it out, and then reaches for a toy several inches away from her. Not being able to reach the toy, Mag returns to the teether in hand. She stares at it for a moment, then places it in her mouth. As she does so, she sees the other toy she had been trying to reach. She again attempts to reach the toy, this time turning over onto her side to lengthen her reach [increased motor accommodation, simple problem solution]. She succeeds now, pulling the toy to her side. She puts it in her mouth and turns back onto her stomach [maintains grasp of two objects at once]. Mag notices that she still has the teether in her other hand and puts both toys down. Lifting her head, Mag looks around at the toys about her and finds a new one.

Mag picks up a cloth that had been near her, puts it down, and then brings it to her mouth. While holding the cloth, she notices one of the toys she just put down. Holding the cloth in one hand, Mag reaches for it with her other hand [beginning secondary circular reaction]. Picking up the toy, she immediately drops it again. In dropping it, Mag turns over an almost empty plastic toy bin while looking at the toy she is dropping. Mag again picks up the toy, drops it, and pulls the plastic bin onto its side. While holding the bin upright with one of her hands, Mag drops the cloth with her other hand, picks up the teether with that hand, and stares at the cloth as she playfully drops the teether into the bin [two independent actions at once, secondary circular reaction].

Moving to the next phase of what seems to have become a simple game, Mag picks up the cloth, brings it to her mouth, and proceeds to throw it onto the floor. Mag bites down on the cloth and brings the hand that had been holding down the bin to the cloth, but in doing so the bin falls down. Out of the corner of her eye, Mag notices that the bin has fallen and restores the bin to its upright position with her hand. Having restored the bin, Mag eyes the teether, drops the cloth in her hand, and grabs the teether [attention to several actions at once]. Dropping the teether too after a moment, Mag seems to be contemplating while she sucks her thumb. She turns to see where some voices are coming from and, in turning back, refinds the cloth lying on the floor. Mag picks up the cloth and simultaneously feels something rubbing against her other arm. Turning back to find out what it is, she sees the teether and raises it off the floor with the same hand that is holding the cloth [beginning secondary reaction]. Mag lifts the teether, drops it by her side, and then puts the cloth down by it as well. With her other hand, Mag erratically pushes the bin away, raises it, and then restores it to its previous position.

While holding the bin upright with one hand, Mag is busy picking up the teether with the other hand. She lets the bin fall down, lifts the cloth, and with the same hand restores the bin to its upright position. Mag continues playing her game of successively dropping the cloth, raising the bin, and dropping the teether [two actions in rotation].

Segment 6 (5 months, 25 days). Mag *sits firmly and well-balanced* on the floor. In one hand she is holding a plastic ring that has several discs strung on it. Mag watches herself jiggle the hoop up and down several times and accidentally drops it. Putting her hand to the back of her head, Mag stares at the ring on the floor [object permanence, stage 3: visual accommodations]. She picks up the ring, holds it in both hands, and gazes about the room. Three bins full of toys behind her catch Mag's attention. Mag looks back at the ring in her hands and transfers it to one hand. She brings the ring to her mouth and chews on it while holding it with both hands [primary circular reaction]. Taking the ring out of her mouth, she rests it on the floor. Crouched over the ring, Mag *glances back over her shoulder* at the toy bins for a moment and then looks back at the ring while she sits up straight again. Bringing the ring back up to her mouth, she gnaws at it while looking up at her mother who is sitting in front of her on the couch. Looking away from her mother, Mag takes the ring out of her mouth and puts her hand in, while still holding onto the ring with her other hand.

Mag *turns and looks back* at the bins once again and stares at them for a second. Her *sit is solidly secure* now. She *turns and glances and turns* back again [it is an easy coordination of movement and attention that is fluid and almost off-hand]. She looks back at the ring in her hand and, having taken her hand out of her mouth by now, puts the ring into her mouth. Mag takes the ring out of her mouth and lets it drop onto the ground. Mag watches her own motions as she lifts the ring off the floor [object permanence, stage 3: visual pursuit]. Having secured the ring in her hands, she *glances back* at the toy bins once again.

She returns to playing with the ring, studying it carefully with her hands and eyes. Mag puts the ring down on the floor and pounds on it several times with her hand. Mag stops pounding on the ring, *looks back at the toy bins and returns* to the ring. She has raised the ring and is now holding it with both hands. Mag lets go of the ring with one hand, expecting it to drop [secondary circular reaction]. She has a surprised expression on her face seeing that it has not fallen. Mag transfers the ring to her other hand and commences playing a game lifting and putting down the ring several times, each time lifting it higher and further back than she had done before [secondary circular reaction].

Mag is smiling and saying, "Ahahah . . ." [bright, alert expression].

Mag stops everything at once and *looks back* at the toy bins, staring at them for two seconds, then turns back to the ring, shakes it, and lets it drop onto the floor [pleasure in own activity].

BIBLIOGRAPHY

FREUD, A. (1965), Normality and Pathology in Childhood. *W.*, 6.

GESELL, A. (1934), *Infant Behavior*. New York: McGraw-Hill.

HOFFER, W. (1949), Mouth, Hand, and Ego-Integration. *This Annual*, 3/4:49–56.

KAPLAN, L. J. (1972), Object Constancy in the Light of Piaget's Vertical Décalàge. *Bull. Menninger Clin.*, 36:322–334.

———— (1976), Elation. Read at the Downstate Medical Center, Brooklyn, New York.

KLEIN, G. S. (1976), The Vital Pleasures. In: *Psychoanalytic Theory*. New York: Int. Univ. Press, pp. 210–238.

MAHLER, M. S., PINE, F., & BERGMAN, A. (1975), *The Psychological Birth of the Human Infant*. New York: Basic Books.

PIAGET, J. (1936), *The Origins of Intelligence*. New York: Int. Univ. Press, 1954.

PINE, F. (1971), On the Separation Process. In: *Separation-Individuation*, ed. J. B. McDevitt & C. F. Settlage. New York: Int. Univ. Press, pp. 113–130.

RESCH, R. C. (1976a), Natural Studies and Natural Observations. In: *Psychoanalysis and Contemporary Science*, ed. T. Shapiro. New York: Int. Univ. Press, 5:157–205.

———— (1976b), On Separating As a Developmental Phenomenon. *Ibid.*, 5: 207–269.

SPITZ, R. A. (1959), *A Genetic Field Theory of Ego Formation*. New York: Int. Univ. Press.

TENNES, K., EMDE, R., KISLEY, A., & METCALF, D. (1972), The Stimulus Barrier in Early Infancy. In: *Psychoanalysis and Contemporary Science*, ed. R. Holt & E. Peterfreund. New York: Macmillan, 1:206–234.

WERNER, H. (1957), The Concept of Development from a Comparative and Organismic Point of View. In: *The Concept of Development*, ed. D. B. Harris. Minneapolis: Univ. Minnesota Press, pp. 125–148.

WHITE, R. W. (1959), Motivation Reconsidered, *Psychol. Rev.*, 66:297–333.

———— (1963), *Ego and Reality in Psychoanalytic Theory* [*Psychol. Issues*, Monogr. 11]. New York: Int. Univ. Press.

WILLEY, I. R. (1978), "Hatching" from Symbiosis and Its Significance for the Process of Separation-Individuation (unpublished MS).

WOLFF, P. H. (1963), Observations on the Early Development of Smiling. In: *Determinants of Infant Behavior*, ed. B. Foss. London: Methuen, 2:113–167.

APPLICATIONS
OF PSYCHOANALYSIS

A. Literature and Art
B. Reactions to Catastrophes

From Preadolescent Tomboy
to Early Adolescent Girl

An Analysis of Carson McCullers's
The Member of the Wedding

KATHERINE DALSIMER, Ph.D.

IN THIS PAPER I SHALL CONSIDER A WORK OF LITERATURE IN LIGHT OF a psychoanalytic understanding of developmental processes. The work, *The Member of the Wedding*, by Carson McCullers, is about a 12-year-old girl. The novel is set in a backwoods Alabama town and is peopled by characters seemingly remote from common experience. Yet the haunting power of this work, about a girl on the threshold of adolescence, depends on its evocation of affective states and of conflicts that are almost universally characteristic of this stage of development. In examining these phase-specific conflicts within the framework of psychoanalytic theory, I shall try to illuminate the power of the novel, and hope that the analysis of the novel may in turn deepen our understanding of the processes of development during this period.

I

Adolescence has been described as "the second individuation process" (Blos, 1967) comparable to the first which takes place

Associate, Columbia College Counseling Service; Lecturer, Department of Human Development, Columbia University.

during the first 3 years of life. The gradual emergence of the infant from the symbiotic matrix with mother to become an individuated, separately functioning young child has been observed and conceptualized by Mahler and her co-workers (1963, 1975). In the earliest years the child becomes more independent of mother's physical presence and ministrations as he develops a constant and reliable internal image of her. Later, in adolescence, the task is that of emotional disengagement from the internalized infantile objects, which frees the individual ultimately to develop new ties outside the family.[1]

Particularly at the beginning of adolescence, there is a heightened experience of separation, as the stirring of new drives necessitates the renunciation of familiar and incestuous objects, and the radical changes of puberty create an estrangement from the familiarity of one's own body. At the outset, the adolescent carries an "enormous burden of the unexpressed" in bewildering new bodily sensations and lone fantasies that he or she is loathe to reveal (Harley, 1971), which therefore intensify the sense of strangeness and isolation. Further, in the shifting alliances of this period, there may be abandonments by friends, real losses in themselves which also potentiate the feeling of loss in relation to parents (Deutsch, 1944). The renewed experience of loss and separation arouses in the adolescent regressive longings for that state of fusion which preceded the first process of individuation.[2]

These states of feeling have been hauntingly described by Carson McCullers in *The Member of the Wedding*. In the spring and summer when she is 12, Frankie Addams feels that she "had become an unjoined person," that she was "a member of nothing

1. Schafer (1973) has questioned the application of the term "individuation" to the giving up, during adolescence, of ties to infantile objects on the ground that one must already be individuated in order to have such ties. He suggests that "it is representational differentiation that must be the core of the separation-individuation concept" (p. 42). The concept of "the second individuation" in adolescence does, however, fulfill this criterion. It not only indicates the disengagement of the adolescent from the matrix of the family, but also connotes the reworking, on a higher level, of the separation of self and object representations.

2. See Geleerd's (1961) observation of a "partial regression to the undifferentiated phase of object relationship" in adolescence.

in the world." The bodily changes of puberty that make her feel freakish, the new estrangement from her father, the loss of friends who are already initiated into the mysteries of sex—all of these changes make her feel suddenly alone and terrified. When her older brother announces that he is to be married, Frankie conceives a fantasy to deny this loss and the cumulative sense of separateness. In this fantasy, she will join her brother and his bride and go everywhere in the world with them, always. She will be a member of the wedding: *"They are the we of me"* (p. 35). This fantasy is an attempt to re-create an infantile state of fusion. Only when the impossibility of this regressive solution becomes apparent does Frankie find an adaptive resolution. Ultimately, she is able to overcome the terrors of her new separateness through the finding of a friend, a close friend of the same sex.

Frankie's development reflects the transition from preadolescence to early adolescence. At the beginning of the novel, in her shorts and B.V.D. undervest, she personifies the preadolescent tomboy described by Deutsch (1944). The tomboyishness characteristic of this period is seen by Blos (1962) as a defense against the regressive pull to the preoedipal mother. In the course of disengagement from parents, the adolescent finally turns toward heterosexual love. Before this, however, in early adolescence, there is a period of close friendship with members of one's own sex.[3] No longer idealizing the parents, the early adolescent idealizes the friend and feels affirmed by the relationship. He chooses someone with qualities he would like to have—or commonly, projects these onto the friend—and thereby possesses them by proxy. The friend, then, is heir to the child's earlier idealization of the parents.

Blos and Deutsch describe early adolescence in girls as being marked by bisexuality. While Deutsch is referring primarily to the bisexuality of the girl's object choices, Blos is referring to that of

---

3. Blos places friendship between members of the same sex in early adolescence, Deutsch (1944) and Sullivan (1953) in preadolescence. Deutsch offers rich descriptions, drawn from clinical work and from literature, of the faithfulness demanded of the friend, the complete partnership in common secrets. Sullivan ascribes critical importance to the relationship with the "hum," which permits modification of the self representation through the intimate disclosures and the experience of seeing oneself through the eyes of the chum.

her self representation. It is the latter sense that is poignantly exemplified by Frankie. In this period, the girl is concerned with the question, "Am I a boy or a girl?" and may maintain the belief that she can decide either way. Thus, early adolescence is a transition between the phallic wishes of preadolescence and progression to femininity.

II

The Member of the Wedding is set in a Southern town during the Second World War, in the oppressive heat of "that green and crazy summer" when Frankie Addams is 12 years old. She has spent most of the summer in the kitchen with Berenice Sadie Brown, the cook, a 40ish black woman with one bright blue glass eye and one sad, dark eye, and with John Henry, Frankie's 6-year-old cousin. Her father, a peripheral figure in the novel, appears abstracted and preoccupied; he is busy much of the time at his jewelry store. Her mother is dead, having died in childbirth with Frankie.

At the opening of the novel, as I have suggested, Frankie typifies the preadolescent tomboy. She is dressed like a boy, has had her hair cut like a boy, and in this first part of the novel she calls herself by a boy's name. Furthermore, her wish to be a boy is suggested by the conspicuously phallic objects of the petty thefts she has committed—stealing her father's gun and shooting it, and taking a three-way knife from a Sears and Roebuck store. When, during the long August afternoons, Frankie, Berenice, and John Henry muse about how each would change the world, John Henry would have rains of lemonade and Berenice a world where there were no separate colored people, but in Frankie's ideal world "people could instantly change back and forth from boys to girls, which ever way they felt like and wanted" (p. 80). It is clear that at 12, Frankie's self representation is bisexual. Its fluidity reflects the propensity for temporary identifications characteristic of this period. It is further suggested by the ease with which she would dress up either in a football suit or in a Spanish shawl when she went into town with her friend, who would just as easily wear the other costume. When the Chattahoochee Exposition comes to town, Frankie is irresistibly drawn to the Half-Man Half-Woman of its sideshow, "a morphodite and a miracle of science. This Freak was divided completely in half—the left side was a man and the right side a woman. The costume on the left was a leopard skin and on the right side a brassiere and a spangled skirt. Half the face was dark bearded and the other half bright glazed with paint. Both eyes were strange" (p. 17). Frankie is afraid of the Half-Man Half-Woman, disturbed by the secret bond she feels with this creature whose freakish split mirrors her own.

Frankie's assertions of boyishness are primitive attempts to deny what the processes of puberty are every day making more apparent: that she is becoming a woman. The anxiety that this holds for her is evident in Frankie's attempt to stop the forward movement of time by clinging to her 6-year-old boy cousin, and regressively taking refuge with him and Berenice in the nurturing locus of the kitchen, whose walls are covered with the "queer, child drawings" of John Henry.

Why is becoming a woman so frightening for Frankie? We are told only that her mother died "the very day she was born," as if it were too terrible to name the connection—that her mother died in childbirth. Frankie's own growth, then, has been conceived by her as murderously destructive. As puberty transforms her body into that of a woman, she becomes frightened of the unspeakable connection. The unconscious equation is fixed: in becoming a woman she is approaching death. As puberty creates the capacity for womanly sexuality and procreation, Frankie is filled with dread of its mortal consequences.

The narrative reflects these unconscious equations. There is a sense of violence and abrupt loss in the description of the spring when Frankie is pubescent, conveyed by the startling choice of words: the wisterias bloomed, and "silently the blossoms shattered":

> April that year came *sudden* and still, and the green of the trees was a *wild bright green*. The pale wisterias bloomed all over town, and *silently the blossoms shattered*. There was something about the green trees and the flowers of April that made Frankie

sad. She did not know why she was sad, but because of this peculiar sadness, she began to realize she ought to leave the town
[p. 19; my italics].

The blossoming of spring that year mirrors the blossoming of
Frankie's own body. The "suddenness" of spring, its "wild bright
green," suggests a bursting forth of something new and uncontrollable, as she felt within her. The fantasies that are awakened
make her feel that somehow she must flee.

On the one side, there is terror in what she is moving toward
and, on the other, the processes of puberty evoke sadness as they
cut her off from the familiar pleasures and safety of the past. This
is suggested metaphorically in Frankie's being unable, now that
she has grown taller, to walk within the protective enclosure of
the arbor, as she had done when she was younger:

> Other twelve-year-old people could still walk around inside,
> give shows, and have a good time. Even small grown ladies could
> walk underneath the arbor. And already Frankie was too big;
> this year she had to hang around and peek from the edges like
> the grown people. She stared into the tangle of dark vines, and
> there was the smell of crushed scuppernongs and dust. Standing
> beside the arbor, with dark coming on, Frankie was afraid. She
> did not know what caused this fear, but she was afraid [p. 7].

"She did not know what caused this fear," just as she did not
know, in the passage quoted previously, what caused her sadness.
We may surmise, though, that at dusk, as darkness comes and
the world of objects begins to disappear, Frankie has a heightened
experience of separation and loss. She asks John Henry to spend
the night with her, projecting onto him her own fear and loneliness. "I am sick and tired of him," she explains to Berenice. "But
it seemed to me he looked scared. . . . Maybe I mean lone-
some . . . I just thought I might as well invite him" (p. 8).

She herself is frightened by the processes that are beginning to
transform her body, processes that seem to be running out of
control:

> She stood before the mirror and she was afraid. It was the sum-
> mer of fear, for Frankie, and there was one fear that could be
> figured in arithmetic with paper and a pencil at the table. This

August she was twelve and five-sixths years old. She was five feet and three quarter inches tall, and she wore a number seven shoe. In the past year she had grown four inches, or at least that was what she judged. . . . Therefore, according to mathematics and unless she could somehow stop herself, she would grow to be over nine feet tall [p. 16].

Her mathematical calculations confirm that she is freakish, and that the changes of her body are propelling her inexorably toward a terrifying fate—that is, "unless she could somehow stop herself," but this she cannot do. Her uncontrollable growth also is a metaphor for the other uncontrollable processes of puberty. "She was in so much secret trouble" at this time. "Besides being too mean to live, she was a criminal. If the Law knew about her, she could be tried in the courthouse and locked up in the jail. Yet Frankie had not always been a criminal and a big no-good. Until April of that year, and all the years of her life before, she had been like other people" (p. 18f.).

That spring and summer, Frankie is "scared and haunted" by the town jail, and she dreads passing it. She feels that its inmates, like the freaks, recognize her as one of them. "It seemed to her that their eyes, like the long eyes of the Freaks at the fair, had called to her as though to say: We know you" (p. 102). Although the primal unconscious "crime" which makes her one of them is having been the cause of her mother's death, the guilt attached to this unspeakable event is in part displaced onto those new "sins" about which she consciously ruminates. She has engaged in some sexual play with Barney MacKean which makes "a shrivelling sickness in her stomach" each time she thinks of it. "She hated Barney and wanted to kill him. Sometimes alone in the bed at night she planned to shoot him with the pistol or throw a knife between his eyes" (p. 21). As mentioned earlier, she has committed some petty thefts, taking her father's gun and a knife, which make her feel that she is a criminal as well as a freak. The upsurge of drives, libidinal and aggressive, makes her feel both estranged from her former self and set apart from other people, as she has not yet shared with anyone else her "lone fantasies" (Harley, 1971).

The ways in which the physical changes of puberty disrupt the accustomed body image and concomitantly the sense of self are nowhere more powerfully expressed than in the following passage:

> It was the year when Frankie thought about the world. And she did not see it as a round school globe, with the countries neat and different-colored. She thought of the world as huge and cracked and loose and turning a thousand miles an hour. The geography book at school was out of date; the countries of the world had changed [p. 19].

The globe is Frankie's body; the neat and different-colored geography book of latency no longer describes it. This book is indeed out of date, for the changes of puberty have transformed her body and with it her sense of self. "Huge and cracked and loose" is Frankie's own body, turning with a terrifying speed.

We see in the character of Frankie that the physical changes of puberty in and of themselves create an estrangement from the past sense of self. The acceleration of growth, the changes in the contours and appearance of the body demand a fundamental revision of the body image; this, in addition to the new and intensified impulses, ultimately contributes to the development of a new sense of self. Before this can crystallize, the young adolescent inevitably feels a loss in relation to the old, a mourning that must occur before the new, more appropriate self representation can be positively invested and enjoyed.

There are other losses attendant upon what Freud (1905) called the "transformations of puberty." The intensification of drive pressures and the change in their quality require that the adolescent renounce the incestuous objects of childhood. It is to this loss that Anna Freud (1958) has ascribed the "state of mourning" characteristic of adolescence. The sense of loss in relation to incestuous objects is expressed in the novel by Frankie's father suddenly telling her that she was now too big to sleep in his bed, and would have to sleep upstairs and alone. From this time, "She began to have a grudge against her father and they looked at each other in a slant-eyed way. She did not like to stay at home" (p. 20).

Sex separates her from other girls, too—those a little older who are sexually more experienced and knowledgeable:

There was in the neighborhood a clubhouse, and Frankie was not a member. The members of the club were girls who were thirteen and fourteen and even fifteen years old. They had parties with boys on Saturday night. Frankie knew all of the club members, and until this summer she had been like a younger member of their crowd, but now they had this club and she was not a member. . . .

"The son-of-a-bitches," she said again. "And there was something else. They were talking nasty lies about married people. When I think of Aunt Pet and Uncle Eustace. And my own father!" [p. 10f.]

The older girls' initiation into the mysteries of sex is a barrier excluding Frankie from membership, for her need still to deny the facts of sexuality, including that of her father, separates her from their circle. In addition, her best friend has moved away, another reflection of the shifting alliances among girls of this age. In contrast, Berenice has her friends, whose presence when they come to call for her intensifies Frankie's feeling of isolation. Even her cat takes off in search of sex and a ladyfriend. "It looks to me like everything has just walked off and left me" (p. 26).

The spring and summer when she is 12 have been for Frankie a season of losses, each resonating with the central event of her life, the death of her mother in childbirth. Her feeling of abandonment is complete when her brother announces that he is to be married. Although he has, in fact, been away for the past two years in the army in Alaska, his impending marriage becomes the focus for all the losses she has suffered. To Frankie, her brother and his bride have no specificity or individuality: in her mind's eye, her brother's face is "a brightness" and the bride "also was faceless." All that is clear is the feeling of being abandoned:

Frankie closed her eyes, and, though she did not see them as a picture, she could feel them leaving her. She could feel the two of them together on the train, riding and riding away from her. They were them, and leaving her, and she was her, and sitting left all by herself there at the kitchen table [p. 24f.].

She tries to deny the pain, busying herself in cutting with a large butcher knife at a splinter in her foot. Proud of having "the toughest feet in town," Frankie asserts with bravado, "That would have hurt anybody else but me" (p. 29), but soon admits her vulnerability, "I feel just exactly like somebody has peeled all the skin off me" (p. 31).

Her attempts at denial fail. Through the cumulative losses associated with puberty Frankie "had become an unjoined person." In preadolescence she does not yet have restitution for these losses, and she turns to fantasy. This has always been a solace to Frankie. In the alchemy of her imagination, her alleycat becomes a Persian; the moths at her window, butterflies. To escape the anguish within she daydreams of being elsewhere. Landlocked in a backwoods town, she holds a seashell to her ear and listens to the ocean. In the oppressive heat of the Alabama summer, she daydreams of Alaska and Winter Hill, and watches in fascination the snow falling inside her treasured paperweight.

When the prospective marriage of her brother makes the sense of loss unbearable, Frankie takes refuge in an elaborate fantasy that she will join her brother and his bride, and go everywhere in the world with them, always.

> They were them and in Winter Hill, together. . . . The long hundred miles did not make her sadder and make her feel more far away than the knowing that they were them and both together and she was only her and parted from them, by herself. And as she sickened with this feeling a thought and an explanation came to her, so that she knew and almost said aloud: *They are the we of me* [p. 35].

"They are the we of me." The underlying wish is to assuage the terror of separateness by regression to an undifferentiated state before there is an "I." It is the wish that Frankie momentarily gratifies when, sitting on Berenice's lap, "She could feel Berenice's soft big ninnas against her back, and her soft wide stomach, her warm solid legs." Frankie slows her breathing in order to breathe in time with Berenice, so that "the two of them were close together as one body" (p. 97f.). The same wish is reflected in her longing to donate her blood to soldiers fighting in the war. "She was not afraid of Germans or the bombs or Japanese. She was afraid because in the war they would not include her, and because the world seemed somehow separate from herself" (p. 20). As her blood mixes with that of the soldiers, she will become part of their bodies and thus dissolve her separateness.

In her fantasy of joining her brother and the bride, they are bound together so that separation is impossible. "The world had never been so close to her" as when, in her mind's eye, she saw "the three of them—herself, her brother, and the bride—walking beneath a cold Alaskan sky, along the sea where green ice waves lay frozen and folded on the shore; they climbed a sunny glacier shot through with pale cold colors and a rope tied the three of them together, and friends from another glacier called in Alaskan their J A names" (p. 59). Frankie sees her brother and his bride not as a man and woman in a sexual relationship, but as undifferentiated from one another. When she conceives the fantasy of joining them, the three form not a triangle but a symbiotic unity. The rope that ties them together, like the umbilical cord that was Frankie's only connection to her mother, is the consummate expression of symbiotic yearning. Further, they are fused with one another through the magic of their J A names: Jarvis, Janice, and now the fantasy name Frankie adopts, "F. Jasmine."

The fantasied regression to a state of infantile oneness assuages her terror at being separate and alone. Now, she is no longer frightened:

> For when the old question came to her—the who she was and what she would be in the world, and why she was standing there that minute—when the old question came to her, she did not feel hurt and unanswered. At last she knew just who she was and understood where she was going. She loved her brother and she was a member of the wedding. The three of them would go into the world and they would always be together. And finally, after the scared spring and the crazy summer, she was no more afraid [p. 38].

The forward movement of preadolescence has brought, so far, only separation and loss. Frankie finds solace in a reparative fantasy, the restitution of an infant's experience with the mothering one. In this fantasy of merging, all the inevitable separations of the "second individuation process" are denied.

The regressive fantasy, assuaging her anxiety, allows Frankie in some ways to move forward. She leaves the protectiveness of the

kitchen, where she has remained all summer with Berenice and
John Henry, and ventures into town. There, "the world no longer
seemed separate from herself and all at once she felt included"
(p. 41). She experiences "a new unnameable connection" with
everyone she sees, a connection "impossible to explain in words"
because it is rooted in the epoch of life prior to the development
of language. Now, walking alone the main street in town, she feels
"entitled as a queen," her power derived from the relationship
to her idealized brother-and-his-bride, whose projected omnipotence she now shares. This idealization is a revival of the young
child's view of the parents (or their surrogates), whose glorified
images are essential to the child's narcissism. Thus, "Under the
fresh blue early sky the feeling as she walked along was one of
newly risen lightness, power, entitlement" (p. 46).

After the fantasy crystallizes that she will be a member of the
wedding, Frankie for the first time enters the Blue Moon cafe,
"a place forbidden to children," where she initiates a flirtation
with a soldier. He is unconsciously equated with her brother, who
has been in the army for the past two years. On her side, it is another attempt at restitution for her loss, and she is made uneasy
and finally panicked by the soldier's sexual intentions.

She is, however, interested for the first time in listening to
Berenice talk about love, when before she would have covered her
ears.

> The old Frankie had laughed at love, maintained it was a big
> fake, and did not believe in it. She never put any of it in her
> shows, and never went to love shows at the Palace. The old
> Frankie had always gone to the Saturday matinee, when the
> shows were crook shows, war shows, or cowboy shows. . . . The
> old Frankie had never admitted love. Yet here F. Jasmine was
> sitting at the table with her knees crossed, and now and then she
> patted her bare foot on the floor in an accustomed way, and
> nodded at what Berenice was saying [p. 82].

The narrative reflects Frankie's unconscious fears: with the forward movement toward femininity and sexuality, death enters the
story. Uncle Charles dies. Although he is only a peripheral figure,
unrelated to Frankie, his dying stirs thoughts of the other deaths

that have touched her life, and finally of the fearful possibility of her own death:

> "It makes me shiver, too, to think about how many dead people I already know. Seven in all," she said. "And now Uncle Charles."
>
> F. Jasmine put her fingers in her ears and closed her eyes, but it was not death. She could feel the heat from the stove and smell the dinner. She could feel a rumble in her stomach and the beating of her heart. And the dead feel nothing, hear nothing, see nothing: only black.
>
> "It would be terrible to be dead," she said, and in the wedding dress she began to walk around the room [p. 77].

Frankie's musing about "how many dead people I already know"— in the present tense—implies that the dead are indeed presences in her inner world, where they continue to live on.

Berenice, in speaking of love, speaks movingly about the death of her first husband, Ludie Freeman. Frankie notices immediately that he died "the very year and the very month I was born," connecting his death, like that of her mother, with her birth—that inseparable unity in her mind. Berenice goes on to describe how she married each of her other husbands—who turned out to be drunk, or crazy, or no good—because each reminded her in some way of her beloved Ludie. One had a thumb mashed like his, another his overcoat. The implication of Berenice's reminiscence is the finality of death, the impossibility—no matter how strong the wish—of reunion with one who has died. Frankie senses that what Berenice is saying has something to do with her plan about the wedding, and at this point she covers her ears to keep from hearing more. Her fantasy of joining with her undifferentiated brother-and-his-bride represents, in part, the "return of the lost parent" (Jacobson, 1965), a fantasy frequently observed in children whose parent has died. The irrevocability of the event is denied, and the child harbors the belief that somehow the parent is still alive and the insistent hope of a future reunion (Wolfenstein, 1966, 1969). When this hope is not fulfilled, there is bitter disappointment and rage, as after the wedding when Frankie is left "wanting the whole world to die."

Until reality forces itself upon her, though, Frankie uses a re-

parative fantasy to assuage her anxiety. The difference between
Frankie in the first part of the novel and F. Jasmine, as she calls
herself in the second, is that the latter is comforted by a fantasy
which denies separation. It is, in a real sense, a "transitional
fantasy" analogous to the early "transitional object" that allows
the child to separate physically from mother so long as he keeps
her symbolically with him. So too, the fantasy allows Frankie to
leave the protectiveness of the kitchen and venture into town, still
feeling a sense of "connection," her word for expressing the overcoming of separation and loss.

She is no longer angry at her father, because she has replaced
his loss with a fantasy. She is no longer envious of soldiers, or of
the girls of 13, 14, and 15. "In the old days that summer she
would have waited in the hope that they might call her and tell
her that she had been elected to the club. . . . But now she
watched them quietly, without jealousy" (p. 79). She can give up
the tomboyishness that she needed and can allow some progression
toward femininity and heterosexuality. The name she adopts for
herself is that of a flower. She enjoys shopping for an organdy
dress for the wedding, and wishes now that her crew cut were
long yellow hair; she will bathe and scrub the brown crust off
her elbows. The transition from tomboyishness to femininity is
reflected in the way she appears before Berenice to show off her
new dress—her cropped head tied with a silver ribbon. The in-
completeness, as yet, of this transition is echoed in the background
music of the novel, the piano being tuned that repeatedly stops
after the seventh note of the scale, without coming to a resolution.

The transition cannot be completed until Frankie gives up her
regressive fantasy. She does not, of course, become a member of
the wedding. Jarvis and Janice go off on their honeymoon, leaving
her sobbing and enraged. Once reality forces itself upon her and
she must relinquish the fantasy of merger, she is left again with
the terror of separateness: "She was back to the fear of the
summertime, the old feelings that the world was separate from
herself—and the failed wedding had quickened the fear to terror"
(p. 128).

To escape this, there is a revival of her fantasies of running
away, again with bisexual possibilities. Either she will take a train

to Hollywood and be a movie starlet, or she will go to New York, dress as a boy, and join the Marines. There is a brief thought of running off and marrying the soldier, but Frankie recoils from sex, frightened by three memories which converge—the silence in the hotel room with the soldier; the nasty talk behind the garage with Barney MacKean; and her glimpse, as a child, of boarders having sex ("Mr. Marlowe is having a fit!"). These memories, real and frightening in themselves, are also more conscious screens for the ultimate consequence of sexuality—death in childbirth. Sex is still too terrifying, yet, "There was only knowing that she must find somebody, anybody, that she could join with to go away. For now she admitted that she was too scared to go into the world alone" (p. 127).

The resolution is in finding a friend, which Blos (1962) considers the hallmark of the early adolescent phase. Friendship allows a sense of "joined-ness" that is neither a regression to a state of fusion, nor yet heterosexual, but which moves forward. In the friendship with Mary Littlejohn, there is mutual affirmation and a sharing both of the outer world and of their inner worlds. They read poetry together, each validating the other's ambitions—Mary to be a great painter, and Frankie a great poet, or else the foremost authority on radar. It is again the season of the fair, but this year Frankie does not go to the Freak Pavilion; no longer feeling a secret bond with freaks, she instead goes on rides with her friend. She gives up her rage at her brother, thinking Luxembourg, where he lives, a lovely name now that she plans to travel there with Mary. Their friendship enables Frankie to give up her regressive longings, and to begin moving toward feminine sexuality: soon after they meet, she reaches menarche.

Through the relationship with her idealized friend, Frankie grows away from Berenice, her mother-surrogate, and from John Henry, her young cousin, her old boyish self. At the end of the novel, John Henry has died, symbolizing the relinquishing of her self representation as a boy, and Berenice is leaving to get married, representing the development of Frankie's autonomy which renders Berenice no longer essential for survival. In the final scene, Frankie and her father are preparing to move. Now, at 13, accompanied by her friend Mary, Frankie is leaving the house where she spent her childhood, the kitchen where she took refuge with Berenice and John Henry from the terrifying sense of loss that accompanied all the changes of puberty. Frankie can now leave behind the tomboyishness that was a denial of her developing femininity, and the regressive fantasy of fusion, which was an attempt to ward off the terrors of separateness and loss. Only through the friendship with Mary does she finally call herself not by the boyish name Frankie, nor by the fantasy name F. Jasmine, but by her real name, Frances.

BIBLIOGRAPHY

BLOS, P. (1962), *On Adolescence*. New York: Free Press.
———— (1967), The Second Individuation Process in Adolescence. *This Annual*, 22:162–186.
DEUTSCH, H. (1944), *The Psychology of Women*, vol. 1. New York: Grune & Stratton.
FREUD, A. (1958), Adolescence. *This Annual*, 13:255–278.
FREUD, S. (1905), Three Essays on the Theory of Sexuality. *S.E.*, 7:125–244.
FURMAN, E. (1973), A Contribution to Assessing the Role of Infantile Separation-Individuation in Adolescent Development. *This Annual*, 28:193–207.
GELEERD, E. R. (1961), Some Aspects of Ego Vicissitudes in Adolescence. *J. Amer. Psychoanal. Assn.*, 9:394–405.
HARLEY, M. (1971), Some Reflections on Identity Problems in Prepuberty. In: *Separation-Individuation*, ed. J. McDevitt & C. F. Settlage. New York: Int. Univ. Press, pp. 385–403.
JACOBSON, E. (1965), The Return of the Lost Parent. In: *Drives, Affects, Behavior*, ed. M. Schur. New York: Int. Univ. Press, 2:193–211.
KAPLAN, E. B. (1976), Manifestations of Aggression in Latency and Preadolescent Girls. *This Annual*, 31:63–78.
MAHLER, M. S. (1963), Thoughts about Development and Individuation. *This Annual*, 18:307–324.
———— PINE, F., & BERGMAN, A. (1975), *The Psychological Birth of the Human Infant*. New York: Basic Books.
McCULLERS, C. (1946), *The Member of the Wedding*. Boston: Houghton Mifflin.*
NAGERA, H. (1970), Children's Reactions to the Death of Important Objects. *This Annual*, 25:360–400.
SCHAFER, R. (1973), Concepts of Self and Identity and the Experience of Separation-Individuation in Adolescence. *Psychoanal. Quart.*, 42:42–59.

* Permission to quote from this book is gratefully acknowledged.

SULLIVAN, H. S. (1953), *The Interpersonal Theory of Psychiatry*. New York: Norton.

WOLFENSTEIN, M. (1966), How is Mourning Possible? *This Annual*, 21:93–123.

——— (1969), Loss, Rage, and Repetition. *This Annual*, 24:432–460.

Michelangelo's Early Works

A Psychoanalytic Study in Iconography

ROBERT S. LIEBERT, M.D.

IN EXPLORING THE CONTRIBUTION THAT PSYCHOANALYSIS CAN OFFER to the understanding of the meaning of an artistic image it is my threefold purpose: (1) to amplify a basic element in the methodology of psychoanalytic iconography that was applied in an earlier Michelangelo study (Liebert, 1977a); (2) to illuminate the representation of certain unconscious and unresolved conflicts, dating back to Michelangelo's early childhood, which were fundamental determinants of both the form and content of images that he created in a single decade of his work—1501–09 (when he was 26 to 34 years old); and (3) to speculate on the developmental process of the "splitting" of the early maternal object representation into, on the one hand, an all-caring, idealized figure (the Madonna), and on the other, an abandoning, murderous figure (the Medea).

With respect to the method, there has long been controversy between art historians and psychoanalysts, largely revolving around the issue of what are to be considered the relevant evidence and methods for interpreting images. For several decades, the principal model in the field of Renaissance art history has been iconography. In this model, interpretation is highly dependent on the

Training and supervising analyst, Columbia University Center for Psychoanalytic Training and Research; and Adjunct Associate Professor, Department of Art History and Archaeology, Columbia University, New York. I would like to express my appreciation to Professor Howard Hibbard and Drs. Robert Michels and Roy Schafer for their helpful suggestions after reading an earlier version of this article.

general system of classification of works of art according to the time and place of their origin. Once the works have been so classified, the researcher knows where to look for the intellectual sources that will yield the meaning of the specific images under consideration.[1] The iconographic approach by itself, however, is of little help in understanding those distinctive and personal aspects of the image that express the unique artistic imagination and particular style of its creator. In my earlier study of Michelangelo's *Dying Slave* (1977a), I developed the argument that the statue represented an artistic resolution to a lifelong conflict between the unconscious meaning of death to Michelangelo and a central, reparative fantasy that served to attenuate his dread. A critical step in the analysis of the form and elusive meaning of the *Dying Slave* was to establish the antique source that was the model for this work. In this instance the source is known to be the younger son in the late Hellenistic marble group, *Laocoön*. Once having traced the earlier source, by examining those aspects of its narrative theme that so deeply touched dominant unconscious themes in Michelangelo, which made it irresistible to him as a model, we understand something about the latent meaning of his derivative later creation, even though it was his conscious intention to produce a visual statement quite different from its progenitor.[2]

For many of Michelangelo's works—both painted and sculptured —a specific work from antiquity, which was known to him, has

1. See Panofsky (1939) for the clearest statement of the iconographic method.

2. Some art historians have been wary of the inferences drawn from this approach, contending, first of all, that Renaissance artists tended to look to antique images as sources for their own artistic solutions. To do so was in keeping with the spirit of the Renaissance—that is, the rebirth and refinding of the idealized ages of ancient Greece and Rome. Second, it is suggested that the magnificence and suitability of the antique image are sufficient to explain utilization by the later artist. The situation is, however, analogous to the explanation for someone saying, "I have nothing but *infection,* I mean *affection,* for my mother-in-law." One could argue that it is sufficient to explain the parapraxis on the basis of the similar structure of the words "infection" and "affection," without the necessity to attend to the unconscious conflict over the meaning of the intended statement. Similarly, with the antique sources, their meaning and form are inextricably linked, and both are necessary determinants of the choice of that work as model by the later artist.

been located and persuasively established as the inspiration for the formal aspects of his creation. In this study of his works from an early decade, I place heavy reliance upon this method to explicate the deeper meaning of the image and thereby to clarify how it evolved in Michelangelo's mind into the final form that we now see.

The second task is to demonstrate not simply the plausibility, but the probable truth of the psychoanalytic assumption that the representation of unconscious and unresolved conflicts from early childhood is a fundamental determinant of both form and content of mature creative images. In this quest, my formulations and conclusions are principally based on the following data about Michelangelo: (1) the wealth of deeply personal statements by Michelangelo himself, which make him unique among artists of the past. These statements are in the form of 480 letters to family, friends, and patrons (Ramsden, 1963) as well as 327 poems (Gilbert and Linscott, 1963) that have been preserved; (2) two biographies by his friends: one by Giorgio Vasari (1568), and the other, published in 1553, when Michelangelo was 78 years old, by Ascanio Condivi, a young assistant to the artist (scholars agree that the Condivi "biography" is largely an "autobiography" based on recollections and letters supplied by the master); (3) lengthy characterizations of him by contemporaries in the literary form of *dialogues:* one by Donato Giannotti (1546), a trusted friend who was a Florentine Republican living in exile in Rome after the fall of the Republic in 1530; the other by Francisco de Hollanda (1548), a Portuguese artist; both dialogues are based on several Sunday afternoon visits with Michelangelo and Vittoria Colonna in 1538; (4) the facts of Michelangelo's infancy and childhood, and of his family, as they are known; and (5) the patterns of child-rearing practices in the fifteenth century in Florence.

In assessing the strength of the propositions with respect to the connection between particular artistic images and specific developmental and psychodynamic forces in Michelangelo's life, we must consider the *repetition* of the same theme and conflict in successive works as a necessary criterion of the validity of these propositions. This position grows out of the assumption that the manifest solution (the work of art) of the latent and unconscious conflict does *not* have the effect of "working through"—that is, of permanently altering the inner constellation of self and object representations, and of bringing about changes in other aspects of intrapsychic organization. Thus, with each artistic endeavor failing in this respect, the underlying conflict will reappear. And, in the creative individual, each artistic solution will emerge somewhat altered from the previous one, still motivated, however, toward a similar end. This study is confined to a relatively brief span of time in Michelangelo's life of creativity.[3] By limiting the time span we can minimize the need to sort out the influence of such factors as sociopolitical change, major leaps in artistic style, and the changing outlook of Michelangelo in his different life stages. It should be emphasized, nonetheless, that the same unconscious conflicts continue to exert their shaping force throughout creative life. The ways in which the conflicts explored in this paper were manifest in the art of the last decade of Michelangelo's life (1555–64) was the subject of another study (Liebert, 1977b).

The third consideration is Michelangelo's "splitting" of the representation of his early maternal imago into contradictory images of the idealized Madonna and the terrifying Medea.[4] The illustrative works of his art from the period of 1501–09 attest to the presence of, and the attempt to reconcile and integrate, these

3. Michelangelo was already uncommonly gifted when he entered the workshop of Domenico Ghirlandaio as an apprentice at age 13. He was productive for the next 76 years and was at work on his *Rondanini Pietà* until eight days before his death, in his ninetieth year.

4. The concept of splitting has been used to convey varied meanings by different writers (see J. Lustman [1977] for a critical review of the topic). Here, splitting refers to the defensive process whereby separate and contradictory aggregates of self and object representation alternate in consciousness. The organizing principle of each of these aggregates is its composition of elements of similar "affective valence" qualities (Kernberg, 1966). For example, the psychic representation of "oneself" or of "mother" can be codified into aggregates that are called the "good me" and "bad me" and the "good mother" and "bad mother," with the appropriate associated affects. Moreover, at any given time, similarly valenced aggregates of self and object representations will accompany each other. The conceptualization of splitting employed in this paper is akin to the Kleinian thesis of the split and alternation between the "depressive position" and the "paranoid position" (Segal, 1964). Stokes (1955) wrote with insight about Michelangelo from the viewpoint of Kleinan theory.

two conflicting aggregates of representation of the mothering figure. This conflict in object representations coexists with a parallel split in Michelangelo's self representation with respect to himself in relation to "mother." This pair of contradictory self representations may be called the "idealized son and victim (Jesus)" and the "matricidal son (Orestes)." It was the tension between these two split representations, particularly the thrust toward subordinating the negative, more violent ones, to those closer to the ego ideal, that left their distinctive imprint on Michelangelo's ultimate artistic solutions in many of his major works.

EARLY MOTHERING

A formidable problem in the psychoanalytic study of Michelangelo is the role of his mother and her surrogates in his early life. It is therefore useful to gather together what is known about his early mothering and speculatively to fill in certain additional pieces. In contrast to the documented knowledge about so many aspects of his life, information about his mother and her relationship with him is virtually nonexistent. All that we know is her name, that she bore five sons, and that she died at age 26, when he was 6 years old. We do not know what she died of, whether her death was unexpected or followed a long illness. We presume the former, since Michelangelo's youngest brother was born that same year. The *only* reference to her in all of Michelangelo's writings is not very illuminating and occurs when the artist was 79 years old, in a letter to his nephew Lionardo (Ramsden, letter 386). There is a question not simply about the quality of the relationship, but whether there was even continuous contact between Michelangelo and his mother during those 6 years.

In the Condivi biography the one reference to mothering concerns Michelangelo's having been boarded at birth with a stonemason's family on the small Buonarroti farm to wet-nurse. Condivi recounts that "Michel Angelo used to say jestingly, but perhaps in earnest too, that it was no wonder he delighted in the use of the chisel, knowing that the milk of the foster-mother had such power in us that often it will change the disposition, one bent being thus altered to another of a very different nature" (p. 5). Thus, Michelangelo depicts himself as the passive object of the mystical power and active force of the milk, which has endowed him as a sculptor, and stands in opposition to his father as his procreative source and identification.[5]

Since Michelangelo's experience of being boarded with a wet nurse is so alien to our century, yet so formative in his life, it is necessary to understand this part of his personal history in the context of the child-rearing practices of the time. In a comprehensive historical study, Ross (1974) established that it was the usual, rather than the exceptional, infant from middle-class families who was boarded with a wet nurse in fifteenth-century Italy. The norm of early childhood experience then is so foreign to us now that Ross's description deserves to be presented in some detail.

> What were the infant's first contacts with the world outside the womb? Birth in the parental bed, bath in the same room, and baptism in the parish church were followed almost at once by delivery into the hands of a *balia* or wet-nurse, generally a peasant woman living at a distance, with whom the *infant would presumably remain for about two years* or until weaning was completed. Immediate separation from its mother, therefore, was the fate of the new-born child in the middle-class families of urban Italy. . . . It became wholly dependent on food, care and affection upon a surrogate, and *its return to its own mother was to a stranger in an alien home, to a person with whom no physical or emotional ties had ever been established* [p. 184f.; my italics].

Unfortunately, we know no more about the stonemason's wife than about Michelangelo's actual mother. So again, we are left with countless questions about her specific influence on Michelangelo and the nature of the maternal care that he received. In answer, we are left only with inferences from his later character

---

5. Vasari attributes a similar statement to Michelangelo: "Talking to Vasari one day, Michelangelo said, 'Giorgio, if I am good for anything it is because I was born in the good mountain air of your Arrezzo and suckled among the chisels and hammers of the stone cutters'" (p. 258). Condivi details Michelangelo's father's fierce opposition to his son embarking on a career as an artist and his contempt for works of art.

structure, relationships with women, sexual orientation, and representations of women in his art—particularly the madonnas and the Virgins with the dead Christ (*Pietàs*). One must bear in mind that the wet nurses were generally lower-class women, initially grieving the loss of their own infants. They nursed on a business basis, often at the insistence of their financially burdened husbands, and had to face the inevitable resentment by her own older children.

As for Michelangelo's actual early situation, we have little more to draw upon than the average expectable circumstances for a Florentine middle-class child. To that extent, my reconstruction is based upon probabilities strengthened by some facts. I assume that he remained with the stonemason's family in Settignano for approximately 2 years, but in some contact with his parents, since it was their farm and just outside of Florence. There is no reason not to conclude that once weaned he rejoined his natural parents, who were then living in the Santa Croce quarter of Florence in a very small communal household with the family of his father's only brother. Michelangelo's mother may be presumed to have been reasonably healthy since she bore three more sons during the 6 years following his birth. With regard to Michelangelo's whereabouts between his mother's death and his father's second marriage, when he was 10 years old, we again have no clear information. His stepmother, Lucrezia, bore no children and died when he was 22 years old. There are no data to suggest that she ever played a significant role in his development.

Upon remarrying, Michelangelo's father and his family continued to share the same household with his brother's family. Although ages are not explicit in Condivi's *Life*, all biographers infer a chronology that definitely places Michelangelo in the home of his father and stepmother from age 10 on. In this hazy early history it is a matter of conjecture where Michelangelo lived between the ages of 6 and 10. Condivi implies that the father placed Michelangelo in a specially selected grammar school (the equivalent of our high school) at about age 10. This leaves open the possibility that he was at the farm in Settignano during the previous 4 years, following his mother's death. If so, however, and the stonemason's family was still there, it would be expected that this information would somehow have entered our body of knowledge through mention in one or another form by Michelangelo. My own conclusion is that he lived with his father and brothers in the collective Buonarroti household in Florence during those years.[6]

To recapitulate my reconstruction of Michelangelo's first 10 years: he was boarded with a wet nurse of unknown character for perhaps as long as 2 years. His weaning from the breast was then associated with an abrupt separation from his mothering one. At this time he returned to his biological mother and father, both of whom were relative strangers to him, as he was to them. His re-entry into his mother's life, particularly as her second son, probably elicited minimal emotional investment inasmuch as she was subsequently pregnant for close to half of the 6 years that remained to her. Thereafter, he was a member of a two-family collective household until 10 years of age, with no known adequate maternal surrogate, and a father who, apart from whatever grief he endured following his wife's death, must have felt his five young sons to be a substantial burden.

We are now faced with the problem of translating this particular childhood history, which was not in any way atypical for the fifteenth century, into the constructs of twentieth-century theory and analysis. It must be assumed that regardless of the norms and prevailing practices during the Renaissance, there are certain invariable laws of human behavior that include, on the one hand, psychobiological impulses and needs that are universal and, on the other, restraints and ethical concerns that are shared by all social orders. In each environment, however, certain predominant pathways of discharge and sublimation of drives and their derivatives are more or less accessible and acceptable. Therefore, some patterns of resolution of conflict and behavior will be facilitated and others impeded (Hartmann et al., 1951). In the case of Michel-

---

6. Tolnay (1943–60, vol. 1) states that it is "probable" that Michelangelo remained with the stonemason family until age 10, at which time he entered his father and uncle's house and began schooling. Tolnay's conclusion, however, is presented without the support of facts or further argument and is therefore unpersuasive. In a recent study of Michelangelo's *Pietàs,* Oremland (1978) assumes, on the basis of psychological reasoning, that Michelangelo was returned to his mother at about age 2.

angelo, even by the standards of the time his childhood was traumatic—marked by inconstant care when he was totally dependent, abrupt losses of the figures responsible for his protection and nurturance, and little experience with continuity in attachments and a dependable and consistent environment that are necessary to provide for the development of stable self and object representations.

SOME OF MICHELANGELO'S WORKS (1501–09)

THE FIRST MADONNA

Having outlined what is known and inferred about Michelangelo's early years, I turn to determining if and how his childhood influenced his artistic images, and whether these artistic solutions in turn yield insight into his inner experience of his personal history. As a preliminary effort in this direction, one of his first pair of sculptured works, *The Madonna of the Stairs* (fig. 1), commands attention for here is Michelangelo's earliest artistic statement about mother and child.

The *Madonna of the Stairs* was completed at age 16 while Michelangelo was living in the household of Lorenzo de' Medici. Art historians are divided as to whether this work is Michelangelo's first or second sculptured work.[7] This low relief is extraordinary in the originality with which he treated the most common subject in Renaissance art. This originality is particularly striking since, at the time, Michelangelo was a student and first learning the technique of sculpturing. Although the work bears a limited resemblance to an earlier fifteenth-century madonna by Donatello

7. I am disregarding a work alluded to by both Condivi and Vasari that was carved at age 14. It was a marble bust of a faun, a simple copy of a work that was available to Michelangelo who was then studying art at the school in the Medici gardens. The faun is lost and the only known "copy" of it is in a seventeenth-century painting by Ottavio Vannini, in the Pitti palace in Florence. It almost certainly represents the artist's fantasy rather than the actual appearance of the faun. According to Condivi, the beauty of the bust attracted the attention of Lorenzo, who, upon seeing the age of the lad who had sculptured it, decided to invite the young Michelangelo to live in his household in the Medici palace.

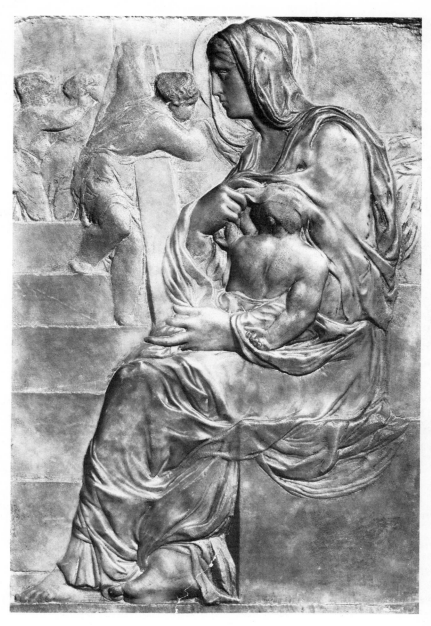

Figure 1. Michelangelo, *Madonna of the Stairs*

Florence, Casa Buonarroti (photo: Alinari)

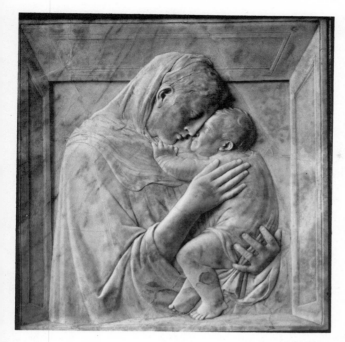

Figure 2. Donatello, *Pazzi Madonna*
Berlin, Staatliche Museen (photo: Museum)

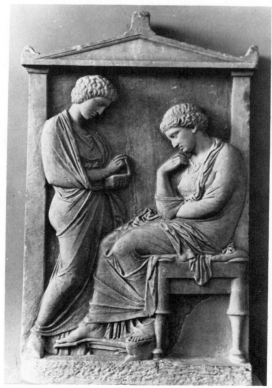

Figure 3. *Stela from Piraeus* (ca. 370 B.C.)

Athens, National Archaeological Museum
(photo: Museum)

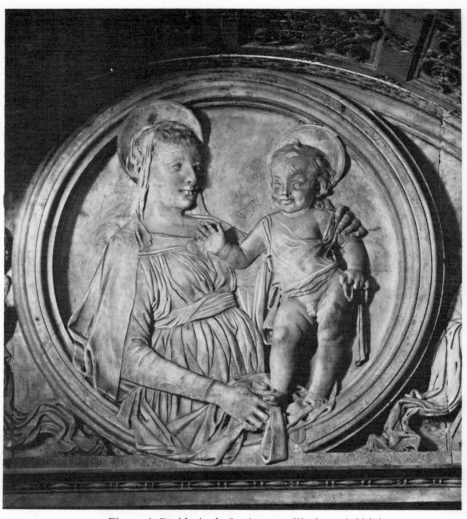

Figure 4. Desiderio da Settignano, *Virgin and Child*

Florence, S. Croce (photo: Alinari)

(the *Pazzi Madonna;* fig. 2), it is most dramatic that Michelangelo drew his primary inspiration from ancient Greek marble grave reliefs such as the *Stela from Piraeus* (fig. 3).

Michelangelo rejected as his model the typical contemporary Tuscan madonna in which she was almost always represented as a young bourgeoise, with Jesus depicted as the blessing saviour (for example, in Desiderio da Settignano's *Virgin and Child;* fig. 4). In these contemporary works the Virgin was rarely presented seated in profile and, with a single exception,[8] never in an upright position. Rather, Michelangelo looked back in time to a special group of works in which a deceased woman is forever commemorated in her image in stone. The stelae, incidentally, often present a dead mother being bid farewell by her child. Michelangelo's *Madonna* shares not only the positional attitude of the women of the stelae, but also their mournful solemnity. Instead of the Renaissance idealized maternal image, who sometimes has her gaze averted in sad foreknowledge of the tragic destiny of her son but is nonetheless in nurturing contact, Michelangelo's *Madonna* is stonelike and detached. Her appearance is all the more striking because of the situation depicted—nursing the child. In this connection, a comparison between Michelangelo's *Madonna* and Donatello's *Pazzi Madonna* (fig. 2) is particularly revealing. In nursing, her hands do not touch Jesus, whereas Donatello's Virgin is not only holding the child, but there is a mutuality both in their gaze and in their touching. Significantly, Michelangelo chose a motif of Jesus nursing at the breast (*Virgo lactans*), which had become quite rare in fifteenth-century Tuscan art.

As one studies this work more closely, several other revealing ambiguities emerge. Jesus appears to rise from her womb to nurse at her breast. However, rather than nurse, he appears to sleep. But it is the sleep of death, which is communicated by the symbolism of his pronated right arm. The arm in this attitude derives its meaning from the iconographic vocabulary of Roman sarcophagi. This pronated arm reappears 60 years later in the dead Christ of the Florence *Pietà,* which Michelangelo intended for his own tomb. Moreover, for the first time in Renaissance art, the child Jesus is shown with his back to the viewer, thereby both

8. The *Madonna of Maestro Andrea* (Rome, Ospedale di Santo Spirito).

increasing his ambiguity and emphasizing the primary role of the madonna in this work.

The interpretation of an artist's motivational currents on the basis of a single work is a hazardous undertaking. Rather, it is more fruitful to consider the single work as just one part of the fabric of attempted solutions to the unconscious challenge of a particular motif. At this point in Michelangelo's adolescence, however, certain lines of thought are suggested by the innovations in the *Madonna of the Stairs* that might tentatively be brought together in the following formulation.

Michelangelo was attracted to the task of creating a figure that embodies the idealized, nurturing mother of the Christian world. In his search for this woman, he is unconsciously compelled to reject the available contemporary repertoire and, instead, seeks the image from the prehistory of Christianity—from a figure of a dead mother, remembered and preserved only by her presence in stone. This is not one of the several traditional Marys—sad yet maternal. Rather, she is cold and stonelike, and strikingly unresponsive to her child. She is manifestly the fused image of Michelangelo's wet nurse and mother, both of whom were forever lost. The yearning to recapture the lost sense of well-being in a symbiotic union with the breast remains an intense force within Michelangelo. This concern is evidenced in the wet-nurse anecdotes in Condivi and Vasari. However, to yield to this regressive yearning is also to risk death—both in the union with the dead mothering one and in the unleashing of the impounded rage connected with the sense of abandonment so early in his life. Thus, it is the strength of these unresolved, traumatic childhood experiences and the continued unconscious attitudes toward his mothering figures and their object representation that found sublimation in this remarkably innovative treatment of the madonna.[9]

9. This formulation disregards the enigma of the four male children (three on the stairs and one almost off the right edge) who appear to be at play, in peculiar counterpoint to the grave image of the Virgin and Jesus. Varying interpretations of their iconography have been offered (see Tolnay [1943–60, vol. 1] for a summary). Two of the boys hold a drapery behind the Virgin, and it is likely that they are connected to the motif of angels holding the holy shroud, which appears in representations of the *Deposition* and *Pietà*. How-

The Holy Family (DONI TONDO)

If the interpretation proposed for the *Madonna of the Stairs* has validity, we would insist on consistent and supporting evidence from later artistic treatments of the same or similar motifs. Hence, to further test my initial hypothesis, I turn to a number of such works—painted, sculptured, and sketched—from the 1501–09 period.

The painted panel of *The Holy Family* (Doni tondo) (fig. 5) is Michelangelo's only painted madonna and is totally different in conception from the Virgin in his five sculptured madonnas.[10] This work, with its seemingly deliberate, enigmatic quality of major aspects, has always defied any agreed-upon, overall interpretation. In its general form in the round, and the separation of the holy family in the foreground and nude youths in the background. the painting derives from Luca Signorelli's tondo of the *Virgin and Child* (fig. 6), which he painted 10 years earlier for the Medici, in Florence. In the Signorelli tondo the background is a pastoral scene with four athletic shepherds in repose. Although Signorelli's shepherds exude a distinctly pagan and sensual beauty, they are there to execute the New Testament theme of the "select" to whom the birth of the Savior was announced and who faithfully watch over their flock as Jesus will come to care lovingly for his

---

ever, how does one explain the two boys at the top of the stairs who are fighting? Is there some private thought that Michelangelo is expressing through these four children? Do these four boys stand in for his four brothers? Are they the children of the stonemason's family at play while he was nursed by their mother? Or do the two that are holding the holy shroud (with which the crucified Christ is later to be wrapped) represent a different focus of identification for Michelangelo, whereby death wishes are expressed toward his younger brothers who were seen as usurping what nurturance was available from his mother upon his return to the family? These passing speculations are, of course, unanswerable. I would suggest, however, that the two boys that are rather incongruously fighting in this holy scene are expressions of the aggressive feelings that were engendered in Michelangelo when he addressed himself to this most maternal of themes.

10. *The Holy Family* was commissioned by Agnolo Doni, the scion of a prominent Florentine family, probably for his wedding.

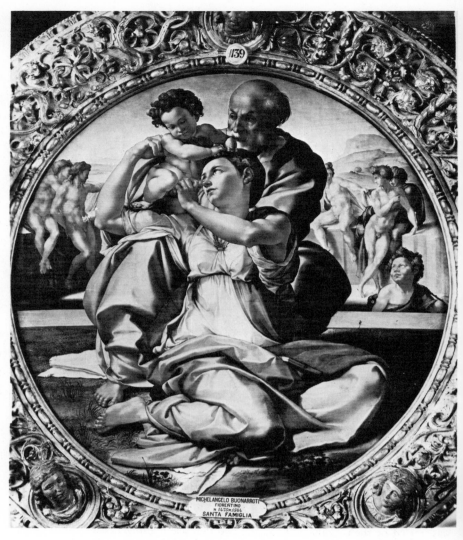

Figure 5. Michelangelo, *The Holy Family* (*Doni Tondo*)

Florence, Uffizi (photo: Alinari)

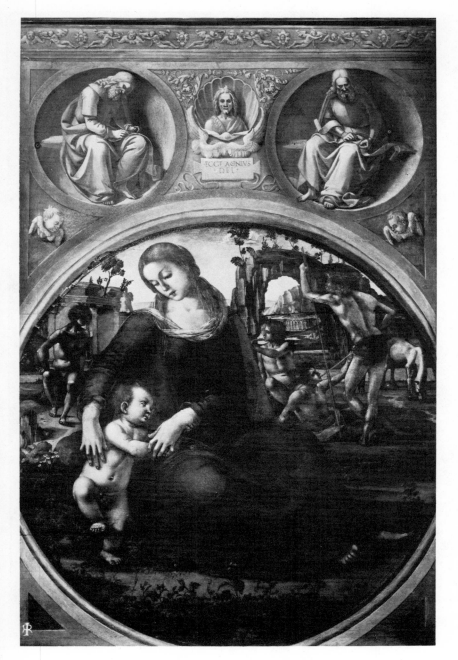

Figure 6. Luca Signorelli, *Virgin and Child*

Florence, Uffizi (photo: Brogi)

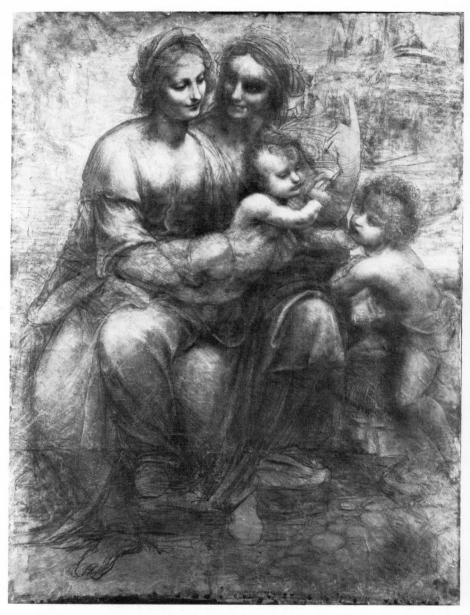

Figure 7. Leonardo da Vinci, cartoon for a *Madonna with St. John and St. Anne*
London, National Gallery (photo: Museum)

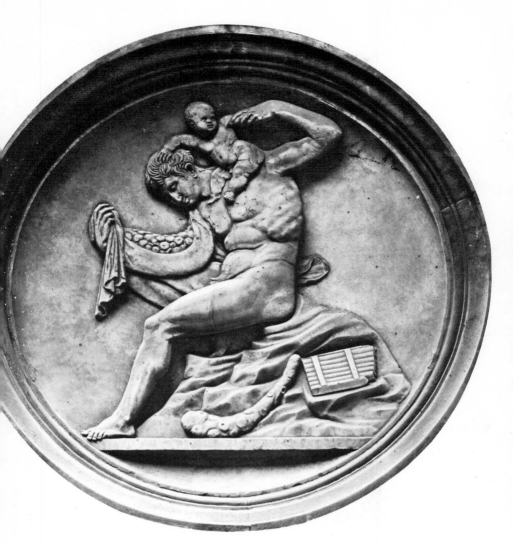

Figure 8. School of Donatello, *Satyr with the Infant Dionysus*
Florence, Palazzo Medici (photo: Alinari)

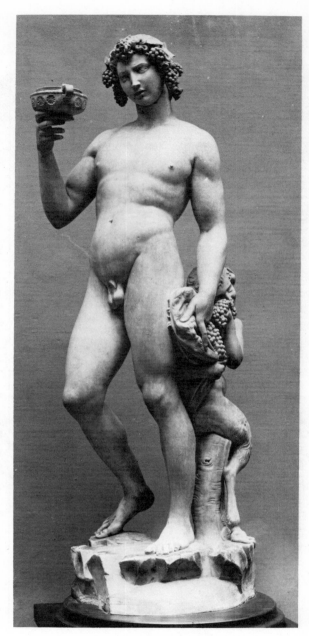

Figure 9. Michelangelo, *Bacchus*

Florence, Bargello (photo: Alinari)

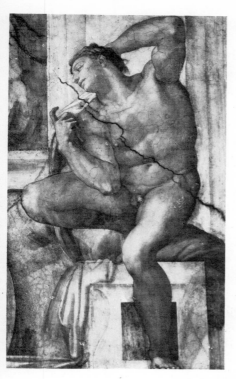

Figure 10. Michelangelo, *Ignudi*
Vatican, Sistine Chapel (photo: D. Anderson)

Figure 11. Roman copy, *Portrait of Euripides* (ca. 340–330 B.C.)

Naples, National Archaeological Museum
(photo: German Archaeological Institute)

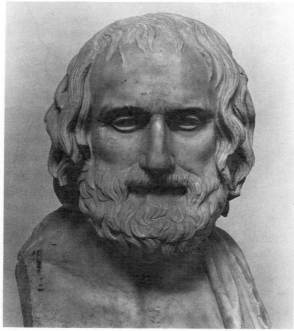

flock. In marked contrast, Michelangelo's background nudes have no such clear meaning or even connection with the primary theme of the holy family in the foreground or the child St. John in the middleground. In the most recent detailed art historical analysis of the work, D'Ancona (1968) concluded that the nudes are "homosexuals," who, as sinners, wait at the baptismal font for purification of their bodies and garments. In Signorelli's tondo, the background is thematically congenial and continuous with the foreground. In Michelangelo's painting, it stands in direct moral antithesis. Signorelli's shepherds have no need for moral redemption, whereas Michelangelo's nudes are sinners awaiting purification. Thus, in a manner that is characteristic, Michelangelo draws directly from an earlier model and then repudiates the inspiration by radically transforming the meaning of the original form.

The Doni tondo is, in a sense, "painted sculpture," in that the Holy Family trio of figures appears to be chiseled out of a marble block rather than created by the manipulation of the brush of color, light and shadow, and atmosphere. In this respect as well as in its rugged intensity, the work represents a direct confrontation with Leonardo da Vinci's prevailing serene and sublime ideal of beauty. In contrast to Leonardo's, Michelangelo's madonna is an earthy, masculinized peasant woman. Her arms are bared for the first time in Renaissance art, revealing their muscularity.[11]

The child Jesus mounts her shoulder like a triumphant Olympian, wearing the traditional fillet of victory around his luxuriant curly hair. Joseph stands behind, handing over but still supporting Jesus. This powerful figure of Joseph, rather than suggesting a simple carpenter, conveys an ancient wisdom and is, in all prob-

11. The great German art historian, Heinrich Wölfflin, refers to the Doni tondo as a "competition piece" (1899, p. 44). Another pathway in the evolution of the Doni panel can be traced by a series of drawings Michelangelo made in response to a particular cartoon of the *Madonna with St. Anne* (lost) by Leonardo (Hartt, 1970, drawings 9–14). Leonardo, after an 18-year absence from Florence, returned in 1500. In 1501, he exhibited the now lost version of the *Madonna with St. John and St. Anne* (fig. 7) for two days. According to Vasari, Leonardo's cartoon met with wild acclaim from huge crowds. We can easily imagine how the 26-year-old Michelangelo, who as yet had no major works in Florence and who had just returned from close to 5 years in Rome, bristled at the triumphant reception accorded the *Madonna* by the 49-year-old Leonardo.

ability, derived from portraits of Euripides from antiquity (Tolnay, vol. 1).

Alone, in the middle plane, stands the child St. John, half-sunken behind the wall of the dry baptismal font. He appears to be embarking on his life of lonely penitence in the desert. His head is positioned to repeat that of the Virgin, and his unearthly expression seems a mixture of awe and sadness. He also bears the crossed reed that foreshadows the Passion of Christ.

In the distal plane are the two groups of nude youths. The homoerotic interplay and competition for favor between the three figures on the right are rather explicit, while the two on the left idly observe them while leaning with easy familiarity against each other. The hairdress of the standing figure on the left gives him a decidedly androgynous cast.

Thus far I have attempted to narrow the issue of why Michelangelo's image of the Doni tondo took the form that it did to the outcome of the dialectic between two opposing impulses. On the one hand, he sought to incorporate something from two contemporary, but older Florentine masters—Signorelli's tondo, which hung in the Medici palace, and Leonardo's cartoon, which was widely celebrated in Florence. On the other hand, he was compelled to repudiate their influence and establish his own autonomy and superiority. Given this conflict, is it possible to be precise about why the Doni madonna became the particular image that it is? Is it an unprecedented creation by Michelangelo, or has he sought the model for the form of the Virgin and Jesus from a more disguised source?

With this work, as with the *Madonna of the Stairs,* the model for the madonna comes from a source with a pre-Christian theme and therefore had originally an entirely different narrative meaning. Smith (1975) persuasively proposed that the source for the image of the Doni madonna was a mid-fifteenth-century marble tondo, in relief, of a *Satyr with the Infant Dionysus* (fig. 8), executed by a follower of Donatello, which stood, as it does today, at the second story level of the courtyard of the Medici palace.[12]

---

12. The image of the Dionysus marble relief was, in turn, taken from a nearly identical image of the same theme in an antique sardonyx cameo that was recorded in the 1465 and 1492 inventories of the Medici collection. This cameo is now at the Museo Nazionale in Naples (Smith, 1975).

There are several parallels between the *Satyr* relief and the Doni madonna: (1) both infants are placed on the shoulder; (2) the near mirror image of the satyr's left arm and the right arm of the Virgin; (3) both infants balance themselves by placing a hand or hands on the head of the supporting adult; (4) the flattened, two-dimensional character of the Virgin's limbs are as if they were carved in relief; and (5) the horizontal band of stone that separates the holy family from St. John and the nudes is close to identical to the base on which the satyr and Dionysus rest.

Michelangelo daily had the opportunity to view the Dionysus relief during the 2 years of his residence in the household of Lorenzo the Magnificent at the Medici palace (1490–92). Moreover, it can be assumed that Michelangelo was extremely knowledgeable about the myth of Dionysus by the time he painted the Doni tondo. During his first stay in Rome (1496–98), he lived in the midst of a cultivated, humanist circle at the palace of Cardinal Riario, where he executed the statue of *Bacchus* (Roman name for Dionysus; fig. 9). We also have additional proof that the image of this particular satyr deeply impressed Michelangelo from one of the *Ignudi* on the Sistine Chapel ceiling, which is again a direct quotation of the same source (fig. 10). It may be further assumed that since this Dionysus marble relief was done by an unknown follower of Donatello, Michelangelo's attraction to the work cannot be ascribed to a special interest in the works of, or identification with, that particular master.

Thus, when Michelangelo made a direct quotation from an antique source, was it simply the unique form of the earlier model that was suitable for his purpose, or was the content or narrative meaning of the image what determined his choice of that one from among an infinite number of images available? If we adopt the latter assumption, we have a possible key to the latent meaning of the final, manifest image to the artist.

Next, I shall attempt to determine: (1) whether the myth of Dionysus as well as the specific element of an athletic young man holding him as an infant have significant features that resonate with Michelangelo's unconscious conflicts and fantasies; (2) whether this connection can be advanced beyond the more general, generic "Apollonian-Dionysiac" inner struggle that has become a tradition to ascribe to all great creative minds; and (3) why Michelangelo utilized this source of inspiration at this particular moment in his life, in the year 1503.

In the myth of Dionysus, several aspects of his birth and childhood stand out as being of possible relevance to the question of why Michelangelo was drawn to the Dionysus tondo.[13] First, there is the story of his birth. Zeus, in the disguise of a mortal, became the lover of the mortal woman, Semele, who became pregnant. Thereupon Zeus' wife, the Goddess Hera, jealously plotted the destruction of her rival by tricking Semele into persuading Zeus to reveal his true divinity. He reluctantly did, but in so doing the blaze of his thunderbolt was more than her human frailty could endure and she burst into flames. The fetus was rescued, however, by Zeus from the dead Semele's womb. He then implanted the fetus in his own thigh, where gestation was completed and from which the birth of Dionysus took place.

Immediately, the infant Dionysus was separated from his "mother-father," Zeus, and delivered to his first nurse, Ino, his dead mother's sister. Ino had to disguise the infant as a girl and keep him in the women's quarters to protect him from Hera's continued vengefulness. Nonetheless, Hera learned of Ino's deed and punished her by driving her and her husband mad. There are several versions of what then ensues. In all, however, the tragic climax is the inadvertent murder by Semele of her own son and her suicidal plunge into the sea—hence, disappearance from the very early life of Dionysus.

The child Dionysus' care was then entrusted to five divine nymphs, who faithfully carried out their charge. However, the child's education and preparation for his mission ahead was given over to an older and particularly debauched satyr, Silenus, who

13. The material on the Dionysus myth in this article is condensed from Apollodorus (50 B.C.–100 A.D.?), Deutsch (1969), Euripides (ca. 415 B.C.), Graves (1955), Guthrie (1950), Ovid (8 A.D.), Pomeroy (1975), and Rose (1959). Deutsch's monograph is particularly rich in psychoanalytic insight. We cannot precisely determine which version of the episodes of the myth were familiar to Michelangelo. The Greek tragic dramatists were not translated into Latin until the middle of the sixteenth century. However, Greek scholars among the humanists knew their works and may have spoken of them to the artist, although Ovid was the general source for pagan myths.

was, at the same time, a repository of liberating wisdom and sobriety.[14]

Consistent with his early cross-dressing and inconstant atmosphere of child rearing, Dionysus reached manhood with a noticeably effeminate bearing. Thus, in Euripides' *Bacchae,* when the young God makes his entry, as a captive, before the adolescent King Pentheus of Thebes, Dionysus asks, "What punishment do you propose?" The King replies, "First of all, I shall cut off your girlish curls" (line 492).

Hera, who personifies the primordial, destructive "witch mother," is unrelenting in her quest for vengeance. Upon discovering Dionysus, she places a curse of madness upon him, causing him to embark on his global wanderings in the company of his mentor and companion Silenus and a faithful following of satyrs and maenads. In the course of his travels he encountered repeated conflicts that ended in his bodily mutilation and death, only to be magically followed by his regeneration. Thus, Dionysus became the symbol of infinite rebirth, foreshadowing the Christian myth of the Passion and resurrection of the also divinely conceived Jesus Christ. It was, incidentally, this aspect of the life of Jesus that intensely preoccupied Michelangelo in the last 20 years of his life. The essence of Dionysus' mission was the uncompromising insistence on the necessity for those who came in contact with him to become aware of the demonic life forces that are the sources of fertility and creativity within all men.

In the best known episode in the myth, which comprises the Euripides tragedy, Dionysus returns to Thebes—his mother's homeland and burial ground. He is intent on the destruction of the Thebians who repudiated Semele for her alliance with Zeus. Here, as throughout the myth, Dionysus' unacceptable impulses are projected onto others, whom he then destroys with a sense of moral justification. In this instance, Dionysus' own rage toward his abandoning mother is projected onto the Thebians. In his coming to Thebes, we intuit Dionysus' quest to refind his mater-

14. The figure of Silenus in the Dionysus relief does not have the usual characteristics of a satyr—goat's legs or other bestial stigmata, or a perpetually erect penis; nor specifically of Silenus, who was traditionally represented as a plump and jovial old man, under the influence of the grape. Rather, the figure in this tondo is a muscular, fully human, young man.

nal origins, and also surmise the substitutive maternal function that is served by the increasingly large following of totally devoted women. The essence of the Dionysiac rituals promised women liberation, but actually involved them as destructive agents or the objects of Dionysus' destructiveness.[15]

The climax of the myth also may have held fascination for Michelangelo. Having established his worship throughout the ancient world, Dionysus was welcomed by Zeus to Olympus, to sit at his right hand. At this point, Dionysus embarks on his ultimate mission—to find and rescue his dead mother from the underworld, Tartarus, where she had been condemned. He succeeds in this mission and returns with her to Zeus' palace at Olympus. Thus, similar to the myth of Jesus and Mary, the eternal reunion of the triumphant son and his lost mother marks the resolution of the central motive of the myth.

Great myths endure through history because of their resonance with the psychological experience of most people of any epoch. Nonetheless, in the myth of Dionysus, there are a number of basic themes that can be thought to have specifically and deeply engaged Michelangelo. With the birth of Dionysus, an essential bisexuality is revealed in Zeus. Here, the most powerful of the Gods unifies the male and female roles in propagation. He is, at first, the agent of destruction of women as sole giver of birth and takes over for himself the functions of gestation and parturition. The birth out of the body of Zeus represents propagation without partnership— thus, the capacity of symbolic immortality. For Michelangelo, at the core of the artistic act, there was a unity of male and female procreative roles. He, too, could provide propagation without partnership and, indeed, looked to his creations as a buffer against his lifelong dread of death.[16] With respect to the nature of

15. Guthrie (1950) has summarized the Dionysiac rituals: "They have one almost universal feature, namely that the god's vengeance takes the form of visiting with madness the women of the land where he has been spurned. This usually leads to their tearing a victim to pieces, either the king himself who has been the opponent, or, when the women themselves have been the offenders, one of their own children. The two motives are combined in the Pentheus story" (p. 165f.).

16. There is almost endless evidence of Michelangelo's obsession with death in his letters and poems. He also openly expressed his concern to friends; Giannotti (1546), for example, attributed the following statement to the artist:

Michelangelo's sexuality, his life was most likely one of manifest abstinence. As a sculptor, which was his primary definition of himself as artist, Michelangelo could balance his maternal creative component with the masculine tools and action of the hammer, chisel, and hand drill. Rarely has there been a clearer monument to the bisexual nature and procreative aspirations of man than in the imagery and conception of Genesis on the Sistine Chapel ceiling.

A parallel exists between Dionysus and Michelangelo in their means of externalizing the feminine components of their self representations. The principal defense that Dionysus employed to ward off his femininity was to project it onto another. Thus, *The Bacchae* involves, in the course of its action, an exchange of masculine and feminine identities between Dionysus and Pentheus. Dionysus, by exciting Pentheus' curiosity about the secret rites in which his mother, Queen Agave, is immersed, is able to persuade him to assume the habitus of a woman. At first Pentheus protests, "I would die of shame," but this temporary renunciation of his masculinity as the price for viewing his mother's orgiastic activity eventually won him over. Once the transvestitic transformation has occurred, the text follows:

> PENTHEUS (coyly primping)
>   Do I look like anyone
>   Like Ino or my mother Agave?
> DIONYSUS
>   So much alike
>   I almost might be seeing one of them. But
>   look: one of your curls has come loose. . . .
> PENTHEUS
>   Arrange it. I am in your hands
>   completely.

Thus, Dionysus for the moment purges his own femininity by the exchange with Pentheus. Having succeeded, he brutally leads

---

"to think on death. This thought is the only one that makes us know our proper selves, which holds us together in the bond of our own nature. . . . Marvelous is the operation of this thought of death; which, albeit death by his nature, destroys all things, preserves and supports those who think on death, and defends them from all human passions" (Symonds, 1893, 2:310).

the King to his destruction at the hands of his mother. Similarly, Michelangelo could externalize this androgynous aspect of himself by the creation of a separate object, born out of his imagination. In this earlier period of Michelangelo's artistic life, the feminine component of his self representation safely finds expression in such androgynous creations as the *Bacchus* (fig. 9), the *Dying Slave*, Adam from the Sistine *Creation of Adam*, and the *Ignudi* of the Sistine Chapel.

Moreover, the theme of abandonment of Dionysus by early maternal figures has a remarkable parallel to Michelangelo's childhood. Both lost their mothers prematurely in death. Dionysus' first maternal surrogate, Ino, through no fault of her own, abandoned him. Similarly, Michelangelo was abandoned by his wet nurse. Out of his history of abandonment, Dionysus's underlying conviction of woman as potentially murderous is not confined to the Goddess Hera. He masters the anxiety associated with his passive position in relation to Hera's murderous intentions by actively staging filicide by mothers, in situations where he is in full control.[17] As I shall show in the analysis of Michelangelo's *Taddei Madonna*, his concern with the danger from a murderous mother, symbolized here by *Medea*, was the controlling unconscious force in the creation of that particular work.

In a sense, Michelangelo was faced with the same choice as Dionysus. If the young God were to accept his father as mother as well, he was left with the representation of himself as both woman and man by virtue of his identification with his bisexual father. The alternative was ultimately to resurrect his mother and bring her into his father's household, thereby establishing the two personae as separate and differentiated, under one roof. In the myth this resolution is achieved. Similarly, Michelangelo's consuming artistic preoccupation in the last two decades of his life was the theme of reunion of son and mother in the figures of the dead Christ and Mary in his final two *Pietàs*, now in Florence and Milan, in the series of drawings of the *Crucifixion of Christ with Mary at His Feet*, and in his last drawings of the *Madonna*.

17. The theme of filicide is dramatized in *The Bacchae* when Dionysus lures the decent Queen Agave into a state of madness during which she unknowingly murders her son, the youthful Pentheus.

In *The Bacchae,* which is an extraordinary explication of the unconscious dynamics of sexual identification, the effeminate Dionysus of the beginning of the play relinquishes this identification only with the liberation of his sadistic and murderous impulses against both a younger male rival, who, at the outset, has all of the trappings of stability and order that are associated with the nuclear family, and his mother. Although there are no descriptions of Michelangelo that suggest an appearance of effeminacy, we do know that he avoided relationships with women until his spiritual friendship with Vittoria Colonna, whom he met when he was 61 years old. From this we can infer that his feelings toward women were distrustful, fearful, and potentially vengeful, and that he defended against these feelings by his social pattern of avoidance.

From the available data about the institution of wet-nursing in general, coupled with Michelangelo's distrust and sense of deprivation, we can surmise that his actual experience of early mothering had been distorted in fantasy and transposed into an idealized form. The tale of the milk from the stonemason's wife endowing him as a sculptor is one element of this idealization. This corresponds with our consistent observation that children who have lost parents early in life, in their later recall, considerably distort, and idealize the parent and their experience with the parent into a wishful fantasy that also serves to deny their rage over the abandonment.

Just as Dionysus was prepared for the world by the sustaining presence of Silenus and other satyr mentors, Michelangelo lived in his all-male immediate family and then moved for the rest of his life from one to another male, mentors at first, and patron-protectors later.

Michelangelo's recollection of the 2 years that he spent in the household of Lorenzo the Magnificent emerges in Condivi's *Life* (1553) as the only years of his life that he came close to feeling unambivalently loved, cared for, and appreciated for his artistic gifts. This island of well-being at the Medici palace ended, however, after 2 years, with the death of Lorenzo in 1492, just as his stay with the wet nurse presumably ended after about 2 years. Both separations were followed by his return to his father's house.

The image of the Medici palace tondo, in which the infant Dionysus is cared for by a youthful, idealized representation of his debauched, old, male companion and mentor may have linked with his unconscious fantasy of Lorenzo as his unitary (i.e., bisexual) parent. Thus, in the stress of the years 1502–03, just prior to his beginning work on the Doni tondo, when Michelangelo was without a powerful male patron or mentor, an image associated with the relatively contented days in Lorenzo's household could have reasserted its power and influence.

For most of the period between 1496 and 1501, Michelangelo was in Rome. In those years he sculptured the *Bacchus* (fig. 9) and the *Pietà* in St. Peter's. Despite his economic hardship he was welcomed into the circle of the worldly Cardinal Raffaele Riario, at whose palace he lived part of the time. In addition, he received the appreciation and patronage of the Cardinal and his wealthy connoisseur friend, Jacopo Galli. There is a 2-year gap in the account of Michelangelo's activities from the completion of the *Bacchus* and *Pietà* in 1499, until 1501, when he returned to Florence, probably to begin the series of statuettes for the Piccolomini altar in Siena. No letters are preserved from those years.

With this background of the first Roman period I return to the question of whether the circumstances in Michelangelo's life during the period just prior to work on the Doni tondo were related to his calling upon the Medici Dionysus tondo as a primary model for the Doni madonna. The period preceding the Doni commission was basically a 2-year period of retrenchment and anxious anticipation. While living in his father's house in 1501, Michelangelo signed a contract for 15 statuettes for the Piccolomini Chapel in Siena. This project held little interest for him and, by 1504, when he dropped the commission, only 4 of the figures were carved. We know of other projects that he began and then turned over to other sculptors (e.g., the bronze *David*, lost), and of some that were never begun (the 12 *Apostles* for the Cathedral in Florence). His consummate endeavor during this period was the carving of *David*, which he began in the autumn of 1501 and completed during April 1504.

Florence itself during those years was in a period of relative stability as a result of its alliance with the French under King

Louis XII.[18] There was, however, no powerful paternal figure in Michelangelo's life such as the Medici, Aldovrandi (in Bologna during 1494–96), and Cardinal Riario and Jacopo Galli had been—and as the popes were to become, beginning in 1505 with Pope Julius II.

The *David,* which would firmly establish Michelangelo's stature in Florence, was yet to be completed. In fact, he worked on the *David* privately, hidden from public view. Thus, in 1503, the *David* was certainly an object of uncertainty and anxiety for him. His relationship with his patron, Agnolo Doni, was uneasy (Vasari, 1568).[19] Moreover, during this period, the nature of Michelangelo's patronage changed significantly. Instead of the powerful secular and papal patrons of before and after, most of the major projects of the 1501–05 Florentine period were municipal or corporate commissions.[20]

In sum, the period when the Doni tondo was conceived was a relatively calm one for Florence, but uncertain and unprotected for Michelangelo. Such a psychological climate would potentiate his yearning to recapture the security he felt when in his teens he lived at the Medici palace in the household of Lorenzo. This looking back carried with it associations to the Dionysus marble relief and the unconscious fusion of Dionysus and Silenus on the one hand, and Michelangelo and Lorenzo on the other.

The discussion of the Doni tondo to this point has focused on the image of Mary and Jesus. The next step is to explore the

18. In 1501, a decision was reached by the *Signoria* to undertake major constitutional changes toward further democratization of Florence. One result was that Piero Soderini, a champion of Michelangelo, was elected in November 1502 to a lifetime term as *Gonfalonieri.*

19. After a squabble over the terms of payment in which Doni tried to acquire the painting at a lesser price than originally agreed upon, the incensed Michelangelo delivered the panel only after forcing the Doni to pay double the original price. Possibly, however, Vasari has made up this tale as a warning to future patrons not to bargain.

20. The Board of Overseers of the Florence Cathedral commissioned the marble *David.* The Guild of the Wool Merchants commissioned the 12 *Apostles* for the Cathedral. The *Signoria* commissioned the bronze *David* and the painting (*The Battle of Cascina*) for the great Council Hall. Of these impersonal group commissions it is significant that Michelangelo completed only one himself—the marble *David.*

other figures as well as the unique composition of the entire panel in order to see if they can be related to Michelangelo's specific conflicts in self and object representations that determined the artistic solution of the madonna. The next figure to be considered is Joseph. Can he be related to the Dionysus myth? Even before Smith connected the Doni tondo to the Dionysus tondo, Tolnay (1:164) stated: "The head of Joseph seems to have been derived from antique portraits of Euripides (c.f. Naples, Museo Nazionale)" (fig. 11).

If this is indeed the source for Joseph, we have additional weight for the argument of a programmed fusion of the Dionysus and Jesus myths, in Michelangelo's own conscious identification with Euripides, the ancient dramatist most associated with the myth of the God.[21]

It is generally assumed from the detail of the book resting on Mary's lap that Joseph is handing Jesus to Mary. Nonetheless, this is unclear from the transaction taking place at her shoulder. Her fingers in both hands are clenched and therefore unreceptive and unsupportive of the infant. If Jesus did not seem to be marching forward, the Virgin might be assumed to be passing him back to Joseph. This ambiguous representation once again bespeaks Michelangelo's conflicted and ambivalent view of mothering figures.

Before turning my attention to the child St. John, I want to say a few words about the formal aspects of the work. The division of the work into three separate planes, each with its own narrative that is only remotely related to the other two, may be considered a parallel to the character of dreams. Further illumination can then be obtained by exploring the work in terms that follow the laws of dream structure. In the three-part organization of the tondo, as in a dream that is manifestly divided into several parts, the artist, like the dreamer, can play out several self representa-

21. Michelangelo's conscious identification with the figure of Joseph is also suggested by an aspect of the *Pietà* in the Florence Cathedral, carved almost 50 years later and intended for his own tomb. In the *Pietà*, the figure of Nicodemus stands in a highly comparable position to Joseph in the Doni tondo. Nicodemus stands behind the dead Christ and Mary, bringing them together for their final union. In the *Pietà*, however, Michelangelo's identification with the figure and role of Nicodemus was explicit, for, as Vasari recognized, it was Michelangelo's self-portrait.

tions through the disguise of the separate characters in each group of figures. Whereas dreams remain in their manifest content private symbols woven into a form that is incoherent unless clarified by knowledge of, or associations by, the dreamer, the artistic image involves the organization of the latent elements of content into a logical and coherent story presented in a recognizable form for the viewer.

What part of Michelangelo's self image is expressed by the child St. John, isolated and half-hidden in the middle plane? Traditionally, he is an integral part of the compositional unit of the holy family (e.g., Leonardo's cartoon; fig. 7). Therefore, the single most striking aspect of this child John is his exclusion from the family group. Moreover, he is presented with Michelangelo's characteristic ambiguity in facial expression and in action (is he departing from the scene?). Regardless of how his facial expression or action is interpreted, John's unprecedented placement in isolation commands speculation. It seems plausible that in this unit of the panel, Michelangelo has identified with the child who was the outsider, unnoticed by the parental figures who are totally engrossed with the other baby. With respect to Michelangelo's relationship with his father and brothers, it is clear that in adulthood he carried the conviction of having been "turned . . . out of my own house" (Ramsden, 1963, letter 238, written at age 69). That the Doni tondo can be regarded as a personal document is further borne out by the resemblance of the back of the font in the distal plane to a stone quarry, which may have been the artist's notation for the atmosphere of the stonecutter's household of his early childhood. Whether this is so or not, John may represent Michelangelo's sense of having been the outsider—the foster child in the family of his wet nurse and then again the outsider upon rejoining his parents, probably about the time of the birth of his brother Buonarroto.

In this connection, a sheet of sketches from the 1501–02 years is revealing (fig. 12). This worksheet of studies for a madonna includes a major figure of the Virgin that evolved into the *Taddei Madonna* (fig. 19) along with variations of the Christ child, including the principal one in the lower left that has the reversed flexed leg position of the Doni Jesus. This sheet, however, is

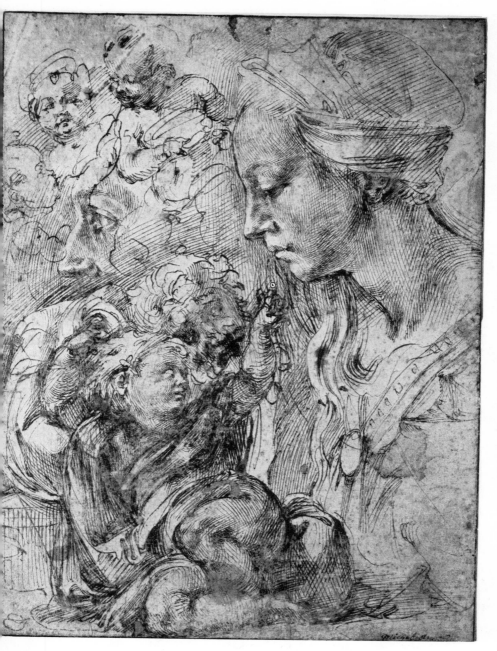

Figure 12. Michelangelo, Sketches and life studies for a *Madonna; Self-Portrait of Michelangelo*

Berlin, Staatliche Museen (photo: Jörg P. Anders)

highly significant because it contains the first self-portrait of Michelangelo. It can be recognized by its broad, low forehead; prominent cheekbones; broken, flattened nose; and short beard—all of which characterized his self-portraits.[22] What bears on my thesis is the placement of this picture of himself on this crowded sheet. He appears between, *but behind,* Mary and Jesus, gazing sideways at Mary with a forlorn, downcast expression. This placement communicates the same poignant longing and feeling of exclusion about himself as that with which Michelangelo endowed the Doni child John.

With respect to a more specific identification by Michelangelo with St. John the Baptist, it is necessary to turn to the myth of the Saint. The childhood of John receives only one sentence (Luke 1:80) in the New Testament texts. It is known to us through the apocryphal literature. According to the fourteenth-century version by Fra Domenico Cavalca, which was the standard for the subject during the Italian Renaissance, John, beginning at age 5, spent more and more time each day by himself in the woods. Then, at age 7, he decided to leave his parents forever and embark on a life of lonely devotion in the desert. The myth of the childhood of John revolves around the universal fear of abandonment or parental loss during the helpless condition of early childhood. Here, John cannot be cast out; he chooses to leave. The anxiety associated with the passive state is mastered by activity. His mortal parents in this process are exchanged for an aura of divine guidance and protection. In addition, his consuming vocation of baptizing converts for the remission of sin suggests the need for a ritual to assuage a body of unconscious guilt, for which expulsion from home would indeed have been an appropriate punishment. Nonetheless, the life of purity and even the performance of the baptism of Christ were insufficient to ward off the destiny that originally spurred his flight. Dionysus spent his lifetime warding off Hera's murderous efforts. John, however, was less fortunate and, in the end, met his death as a consequence of the murderous wishes of the reigning Queen Herodias, through the agency of her daughter Salome. Michelangelo may have easily

22. Hartt (1970) was the first who convincingly argued that this head was Michelangelo's self-portrait (drawing 10 in Hartt).

identified with the child John in the temptation to a lonely existence as well as the struggle between self-sufficiency and reliance on higher power (e.g., the Popes and the Medici). Both of these trends certainly did characterize Michelangelo.[23] None of the external glory that befell Michelangelo or the celebration that he encountered in the Papal courts could still his unrelenting state of loneliness. Like the odd child John, who left his parents to be a wanderer, Michelangelo also was a wanderer. Although sometimes compelled to move by the orders of popes or because of the prevailing political situation, he eventually chose to live the last 30 years of his life in a state of self-exile in Rome, separated from his family and roots back in Florence. Not even once did he visit.

John's mission in the wilderness illustrates the dynamic in the young child and adolescent where the choice of seclusion and penitence effectively functions as a defense against impulses of destructive rage toward the parents. This dynamic may well have unconsciously drawn Michelangelo to the myth of John. It is of interest that on five occasions during his life Michelangelo precipitously took flight from where he was to another city. All five flights are best understood as related to his fear of the eruption of unmanageable aggressive impulses at those moments. Moreover, an examination of the *Taddei Madonna* and the Sistine Chapel *Expulsion from Paradise* will provide more compelling evidence of the strength and influence of Michelangelo's unconscious struggle with the theme of a murderous contest between mothers and children.

The Doni tondo John's general expression reappears several decades later in the faces of the two young Medici dukes—*Giuliano* (fig. 13) and *Lorenzo,* in Michelangelo's Medici Chapel. From their tombs they both gaze across the silent space, looking at the image of the *Medici Madonna* (fig. 14). While this device functions effectively to unify the separate sculptural units in the Chapel into a cohesive whole, it also conveys the lonely and iso-

23. In 1495–96, several years before he began to work on the Doni tondo, Michelangelo carved a small statue of St. John as a child that was commissioned by a minor Medici, Lorenzo di Pierfrancesco. Whether the subject was dictated by the patron or was of special interest to Michelangelo is not known. In any event, the statue is lost and no copy exists.

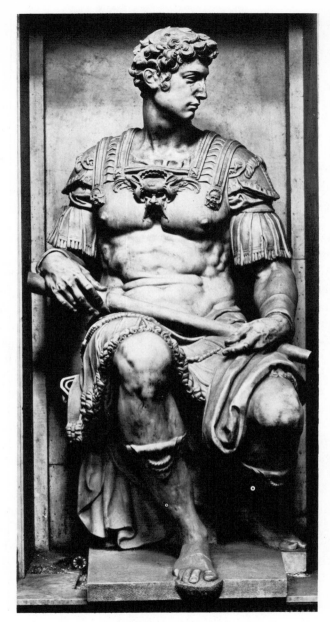

Figure 13. Michelangelo, *Giuliano de'Medici*

Florence, Medici Chapel (photo: D. Anderson)

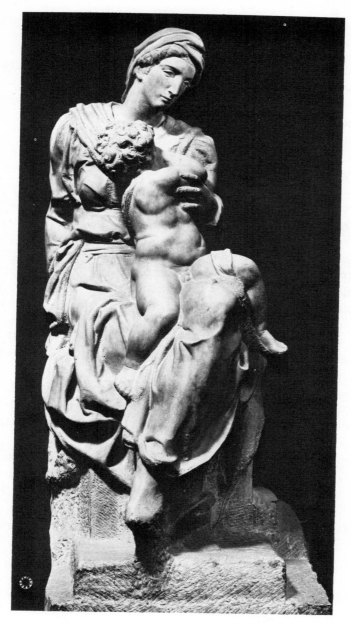

Figure 14. Michelangelo, *Medici Madonna*
Florence, Medici Chapel (photo: D. Anderson)

lated quality of two young men, prematurely dead, trying to make visual contact with the madonna, who is conspicuously oblivious to their plea. In addition, she offers little support to Jesus. Her right arm hangs limply at her side, while the seemingly self-sufficient, Herculean Jesus turns in vain to her clothed breast.

To recapitulate: in the near and middle planes of the Doni *Holy Family* there seems to be a consistency in two separate projections of Michelangelo's self representation and the object representation of his mother and her surrogates, growing out of their earlier complex interaction, and elicited by the subject matter of the painting.

Moving to the rear plane with the five androgynous youths in homoerotic interplay, I assume that the iconographic program was to create a moral contrast between the holy family (the world redeemed from sin by the triumphant arrival of Christ) and the world of sinners before redemption. The sinners that Michelangelo has selected, who appear to await cleansing at the baptismal font, are presumably homosexual. In terms of the overall formal demands of the tondo's composition and spatial organization, these nudes serve an integrating function, but no more so than landscape, a procession of magi, or shepherds could have. Therefore, why did Michelangelo give a homoerotic cast to his classical nudes? His ambivalence on the subject of their sin is clear. The official iconography designates them as "sinners," but, at the same time, they are drawn with a sensual abandon and dramatic style that could only be called "camp" in today's popular vocabulary (fig. 15). Moreover, they hardly seem penitent as they await baptism. In view of the strikingly unusual character of this part of the Doni tondo, we are led to wonder whether these nudes represent an image that was a central element in Michelangelo's fantasy life.

In an earlier study (1977a), I explored the presentation drawing of *The Rape of Ganymede* for Tommaso de' Cavalieri as well as Michelangelo's relationship with Tommaso. I concluded that, for Michelangelo, respite from the earthly terror of death and the anxieties of daily existence was invested in fantasies of a beautiful young male lover of an all-protective, powerful, older man. It should be emphasized that the fluidity of his fantasy life and mental organization enabled Michelangelo's genius to flower in many realms and also provided for several different, indeed contradictory, themes of fantasy as pathways for escape from the dreads that beset him.

In the Doni tondo, the motivational basis for the homosexual motif might be formulated as follows: the excluded child (John) attempts to cope with his inner rage at the rejection by his parents, particularly his mother, through a life of seclusive self-sufficiency and expiatory good works. Nonetheless, destiny cannot be altered and he ends up beheaded because of the vengeance of an evil queen-mother. Since the "John solution" does not succeed, a more narcissistic organization of defenses and behavior is required. Thus a world is created in which woman does not intrude and man is not vulnerable to her power to wound and betray. Such is the world of the distal plane of the Doni tondo. Parallel to the appeal of the bisexual aspect of Zeus in the Dionysus myth, these Doni tondo youths are conspicuously androgynous—that is, they have internalized and, to that extent, "become" the female. Hence, they neither need nor wish for females as real beings in their life space.[24]

Artists' sketches often serve as unguarded "associations" to the more finished paintings and statues and therefore are of considerable value. A series of drawings from the years 1501–02, the period

24. A connection with the theme of death and loss, which is the traumatic origin of the development of Michelangelo's homosexual self representation, can be found in the first reappearance of these youths after the bravura artistic exercise of the *Ignudi* on the Sistine Chapel ceiling. These figures reappear in an early drawing of the plans for the Medici Chapel, sketched in 1520–21 (fig. 16). In this drawing the slender nudes are in comparable postures, leaning on a cornice, but *here cast as mourners*. In the original plan for the tombs there were to be two double-wall tombs: one for Lorenzo the Magnificent and his assassinated brother Giuliano. The other was to be for the two Medici dukes—Lorenzo the Younger, Duke of Urbino, and Giuliano the Younger, Duke of Nemours. However, the tombs for Lorenzo the Magnificent and his brother were never executed. It is therefore equally possible that this drawing of the double tomb was the one intended for Lorenzo the Magnificent and that these androgynous youths from the Doni tondo reasserted their presence in Michelangelo's creative imagination when he searched for mourners for Lorenzo, the parental figure whom he remembered for the rest of his life with a singular warmth of feeling.

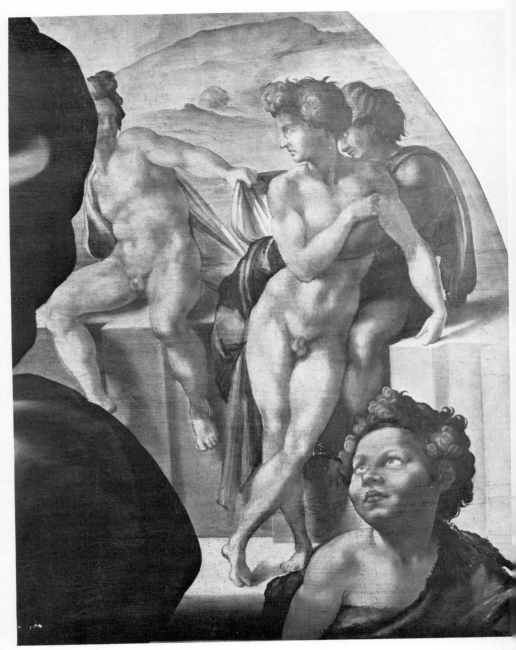

Figure 15. Michelangelo, *The Holy Family* (detail of St. John and background nudes)

Florence, Uffizi (photo: Alinari)

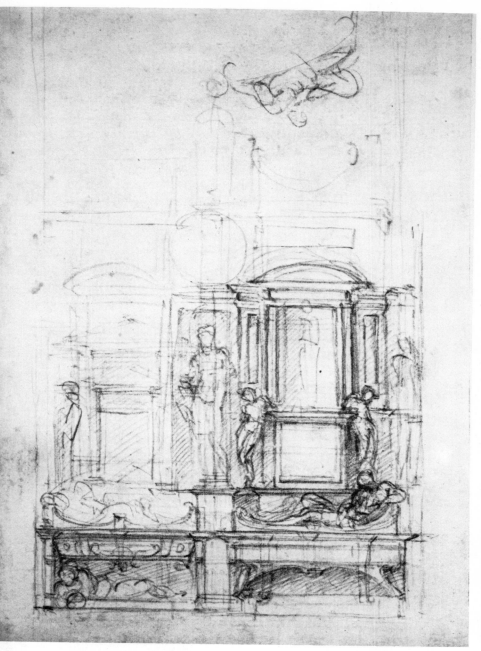

Figure 16. Michelangelo, Study for the *Medici Tombs*

London, British Museum (photo: Museum)

just before work on the Doni tondo, reveals parallels in the evolution from a position of being a frightened, excluded child in a family to a homosexual adaptation. I noted the placement of Michelangelo's first self-portrait between, but behind, Mary and the child Jesus (fig. 12). His next self-portrait appears in a *Study of a male back, four heads, and a self-portrait* (fig. 17). (The self-portrait is in the center when the sheet is rotated 90° clockwise.) Also on this sheet is a study of a young man, nude to his waist, with long curls. Significantly, he appears to be the model for both the madonna in the drawing in figure 12 and the profile of the face of the standing nude on the right in the Doni tondo. This same adolescent model, according to Hartt (1970), is used again in the drawing of *A nude youth, and two self-portraits* (fig. 18). In this study his nude body is fully revealed. However, Michelangelo has inexplicably tapered all four limbs into a triton's serpentine fins. A youth's face has been supplanted by that of a craggy, middle-aged man wearing a winged helmet. These two self-portraits are extraordinary in the frankness of their path of advance, so that the chin of one rests at the crotch of the youthful male body.

In these sketch sheets containing self-portraits from the 1501–02 period, there are two relevant lines of development. First, the model for the androgynous nude in figure 17 is used for the madonna in figure 12, a Doni tondo nude, and the nude triton with Michelangelo's self-portrait approaching the youth's crotch (fig. 18). Secondly, Michelangelo's head, with its taut and depressive set, moves sequentially from a position close to the breasts of the madonna in figure 12 to near the underdrawn penis of the triton in figure 18. This change in placements suggests a renunciation of the breast and women as sources of nurturance and a tentative movement toward the penis and men as more reliable and satisfying providers. Finally, the figure of the triton bears striking similarities to Silenus of the Medici Dionysus tondo (fig. 8). The three-quarter presentation of the muscular torso of the triton with the upraised, right, lower extremity, the knee acutely flexed, and the downward oblique cast of his left thigh is identical to the image of Silenus. This worksheet suggests, once again, Michelangelo's feeling of kinship with Dionysus, but now in the context of a clearer emergence of sexual elements. Goldscheider (1951) and Parker (1956) concluded that Michelangelo added the fins as a later afterthought, which is most apparent in the left arm. Perhaps Michelangelo introduced this bizarre bit of whimsy to divert and even ridicule the homosexual implications in the drawing. In the utilization of self-portraits in this manner, there is always the methodological issue of selective use to fit a hypothesis. In this case, however, the three drawings are widely accepted as authentic and there are no other drawings from this Florentine period that have been proposed as self-portraits.

A final important point concerning the nudes in the Doni tondo needs to be made. The haunting specter of painful exclusion persists in Michelangelo's contemplation of the homosexual solution. If one looks at the three figures in the group on the right, the two that are in embrace appear to be lovers, while the third glares at them and agitatedly tugs at the shroud that is connected to them. Thus, he too is alone and jealous. Perhaps the awareness that the insistent power of the identity as the abandoned and excluded one was such that it would pervade any attempt at a committed and sexual relationship was one of the principal determinants of Michelangelo's abstinence from a manifestly homosexual adult life.

Madonna and Child with St. John (TADDEI TONDO)

I have postulated that if an unconscious conflict is sufficiently strong to be a major determinant of the distinctive aspects of any particular work of art, it will reappear as a discernible influence in other works by the artist. Unconscious conflict fires great art but is rarely resolved by a successful artistic sublimation and solution for longer than the moment. In the discussion of the Doni tondo, I referred to the themes of filicide and matricide as underlying concerns of Michelangelo. These themes reappear in the marble relief of the *Madonna and Child with St. John* (fig. 19), which was executed for a Florentine patron, Taddeo Taddei, shortly after the completion of the Doni tondo, sometime during 1503–05.

In the Taddei tondo the child John holds a goldfinch before the child Jesus. The goldfinch foretells the Passion of Christ. Here, however, for the first time in Renaissance art, Jesus is clearly

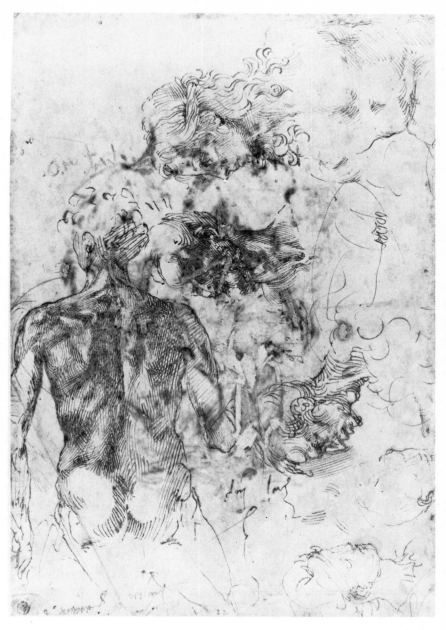

Figure 17. Michelangelo, Study of a *male back, four heads, and a self-portrait*
Oxford, Ashmolean Museum (photo: Museum)

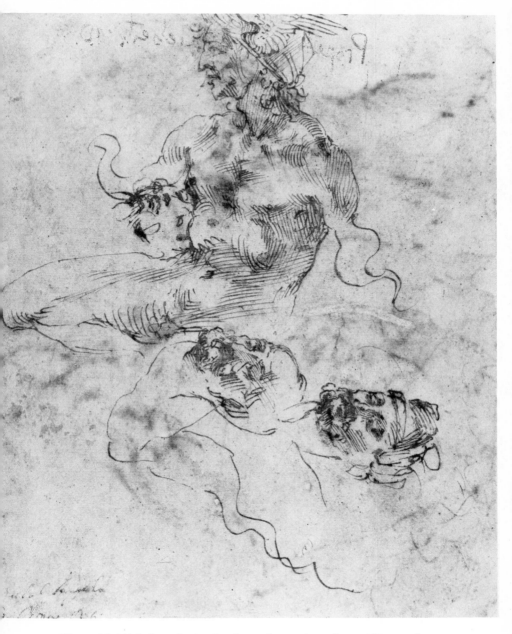

Figure 18. Michelangelo, Study of a *nude youth, and two self-portraits*

Oxford, Ashmolean Museum (photo: Museum)

frightened by the symbolic bird and tries to climb into Mary's lap for protection and comfort. Her facial expression is not the traditional, sadly averted gaze that conveys her own premonition of her son's tragic fate. Rather, her detachment has the same quality as that in the *Madonna of the Stairs* (fig. 1) and the *Medici Madonna* (fig. 14). Again, Michelangelo's need to integrate his conflicted inner representation of his experiences with his mother and wet nurse in this work is illuminated by tracing its sources. It has been proposed that the Taddei Jesus and John derive much of their compositional basis from the antique Roman *Medea Sarcophagus* (fig. 20), in which Medea's two sons are depicted trying to escape death at the hands of their mother.[25] The Taddei tondo is an example of Michelangelo's attraction to a manifestly terrifying narrative and subsequent transmutation into a work that is closely related in form, but opposite in motivational intent.[26] Although Michelangelo has attempted to deny the concept of the murderous mother of the Medea myth by transposing it into a narrative of a traditionally nurturing mother-child relationship, the defensive aspects of the sublimation are incomplete. The anxiety connected with the original filicide myth-fantasy persists and is reflected in the distinctive features of the Taddei tondo.

Thus, the Taddei tondo represents an attempt at resolution through creativity of one of Michelangelo's primary childhood conflicts. The child, terrified of death, seeks comfort, but in vain, from an emotionally unavailable mother. However, the anxiety remains manifest and therefore gives rise to an innovative artistic treatment of a most common subject.

A comparative dimension to the issue of the relationship of an artist's childhood experience to his later artistic treatment of a common motif can be gained by contrasting the Taddei tondo with Raphael's *Madonna of the Goldfinch* (fig. 21). Raphael painted this madonna in Florence, about 2 years after Michel-

25. Panofsky (1939), Pope-Hennessy (1970), and Tolnay (1943–60, vol. 1) are in agreement that the Taddei Jesus and John derive from the *Medea Sarcophagus* at Mantua, which was presumably known to Michelangelo.

26. The same process operated in Michelangelo in his conversion of the terrifying narrative of the antique *Laocoön* into the sensual, dreamlike *Dying Slave* (Liebert, 1977a).

angelo carved his Taddei tondo. Raphael, who was 8 years younger than Michelangelo, was in his early 20s at the time and in Florence was busy assimilating and condensing the art of Leonardo and Michelangelo into his own distinctive style. That Raphael had studied the Taddei tondo is clear from several of his drawings and from his painting, *The Bridgewater Madonna.*[27]

In Raphael's *Madonna of the Goldfinch,* Jesus tentatively investigates the goldfinch while sideling against Mary for reassurance of her presence. This Mary, however, in contrast with Michelangelo's, exudes an easy and natural warmth and sentiment that characterize Raphael's many paintings of the madonna. As in Leonardo's paintings, the delicate and harmonious background landscape sustains the tenderness of the mother-son relationship.

Can Raphael's treatment of this goldfinch motif be explained in terms of his personal history? A brief description of his infancy and later personality argues persuasively for the relationship between these forces and the painting style that is so distinctive of Raphael in his Madonna series.

Probably because it was so exceptional, Vasari (1568, vol. 2) wrote of Raphael having been nursed by his own mother due to his father's deep concern for his welfare, in opposition to the prevailing practice of foster-mother wet-nursing:

> He [Raphael's father] knew how important it is that a child should be nourished by the milk of its own mother, and not by that of the hired nurse, so he determined, when his son Raphael . . . was born to him, that the mother of the child . . . should herself be the nurse of the child.
>
> Giovanni [Raphael's father] further desired that in his tender years the boy should rather be brought up in the habits of his own family, and beneath the paternal roof, than be sent where he must acquire habits and names less refined, and modes of thought less commendable, in the houses of the peasantry [p. 20].

This passage is remarkable in that despite wet-nursing being the standard for the middle class in the Renaissance, Vasari con-

27. The drawings are: Raphael's *Sketches for a Virgin and Child* (Florence, Uffizi) and Copy after Raphael, *Virgin and Child* (Paris, Louvre). *The Bridgewater Madonna* is in the National Gallery of Scotland in Edinburgh. Taddei was also a patron and friend of Raphael.

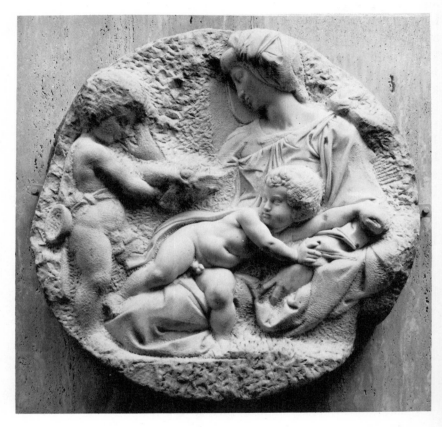

Figure 19. Michelangelo, *Madonna and Child with St. John (Taddei Tondo)*
London, Royal Academy of Arts (photo: Academy)

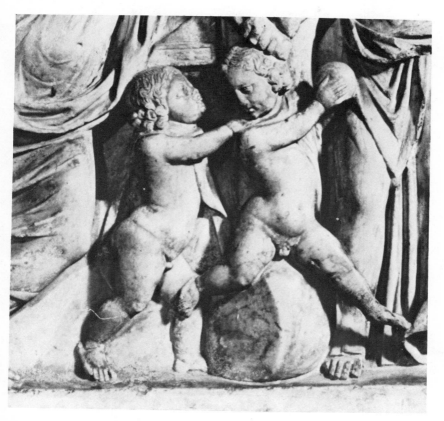

Figure 20. Early Roman *Medea Sarcophagus* (detail of fleeing sons of Medea)
Mantua, Palazzo Ducale (photo: Department of Art History, Columbia University)

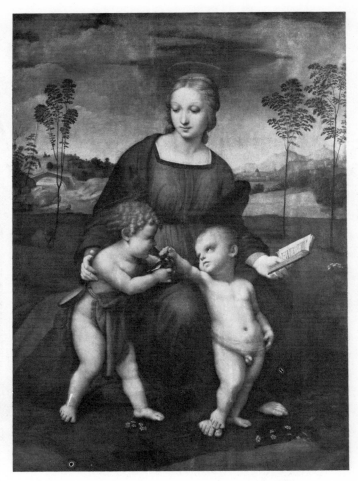

Figure 21. Raphael, *Madonna of the Goldfinch*

Florence, Uffizi (photo: Alinari)

veys Raphael's father's—as well as his own—awareness of the desirability of having the infant nursed by his own mother and of consistent maternal care.[28]

With regard to the linkage of early mothering, later character structure, and artistic style, it is informative to quote Vasari again in relation to Raphael's character:

> No less excellent than graceful, he was endowed by nature with all that modesty and goodness which may occasionally be perceived in those few favoured persons who enhance the gracious sweetness of a disposition, more than usually gentle, by the fair ornament of a winning amenity, always ready to conciliate, and constantly giving evidence of the most refined consideration for all persons and under every circumstance [p. 19].

Vasari's flowery prose is actually consistent with the gracious and amiable picture that we have of Raphael from other of his contemporaries. It is a picture that stands in dramatic contrast with the descriptions of Michelangelo, which were condensed in the term *terribilita* that became attached to him, communicating his unapproachability because of his awesome and frightening nature.

It has been the purpose of this brief comparison of the approach to the identical motif by Michelangelo and Raphael, executed at essentially the same time, in the same place, and in the early period of each of their careers, to demonstrate the relationship between the radically different artistic solutions and the equally radically different early histories of mothering and subsequent character development.

The Expulsion of Adam and Eve from Paradise

For Michelangelo, the subject of murderous impulses of mothers toward sons and sons toward their mothers continued as a con-

28. Vasari goes on to describe how Raphael's father took him to study painting with Pietro Perugino "though not without many tears from his mother, who loved him tenderly" (p. 20). This is, no doubt, a typical liberty that Vasari has taken with facts inasmuch as Raphael's mother is known to have died when he was 8 years old. His father did, however, remarry the next year. Nonetheless, as the information filtered down to Vasari (who was 9

flicted issue that significantly informed his art. Up to this point I have emphasized the child's fear of abandonment and the destructiveness of the mother. In the actual psychic life of a child, however, such fantasies are invariably only one component in the splitting of self and object representations; it also includes fantasies of oneself as destructive and responsible for the loss of the mother if that event has indeed occurred. This rage at the mother was suggested as one current of the defensive motivation underlying St. John's boyhood retreat to a life of penitence in the desert.

That the theme of his own matricidal impulses remained a powerful unresolved conflict for Michelangelo can be demonstrated in another work of this 1501–09 period—*The Expulsion of Adam and Eve from Paradise* (fig. 22). The *Expulsion* is actually only half of the panel of *The Fall of Man,* which was the fourth of the nine "histories" painted on the ceiling of the Sistine Chapel (probably in 1509). The left side of the panel depicts *The Temptation of Adam and Eve,* in which they reach for the forbidden fruit from the Tree of Knowledge at the beckoning of the Satan-serpent.

The *Expulsion* stands as Michelangelo's least original conception among any of the sections of the nine ceiling histories. It has long been recognized that it derives primarily from Masaccio's *Expulsion* (fig. 23), in the Brancacci Chapel in Florence, where Michelangelo spent long hours during his boyhood assiduously copying the earlier Florentine master's monumental frescos of 1427–28. Interestingly, Masaccio's image of Adam and Eve seems more dynamically communicative of the remorse and anguish of Adam and Eve at that irreversible moment than does Michelangelo's. Of critical importance, however, are some of the seemingly minor differences between the two works. In Michelangelo's *Expulsion,* Adam and Eve, apart from a slight rotation of their bodies, and a shift in the positioning of the legs and head of Eve, differ from Masaccio's in the defensive gesture of both of Adam's arms—as if he is warding off the unrelenting banishing angel.

---

years old when Raphael died in 1520), the impression of nurturing maternal care was well established. Perhaps it was the Renaissance intuition that anyone who could paint such tender madonnas as Raphael did must have been well mothered.

If one disregards the comparison with Masaccio's rendering of the figures, the face of Michelangelo's Adam expresses greater intensity and more inward torment than are to be found in any figure that he had created up to that time. Michelangelo's elevation of man through his Fall to the stature of a moral and psychological being has led Tolnay to observe: "Adam flees, pursued not by the angel, but by his own inner remorse; the movement of his arms is a form of defense against the furies of his own conscience" (2:32).

What "sin," i.e., what elements of troubled conscience, could Michelangelo draw upon from within himself to create so compelling an image? Part of the answer to this question may be advanced by once again locating the formal source for the Adam of this panel and then examining its narrative meaning. Simply to note that Michelangelo's *Expulsion* derives from Masaccio and, to a lesser extent, from Jacopo della Quercia's *Expulsion* in Bologna really adds little illumination to the creative process in Michelangelo since the theme of these earlier works is identical. In one crucial aspect, however, Michelangelo has not drawn his image from the earlier Italian *Expulsions*—the defensive gesture of Adam's arms, which are again rather direct quotations from a pagan source. In this case it is an antique Roman *Orestes Sarcophagus* (fig. 24).[29]

In the sarcophagus narrative, Orestes is attempting to fend off the furies, who accuse and torment him for the murder of his mother, Clytemnestra. In examining the position and gesture of Orestes' arms, we become aware that Michelangelo has virtually copied them for his Adam. The moment represented on the sarcophagus comes from the end of the second play of the *Oresteia* trilogy by Aeschylus—*The Choephoroe*.[30]

29. The derivation of Michelangelo's *Expulsion* from the *Orestes Sarcophagus* was first made by Walter Horn (cited in Tolnay, 2:134). Tolnay himself as well as Hartt (1964) support Horn's thesis.

30. In the sarcophagus, Orestes appears to be represented at the following point in Aeschylus' text:

ORESTES

> Look! Do you see those women, like Gorgons.
> All clothed in black, their heads and arms
>   entwined
> with writhing snakes! How can I escape?

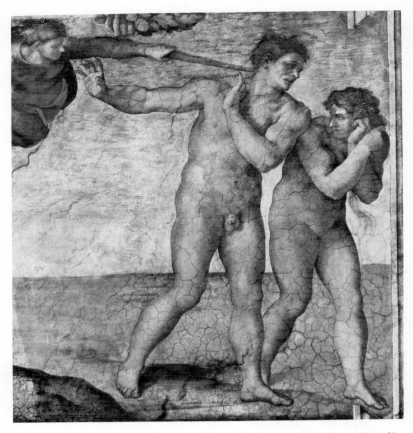

Figure 22. Michelangelo, *The Expulsion of Adam and Eve from Paradise*
Vatican, Sistine Chapel (photo: D. Anderson)

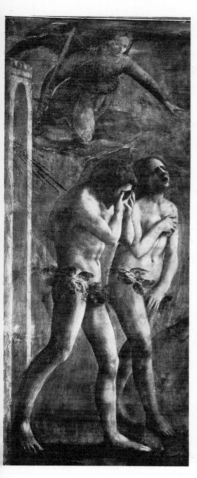

Figure 23. Masaccio, *The Expulsion of Adam and Eve from Paradise*

Florence, S. Maria del Carmine (photo: Alinari)

Figure 24. Early Roman *Orestes Sarcophagus* (detail of Orestes fleeing the furies)

Vatican, Museo Laterano (photo: German Archaeological Institute, Rome)

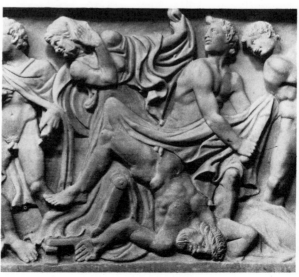

The trilogy begins with a social code of vengeance, in which the *Orestes Sarcophagus* partakes, and evolves by the end into a code of social and individual responsibility, aided by divine guidance, which allows for full forgiveness of Orestes' murder of his mother. Thus, the resolution of the *Oresteia,* with its justification and forgiveness of the murder of a mother, makes comprehensible Michelangelo's attraction to and use of this particular sarcophagus as a counterforce to the Old Testament verdict of banishment that is represented in the Sistine Chapel *Expulsion.* Michelangelo's drawing upon the *Oresteia* lends strong support to the conclusion that his own unconscious source of inspiration for the motif of the *Expulsion* was the unresolved and unneutralized residue of murderous impulses that he harbored toward his abandoning wet nurse and mother.[31]

SUMMARY

We cannot account for Michelangelo's endowment as a sculptor, painter, architect, and poet. No one in the Buonarroti family line

---

CHORUS
What imaginings are these. . . .
ORESTES
Imaginings! They are real enough to me.
Can you not see them? Hands of a mother's
curse!
CHORUS
It is the blood still dripping from your hands
That confuses your wits, but it will pass.
ORESTES
O Lord Apollo! See how thick they come
and their eyes are oozing gouts of blood! . . .
You cannot see them, and yet how plain
they are!
They are coming to hunt me down. Away, away!

31. A further theme in the *Oresteia* that may well have connected with Michelangelo's earlier wishful fantasies is that in the course of the third play of the trilogy, *Eumenides,* by virtue of Athena's divine intervention and persuasion, the furies who have vengefully tormented Orestes are transformed into benevolent deities—the Eumenides. The murderous women of earlier consciousness become the source of blessing and, indeed, the protectors of the lives of young men.

had ever been concerned with such matters, and his early inclinations toward art were actively opposed by his father. We can, however, address ourselves to the content and form that his art assumed by reconstructing his childhood and its later psychic representation. Michelangelo was profoundly shaped by the early terror with which he filled the void left by maternal disappearances. The bewilderment of what happens to the body—to his own as the abandoned, helpless one and after death—haunted him and, in time, became translated into an artistic vocabulary by which all meaning was expressed largely through the representation of the nude male. In contrast with the spirit of these Herculean beings, he suffered an unrelenting preoccupation with death. His hope, and sustaining unconscious belief, which informed so much of his art from the first to the last, was the reconciliation of son and mother. From the *Madonna of the Stairs* to his final *Rondanini Pietà,* waves of yearning, pity, and rage coalesced and broke forth in creative rushes, only then to recede. When they returned, it was with renewed intensity, artistry, and wisdom.

In this study I have attempted to isolate the representation of certain unconscious and unresolved early conflicts in Michelangelo that were among the basic determinants of the form and content of a group of paintings, sculptures, and drawings from an early period in his career. The first requirement in this task was a partial reconstruction of his childhood on the basis of those facts that are known about his particular developmental history as well as the usual child-rearing practices of the late fourteenth century in Florence. In this connection two special concerns were: his experience of boarding with a wet nurse from birth to about 2 years of age, and then, following his return to his natural parents, the death of his mother at age 6. The unconscious meaning and formative effects of those experiences were somewhat clarified by his own writings, other contemporary descriptions of him, and the nature of his adult relationships. Insofar as we are interested in the man because of his creativity, it becomes important to find from within the products of this creativity an independent method for revealing the conflicts and fantasies that compose the latent meaning in his artistic statements.

Inasmuch as the works of art tend to repeat in content the vocabulary of conventional motifs and stylistic conceits of the time, only limited conclusions can be drawn from the representation of a popular theme itself. Could one say much about a Renaissance artist because he painted many madonnas? Clearly not on that basis alone. With Michelangelo, however, in the case of many of his works, by locating the earliest source from which he derived aspects of the form of his own later creations, we have a promising starting point for understanding the distinctive and innovative qualities of his art. This is particularly true when the narrative of the early source is entirely different from the theme of his later derivative work. It has been my assumption that when Michelangelo was drawn to a specific antique work as a source for his artistic solution, it was not simply because of the magnificence and suitability of the antique image. It was, in addition, because the narrative theme of the early work deeply touched dominant unconscious themes in Michelangelo which made it compelling as a model. Moreover, the conflict in the original work was sufficiently disturbing that he was impelled to master the anxiety inherent in the conflict by transposing it into a theme that was manifestly quite different. Thereby, Dionysus and a satyr could become Jesus and Mary, Medea could become the Virgin Mary, and Orestes could become Adam. To what extent this process operated consciously or unconsciously in Michelangelo we cannot say. However, the content of the pagan themes that he transposed into sacred art informs us in a more specific and hierarchically organized manner of the conflicts bearing on his creative outflow.

The works that have been explored in this study emphasize the importance of splitting as a defensive operation in Michelangelo for coping with the potentially disruptive affects connected with contradictory primitive representations of early maternal imagos. The representations are, on the one hand, an idealized, all good image (the Madonna) and, on the other, a murderous and terrifying one (the Medea). The view of his mother as a Medea carried with it a complementary, affectively valenced self representation as the murderous, avenging son (Orestes), just as the view of his mother as Madonna was accompanied by an identification with Jesus—the martyred son who, resurrected, will rejoin his mother in the kingdom of God. On the basis of our clinical work, we may conclude that the 6-year-old Michelangelo conceived that his mother died *because* of his rageful thoughts and feelings, stemming largely from his early experiences of traumatic abandonments and sibling displacements. We may further venture that had his mother not died when he was so young, there would not have been the developmental arrest that occurred in the progressive integration of diverse constituents comprising the representation of mother and himself and, along with this, an integration of the clusters of affect, motoric discharge patterns, and particular behaviors associated with each part representation. These primitive formations would have become more completely repressed, and their associated affects would have been neutralized in the face of the corrective reality of his mother's living presence. Splitting would have yielded to repression as a more effective defense against the dangerous ideational and affective components of his early drive states. Central to Michelangelo's creativity was a fluidity in the level of organization of the inner representations of himself and objects, and in the range of affects associated with these part representations. This fluidity was the essence of Michelangelo's capacity to master and transform his tormented inner drama into art.

BIBLIOGRAPHY

AESCHYLUS (ca. 458 B.C.), *The Oresteia Trilogy,* tr. G. Thomson. New York: Dell, 1965.

APOLLODORUS (50 B.C.–100 A.D.?), *The Library of Greek Mythology,* tr. K. Aldrich. Lawrence, Kansas: Coronado Press, 1975.

CAVALCA, D. (1320–42?), La Vita di San Giovanni Battista. In: *Biblioteca scelta di opere italiane antiche e moderne,* ed. D. Manni & A. Cesari, vol. 4, Milan, 1829.

CONDIVI, A. (1553), *Michel Angelo Buonarroti,* tr. C. Holroyd. London: Duckworth, 1903.

D'ANCONA, M. L. (1968), The Doni Madonna by Michelangelo. *Art Bull.,* 50:43–50.

DEUTSCH, H. (1969), *A Psychoanalytic Study of the Myth of Dionysus and Apollo.* New York: Int. Univ. Press.

EURIPIDES (ca. 415 B.C.), *The Bacchae,* tr. W. Arrowsmith. Chicago: Univ. Chicago Press, 1959.

GIANNOTTI, D. (1546), *Dialogi di Donato Giannotti.* Florence: Sansoni, 1939.

GILBERT, C. & LINSCOTT, R. (1963), *Complete Poems and Selected Letters of Michelangelo.* New York: Random House.

GOLDSCHEIDER, L. (1951), *Michelangelo Drawings.* London & New York: Phaidon.

GRAVES, R. (1955), *The Greek Myths,* 2 vols. Baltimore: Penguin.

GUTHRIE, W. K. C. (1950), *The Greeks and Their Gods.* Boston: Beacon Press.

HARTMANN, H., KRIS, E., & LOEWENSTEIN, R. M. (1951), Some Psychoanalytic Comments on "Culture and Personality." In: *Psychoanalysis and Culture,* ed. G. B. Wilbur & W. Muensterburger. New York: Int. Univ. Press, pp. 3–31.

HARTT, F. (1964), *Michelangelo.* New York: Abrams.

——— (1970), *Michelangelo Drawings.* New York: Abrams.

HOLLANDA, F. DE (1548), *Michel Angelo Buonarroti,* tr. C. Holroyd. London: Duckworth, 1903.

KERNBERG, O. F. (1966), Structural Derivatives of Object Relationships. *Int. J. Psycho-Anal.,* 47:236–253.

LIEBERT, R. S. (1977a), Michelangelo's *Dying Slave. This Annual,* 32:505–543.

——— (1977b), Michelangelo's Mutilation of the Florence *Pietà. Art Bull.,* 59:47–54.

LUSTMAN, J. (1977), On Splitting. *This Annual,* 32:119–154.

OREMLAND, J. (1978), Michelangelo's *Pietàs. This Annual,* 33:563–592.

OVID (8 A.D.), *The Metamorphoses,* tr. H. Gregory. New York: Viking Press, 1958.

PANOFSKY, E. (1939), *Studies in Iconology.* New York: Harper & Row, 1972.

PARKER, K. T. (1956), *Catalogue of the Collection of Drawings in the Ashmolean Museum,* vol. 2. Oxford.

POMEROY, S. (1975), *Goddesses, Whores, Wives and Slaves.* New York: Schocken.

POPE-HENNESSY, J. (1970), *Italian High Renaissance and Baroque Sculpture.* London & New York: Phaidon.

RAMSDEN, E. H. (1963), *The Letters of Michelangelo,* 2 vols. London: Peter Owen.

ROSE, H. J. (1959), *A Handbook of Greek Mythology.* New York: E. P. Dutton.

ROSS, J. B. (1974), The Middle-Class Child in Urban Italy, Fourteenth to Early Sixteenth Century. In: *The History of Childhood,* ed. L. de Mause. New York: Harper & Row, pp. 183–228.

SEGAL, H. (1964), *Introduction to the Works of Melanie Klein.* New York: Basic Books.

SMITH, G. (1975), A Medici Source for Michelangelo's Doni Tondo. *Z. Kunstgeschichte,* 38:84–85.

STOKES, A. (1955), *Michelangelo.* London: Tavistock.

SYMONDS, J. A. (1893), *The Life and Work of Michelangelo Buonarroti,* 2 vols. London: Scribners.

TOLNAY, C. DE (1943–60), *Michelangelo,* 5 vols. Princeton: Princeton Univ. Press.

VASARI, G. (1568), *The Lives of the Artists,* 2 vols. New York: Hermitage Press, 1967.

WÖLFFLIN, H. (1899), *Classic Art.* London & New York: Phaidon, 1952.

The Psychological Effects of
Mutilating Surgery in
Children and Adolescents

ELSPETH M. EARLE, M.B., B.S., M.R.C. Psych.

MODERN MEDICAL AND SURGICAL TECHNIQUES HAVE DEVELOPED TO such an extent that children who would previously have died may now be kept alive, but at a cost to the emotional development of each individual. There is an increasing literature on the psychological meaning of even apparently minor investigations as well as major surgery to children. In this paper I want to concentrate on a group of children who had to have a limb amputated. Fortunately, this is not a very common procedure, so that the number of children in this group is small. I am concentrating on these because there is relatively little in the literature about children requiring amputation of a limb, and even less about its psychological effects on young adolescents.

These children must face and come to terms with problems in at least four areas: (1) the effects of being in the hospital and being subjected to investigations; (2) the anticipation, and in most cases the actuality, of having a limb amputated; (3) the effects of long-term chemotherapy; and (4) the anticipation, and in some cases the reality, of death. These four areas are, of course, closely interrelated, but I shall concentrate on the second and third be-

The author is Clinical Assistant in the Department of Child Psychiatry, The Middlesex Hospital, London, and Child Psychiatrist at the Hampstead Child-Therapy Clinic.

This paper was presented at the Wednesday Conference of the Hampstead Child-Therapy Clinic, London, June 1978.

cause it was problems in these areas which led to my being asked to see the children. My contact with them was based on their need and was not planned as a research project. I also cannot fully discuss the reactions of the parents or the staff, important as these are. Nevertheless, the observations I made pose significant questions, only some of which have been raised in the literature.

REVIEW OF THE LITERATURE

THE EFFECTS OF HOSPITALIZATION

Anna Freud (1952) described the effects of various nursing, medical, and surgical procedures on the child. The physically ill child has to renounce ownership of his own body and permit it to be handled passively, a condition that may exert a regressive pull toward earlier levels of infantile development. Those children who have built up strong defenses against passive leanings oppose this enforced regression to the utmost, becoming difficult and intractable patients; others lapse back without much opposition into a state of infantile helplessness. According to their interpretation of painful investigations and procedures, young children react to pain not only with anxiety but with other affects appropriate to the content of the unconscious fantasies—on the one hand, with anger, rage, and revenge feelings; on the other, with masochistic submission, guilt, and depression. Anna Freud also discusses the psychological meaning of pain and explains why doctors and other inflictors of pain are not merely feared but in many cases highly regarded and loved by the child.

Thesi Bergmann and Anna Freud (1965) describe how frequently children view surgery as a punishment and as a consequence of their own naughtiness. They note that, whether major or minor, surgery is likely to arouse the child's fantasies and fears with regard to being attacked, mutilated, and deprived of a valuable part of his own self. They also discuss the case of a 4-year-old who, despite preparations for amputation of her limb, reacted with despair and appeared lost and forlorn, grieving like a child who has lost a beloved person. They add that there is no adequate preparation for shocks and losses of this kind. Plank and Norwood

(1961) describe a girl of 4½ years who with the help of doll play was prepared over a period of 3 weeks for the amputation of part of both legs. The specially constructed doll could undergo the same medical and surgical procedures as the child, and the child could control these procedures. Healy and Hansen (1977) report similar work with a 2½-year-old boy in which they used a "like me-not me" doll to enable the child to master his fears; the doll also served as a means of communication for those who cared for him.

Becker (1972) reviewed the recent literature on doll play as preparation for surgical procedures and concludes that these play activities may, if used indiscriminately, have paradoxically countertherapeutic effects on some children. He suggests an alternative clinical model for direct psychotherapeutic presurgical and postsurgical intervention—the use of a mutual storytelling technique devised by Gardner (1971). The upper age limit for this projective technique is considered to be 11 years.

LOSS OF LIMB AND GRIEF REACTIONS

Kessler (1951) states that the "emotion most persons feel when they are told they must lose a limb has been compared with grief at the loss of a loved one. A part of one's body is to be irrevocably lost, the victim is incomplete and no longer a whole person" (p. 107f.).

Freud (1917) described the mood of mourning as a painful one. Reality testing shows that the object no longer exists and libido has to be withdrawn from that object. Parkes (1975) notes that adult amputees only occasionally pine for the lost limb; more often they pine for aspects of the world which are lost. I would add that in early adolescence the grieving is over the loss of the image of the self as a complete adult. Parkes found that in adult amputees interviewed 4 to 8 weeks after the loss, 10 percent of female amputees became tearful and half were preoccupied with thoughts of loss, had difficulty in believing the fact of the loss and avoided reminders. In comparison with widows, amputees were not expected to grieve, and friends and staff did not mention the loss or disposal of the limb. While the amputees had no visual or auditory illusions, 85 percent reported experiencing painful or other unpleasant sensations in their phantom limb at some time.

Gilder et al. (1954) describe the meaning of amputation to the patient in terms of threat to total body integration, phantom sensations, and the body image; they also discuss the effects of emotions on phantom behavior and the emotional reactions of others on viewing amputees. In two detailed case presentations, Gilder et al. demonstrate how important it is for patients to know whether the amputated limb has been cremated or buried. They also show that psychotherapy can help patients to get over the effects of painful phantom limbs.

BODY IMAGE AND PHANTOM LIMBS

According to Bailey and Moersch (1941), the occurrence of a phantom limb after amputation is almost universal, but Ewalt et al. (1947) noted that a painful phantom is infrequent. The occurrence of the phantom is explained as the patient's enduring concept of his total body image after the loss of a part. However, Kolb (1952) maintains that phantom limbs are not a problem in patients who sustained a congenital amputation or who underwent amputation in infancy. Kyllonen (1964) noted that if an infant under 1 year of age is fitted with a prosthesis, it becomes incorporated into the body image. Kolb (1952) believes that the shrinking away of the phantom demonstrates the modification of the body image which occurs as a result of the amputee's new sensations. The phantom shrinks away in an order reverse to that in which the impression of the body image was successfully built up through childhood. Pain in the phantom appeared to represent an emotional response which was psychologically unhealthy and maintained in reaction to anxiety or unresolved hostility.

Most of the above work was done with adults, but Kagen-Goodheart (1977) described the specific problems which adolescents have in "reentering" society and facing family, friends, and the community with a prosthesis and also while undergoing rigorous medical treatment. She describes a 16-year-old girl who was particularly sensitive about her appearance and was fearful of rejection.

Relatively little work seems to have been done by psychologists using projective tests with amputees. Two analysts, however, Silberpfennig and Mahler-Schoenberger (1938) recorded the responses of 17 amputees to the Rorschach test. Twelve still complained of phantoms and seemed preoccupied with restitution of the integrity of the mental image of their bodily representation. The amputees gave up 100 percent responses which had anatomical structures of the body as their content. Mahler (1968) suggests that the permanent trauma to the integrity of the body triggered a kind of permanent feedback to castration anxiety.

Jorring (1971) found that some patients, after the prosthesis had been fitted, continued to dream that they were walking on their own legs; but after they had accepted their handicap completely, they were using their prostheses even in their dreams. He also demonstrated that phantom-limb pains were immaterial if amputation dated back to childhood, in contrast to Lunn (1948), who found that 20 percent of child and adult patients experienced phantom pain. Noble et al. (1954), using the Draw a Person test in amputees, found that those patients who were adapting favorably often drew the amputated extremity smaller or omitted it, while those who were adapting poorly drew the missing extremity larger than the opposite limb or with increased markings.

Kaufman (1972) studied the body-image changes in physically ill teen-agers with the help of interviews designed to elicit fantasy material and the children's drawings depicting their illnesses and internal bodily functions. In all children the changes in the body were trivial in comparison to the changes in the drawings, although those related to internal and not external body change. Sandler and Rosenblatt (1963) describe how the child has to create a representation of that which is outside himself as part of his representational world. Sensations arising from the child's own body and its interaction with the environment result in the formation of a body representation. This self representation plays an important part in self-esteem.

COPING MECHANISMS

Lussier (1960) analyzed a 13-year-old boy with congenital abnormalities of both arms. This boy coped primarily by denying the reality of his handicaps, building a fantasy world from which the handicap was excluded and by resorting to reaction formations as defenses against insecurity and inferiority. He suggested that physically disabled people can be divided into two categories—the active and the passive ones. The passive individuals preserve the conviction that they could accomplish great things by avoiding test by action. The "active disabled" do not usually seek psychiatric help, and their reactions are usually dismissed as normal. This boy fell into the latter category; he overcame great obstacles, and his activity appeared to be creative and sublimatory.

Solnit and Priel (1975) studied young soldiers with burns leading to scarring of the hands and face. The appearance and competence of the hands are crucial for a sense of intactness. They also noted that the soldiers' returning interest in the outside world was often ushered in by demands, irritability, behavior that doctors and especially nurses experienced as lack of gratitude for the care provided by them. The unmarried soldiers' reactions to injuries were exaggerated by the apprehension that they would not be able to function socially, to have satisfactory sexual relations, and to find desirable young women to marry.

Norton (1965) described the management of catastrophic reactions in children. He postulates that the catastrophic reaction is a complex of defense mechanisms designed to ward off the profound anxiety which a person experiences when massive forms of bodily insult threaten the whole structure of his lifelong adaptive and defensive patterns.

DESCRIPTION OF TREATMENT

The Middlesex Hospital has become an oncology center and is admitting all children with bone cancer from the South of England. The Medical Research Council is supporting a new treatment regime which they hope will increase the child's chance of living. During a 2-year period 13 children ranging in age from 8 to 16 years were admitted with bone cancer. Ten of these— 7 boys and 3 girls—had an arm or leg amputated. The 3 who did not have a limb amputated already had secondary spread and subsequently died. Two others also died. The child who survived longest had her operation 36 months ago. The previous treatment for osteogenic carcinoma involved radiotherapy to the tumor and, if there was no spread, amputation after 6 months. The 5-year survival rate was less than 20 percent; it is hoped, however, that with the new regime, the 5-year survival rate can be improved to 50 percent.

The children usually contact their physician because of pain in a joint or bone. An X ray at their local hospital leads to a suspicion of the diagnosis of bone cancer. This diagnosis cannot be confirmed without a biopsy for which the child is usually referred to the Middlesex Hospital. During admission various procedures have to be carried out. After the diagnosis has been confirmed, the child must have full body scans and bone scans to prove that there is no secondary spread of the tumor. They also must have kidney tests to confirm that their bodies can deal with the cytotoxic drugs which will be prescribed. These tests take about 2 weeks. During this period I had some contact with the children, but only on a casual basis. I was not able to discuss the diagnosis or treatment because these had not yet been confirmed, but I was able to explore the child's fantasies.

It is important to realize that at no time were any of these children in psychotherapy with me. I was part of a team of doctors trying to care for them, but interviews were often not private or were interrupted by other ward events.

Once the diagnosis and treatment are confirmed, the parents are told that the child's limb will be amputated and that chemotherapy will follow. The child is usually told in the presence of his parents on the day before the operation will take place, and at the same time he may or may not be told about chemotherapy. If possible I saw the children on the day before surgery to give them the opportunity to share their feelings and distress. I also saw them immediately postoperatively and at frequent but irregular intervals during the 3 to 4 weeks they remained on the ward. During this time chemotherapy was started. This requires an intravenous injection or drip; the drugs induce nausea, and the child often vomits for the next 24 hours. The longer-term side effects include the loss of head and body hair, usually about 3 months after the initiation of the drugs. The drugs must be administered at 3-week intervals over 18 months. A child who may be feeling quite well must be readmitted to the hospital and made to feel ill, which makes it hard for both the child and the adults around him to continue their attendance at the hospital.

The children are primarily under the care of the orthopedic surgeon. However, because they are admitted to the pediatric ward, the day-to-day management is carried out by pediatric nurses, and day-to-day treatment is implemented by the pediatric medical staff. As a child psychiatrist, I was closely allied to the pediatric staff. I would see any child that they felt needed to be referred. Because I was on the wards most days, I would also know most of the admissions. At the time that this work was done we did not have a social worker specifically attached to pediatrics, but one of the social workers attached to child psychiatry would see the parents and other relatives of any child I was seeing if I felt that this was necessary. Either preoperatively or immediately postoperatively the radiotherapist would also see the child and the parents to decide on what chemotherapy had to be instituted. However, the treatment on each visit to the hospital was actually given on the pediatric ward by the pediatric medical staff. The fact that four different disciplines were involved in the management of each child and his family did, of course, at times lead to difficulties.

CASE DESCRIPTIONS

I want to describe briefly one child who slipped through the net before her surgery and was referred to me only after surgery: Mary was 8 years old, and had a tumor in the bone just above her left elbow. This was thought not to be malignant, and on two previous occasions she had had surgery in which the tumor was scooped out but the arm was saved. On her third admission to the hospital, the surgeon was not sure whether he would be able to save her arm or would have to amputate. This was discussed with Mary's mother, and it was decided not to tell Mary about the possibility of amputation because if it did not happen, she would have been unnecessarily worried. However, at surgery, it was decided that there was no way to save the arm and Mary had an above-elbow amputation. When she came round from the anesthetic, she did not at first realize that the arm had been amputated because she still had sensations in her phantom limb. However, very shortly she looked down and realized that she had only a stump, and then she reacted, I think appropriately. She was furious. She did not show her anger with her mother, who had stayed with her throughout, nor with the surgeon—she may have realized that her life depended on him—but she was angry with the nurses. She refused to let anyone of the nurses touch her, shouting that she would chop off their arms if they came near her. It was at this point that I was asked to see her. On the first occasion I talked only briefly to Mary. I acknowledged how angry she must be, at having been tricked, not having been told what was happening, and that naturally she wanted to get back at the grownups who had so badly let her down. She talked quite freely about her anger and also asked a number of questions about her arm and how she would manage without it. I felt that my main task was not so much direct work with Mary but helping the staff and her mother manage Mary. Her mother was very sensible and was able to answer some of Mary's questions, and when she did not know the answers, she checked with the nurses. However, it was the nurses who had the main problem. They are used to doing good work and being appreciated by their patients; they found it very hard to accept that a child may feel angry and not allow them to help. As Mary's defense of identification with the aggressors slowly diminished, she was able to talk with the nurses and begin to accept her disability, and when she was fitted with a prosthesis, she began to be able to use it. The splitting mechanism which she showed persisted—she was at no time directly angry either with the surgeon or with her mother.

Two years after surgery, I saw Mary on the ward. She was a happy little girl, who talked quite cheerfully with the nurses and demonstrated how her prosthesis worked.

Sharon, age 14 years, was admitted to the ward from another hospital, where she had been told that she probably had cancer and was coming to a specialist center for diagnosis and treatment. During the 2 weeks when investigations were being done, I got to know Sharon and spoke to her briefly on many occasions. However, when I tried to settle down with her to discuss the possible outcome of the investigation and what she thought might happen in treatment, she was unable to discuss this. There were no other children on the ward who had had an amputation, yet I suspected that this was on Sharon's mind. However, when her parents were told on the day before surgery that she would have to have her leg amputated, and Sharon was told about it in the evening, she shed no tears, and apparently was relieved that the painful limb would be cut off. When I spoke with her about the possible consequences of losing a limb and the sort of feelings she might have, she denied them, saying that she had helped her mother to get used to the idea, but that she herself was looking forward to getting rid of the pain and was sure that she would be able to manage with the prosthesis. This denial and cheerfulness were maintained through the immediate postoperative period. Sharon got hold of Douglas Bader's book *Reach for the Sky* and also wrote to Douglas Bader who became her hero. If he could fly again with two artificial limbs, she could lead a normal life with one, and she certainly appeared to prove this. Only 2 months after the surgery, Sharon completed a 20-mile charity walk on her crutches and earned money for other people who she felt were worse off than she.

In the immediate postoperative period, she asked very few questions about her artificial limb, but the questions did begin to focus on the side effects of the cytotoxic drugs. While she was in the hospital, she had the first two doses of drugs, and was told that her hair might fall out, and because of this she was measured for a wig. During these 3 weeks and on her subsequent visits to the hospital for chemotherapy, Sharon was preoccupied with fears of her hair falling out; what it would mean in terms of having boyfriends; whether she should tell her boyfriend that she had a wig; whether he would notice; whether anybody would be able to care for her if she did not have her own hair. She also asked if her pubic hair would fall out, and whether her periods would stop. We did not know the answer to her last question because none of the adolescents on the ward was receiving high doses of the drugs. We had to ask Sharon to record her periods and let us know about that. Although the threat of losing her hair was a reality, I tried to link it with her feelings about losing her leg, and the revival of more primitive fears—fear of loss of the object, fear of loss of love, and castration anxiety. Sharon continued to use denial in relation to her leg, but she did mourn as she began to lose her hair. She had beautiful long hair, and about 3 months after surgery, it began to fall out; as she sat brushing it, handfuls came away. During the ensuing admission to the hospital I helped her to grieve, not only over the loss of her hair but also over the loss of her previous image of herself as a girl with two legs who was physically active. Gradually she was able to accept herself as a girl who had some physical changes in her body but could still be active and could still be attractive to boys. Sharon returned to school at the earliest possible opportunity. She sat her "O" levels and is now studying for "A" levels. Since she has stopped her cytotoxic drug treatment, her hair is growing back, and she is able to accept her artificial limb in a more healthy manner. She does not deny its existence, but laughs, saying that she hangs it up at the end of the bed at night. She is not ashamed to tell people that she has an artificial limb, and she is able to look at her stump and deal with her limb entirely on her own.

John was 13 years old when he was admitted to the ward, having had a mid-thigh amputation of his right leg at another hospital one week previously. He was given a first dose of cytotoxic drugs and quite quickly discharged home. However, within 4 days he was back in the hospital with symptoms of nausea, vomiting, and general malaise. I was asked to see him and went over to the ward one evening. I found a tall, good-looking boy who was in early adolescence. As I sat talking to him, it became clear that he was having a panic attack, and I slowly tried to unravel with him what was going on in his mind. It seemed that the next day he was due to go to the limb-fitting center for his first appointment for a prosthesis. In his fantasy, he was going to be fitted the next day with a bionic limb. In spite of his positive identification with the "Six Million Dollar Man," he was panicked by the thought. Apparently he feared that the bionic limb would not be under his control but would have a life of its own and lead him into all sorts of difficulties. I asked John about his phantom limb and what sensations he had in it. He seemed relieved to be asked about this, and implied that nobody had warned him about the phantoms and he did not know that it was normal. He described the feeling that he could wiggle his toes, although when he looked down he knew that his leg was not there. This was thoroughly confusing to him. He also told me that he could feel his foot at about the level his ankle ought to be, and this also seemed strange, since it must mean he would walk with a limp if his limb were there. John was relieved when I told him that all these sensations were normal and that the fitting of an artificial limb did not mean screwing a bionic limb into the socket; it meant that he would have a leg which he could stand on, which he could put off and on at his convenience, and which he could learn to use in conjunction with his own leg. We canceled his appointment for limb fitting the next day and decided to keep him in the hospital for another 2 weeks to try to work through some of these feelings. Over the next 10 days I saw John daily. He told me how his foot was slowly moving nearer and nearer to his stump. Although this is the commonest way in which a phantom disappears, it seemed to me that John was using this as a way of controlling the loss of his limb, so that he gradually came to terms with the loss and with the change in his body image, until he was able to face the thought of having an artificial limb.

John's response to his amputation was also colored by his previous experience. His parents had separated when he was 7 years old. His father was living abroad, and John saw him infrequently. He resented his mother's new boyfriend and the fact that he had been sent to a boarding school. However, he had found a place for himself at school where he gained respect from both the boys and the masters by his achievements in cross-country running; he was scheduled to represent his county as a junior runner. Thus the amputation not only was catastrophic in terms of his loss of image of himself as an athlete, but it also revived castration anxiety and the loss of his father.

His father flew in from abroad to visit him, and John had the fantasy that perhaps he could bring his parents back together again and remove mother's boyfriend. John displaced some of his own fears about cancer onto his mother and became worried that her smoking would give her lung cancer and that she would die. Unfortunately, within a few months of his surgery John had secondary spread of the tumor and died.

For Catherine, too, coming to terms with the loss of her limb was colored by a previous loss. Because of the size and site of her tumor, there was some delay in deciding whether the leg could be amputated and how radical the surgery would have to be. During the time that this decision was made, Catherine's parents took her to Lourdes, in the hope that she would be helped in this way. Catherine was told 24 hours before the surgery that her leg would be amputated and that part of her hip removed. During that day Catherine regressed from being a fairly adult 15-year-old to a small baby, who clung to her father, had her arms around his neck, and sobbed silently most of the day. I saw her several times during that day, and on each occasion she asked not about the amputation but whether she would die under the anesthetic. She clearly felt that death was the punishment which she deserved, but I could not understand what she felt she had to be punished for until her father left the hospital that evening. Then I sat with Catherine and the story slowly emerged.

The person whom we saw with her father and assumed to be her mother was in fact the stepmother. Her sister was only a half sister. Catherine's mother had left home when Catherine was only 2½ years old and had not been heard of since. Her stepmother had moved into the house soon afterward, and the mother was never talked about. In fact, Catherine said that her father would be furious if he knew that she had told me about her own mother. Clearly, denial of the loss of her mother had not worked for Catherine, and she did not use it in relation to the loss of her leg; rather, she resorted to displacement.

Because the surgery involved more than the removal of the leg, Catherine had a stormy postoperative period, and I saw her frequently. She was relieved that she had not died, and slowly began to think about how she would live with an artificial limb. Catherine needed to know what had happened to her amputated limb. Her fear was that it had been discarded. Her wish was that it should be buried somewhere safe, so that she could go and see where that part of herself was. I linked this with her difficulty in getting used to her mother's absence when she did not know where her mother had gone. Finally, Catherine decided that her limb should be in a museum where everyone could see it. This was, perhaps, a grandiose idea, to defend against her loss, but it helped Catherine to give up her limb. Her fear for the intactness of her body was very clear. Because she had lost some of her hip-bone she was afraid some of her internal organs would somehow come out through the wound. She did not feel safe. She said that her sister did not want to come and visit her because she did not want to see her without a leg, and this was Catherine's attitude toward her discharge from the hospital—that nobody would want to see her and that there was no way in which she could lead any kind of normal life. There were many practical difficulties in fitting a limb, since there was no stump to fit it on; she had to have a complicated system of straps over her shoulder, which would help her to lift the limb. When Catherine was in the ward, a number of other children who had had amputations came up for their cytotoxic drug treatment, and they were able to answer many of her questions and show her how they fitted and used their prostheses.

Here I briefly mention Anthony, who was 12 years old when he had his leg amputated. He was extremely distressed in the postoperative period, but did go through a mourning process and apparently came to terms with a changing body image. His parents were very supportive, as was his boarding school to which he soon returned. Using his artificial limb, he played cricket and got some dents in his prosthesis, which then needed repairs. Six months after his operation Anthony went to the limb-fitting center, but on this occasion did not allow the doctor to examine his stump. This made fitting difficult, and Anthony was sent to a psychologist. He did not talk to her, claiming that she was more mutilated than he. On his next admission to the Middlesex Hospital for cytotoxic drugs I saw him. He was shy and embarrassed where previously he had been forthcoming. The nurses noted that, unlike during his previous admissions, he was secretive and would not let them see his stump. It slowly emerged that he was entering puberty; he was developing pubic hair, but thought the nurses and doctors would laugh at its scantiness. His penis was enlarging, but he had become preoccupied with fears of castration. It appears that both the dents in his artificial limb and his pubertal changes had rearoused castration anxiety, which he had mastered postoperatively but not adequately defended against. Over the ensuing weeks we worked through some of this anxiety and once again Anthony was able to work and play.

David was one of the few children who had been tested by the psychologist. During the year following his leg amputation he prepared a scrapbook containing drawings of the church adjacent to the hospital, the hospital itself, and his experiences in it. Under each picture was a description of the structural changes the buildings had undergone. It was striking to learn of the contrast between his pleasant and compliant manner to external situations and objects and his internal situation. In his human figure drawings he depicted blatant castration anxiety—fear and anger provoked by his surgery. His first attempt showed a boy with one eye missing and a deformed leg. He abandoned his second drawing when the parting of the hair further raised his castration anxiety. Finally, he produced a third drawing which not only looked normal but actually bore a remarkable resemblance to him.

DISCUSSION

Due to the particular circumstances of the hospital and the urgency of implementing the decision to amputate a limb, once this decision has been reached, there is very little time for preparation for surgery. It is difficult to know what would be an optimum time for preparation, particularly in preadolescence and early adolescence. With small children play methods can be used, but in one recorded case this did not appear to be adequate. Perhaps the consequence of major surgery cannot be fully anticipated and worked through in fantasy. Although some grieving can be achieved in anticipation, the reality has to be faced directly. The ways of grieving and the capacity to work through depend on the child's previous life experiences. In two of the cases described, the surgery revived grief feelings which had been inadequately coped with and the previous defense of denial broke down. Although I do not have enough information on the children, it is probable that Catherine's development had been severely interfered with by the loss of her mother at the age of 2½ and, confronted with the surgery, she regressed to a previous fixation point. She certainly behaved like an oedipal child in her relationship to her father and stepmother.

Anna Freud (1956) pointed out that in cases of minor surgery the child's fantasies about what will be done to his body outweigh in importance the reality of the operation. However, in major surgery of the nature described here, the child cannot anticipate the awful reality and his anxiety is relatively low.

The material which I have selected to discuss confirms the findings of other writers, but also adds something to them. It is unusual for children to have painful phantom limbs. Although all of the children had pain in the limb before amputation, none complained of a persistent painful phantom. The way in which the phantom was used, particularly by John, to have some control over a massive assault on the body, is also interesting. Many of the young adolescents who had an amputation were ashamed to let their family or friends see them at first. However, those, like Sharon, who previously had been secure in their image of themselves, were most able to overcome the shame. Siblings and school friends can be helped to accept the amputee, and visits in the postoperative period are important in helping the children feel accepted.

With regard to the body image, it is perhaps surprising to see the relative ease with which these young adolescents accept their mutilated bodies. We know that adolescence is a dynamic phase in the continuum of life, during which profound changes take place in physical, physiological, biochemical, and personality development. These changes normally lead to a person's feeling that he or she is a sexually attractive adult capable of reproduction. The body image is dependent on the impression a person makes on others and how his body appears to him. If a child has had a limb amputated, then others will notice and will react to him with horror, fear, sympathy, or indifference. The adolescent interprets anything that makes him feel different as being inadequate, which has to be defended against. His self-esteem is very vulnerable, and he needs constant reassurance from external sources.

I gained the impression that these adolescents were able to

value themselves. We know that amputations performed under the age of 2 years can be accepted into the body image. It seems to me that the early adolescent who is undergoing other bodily changes may be better equipped than an adult to accept this change. Provided that other physical changes progress normally, these young amputees can view themselves as sexually active adults. In this area the fact that our 13 patients all knew each other was helpful. At first we tried to keep them apart, fearing that if one died the others would become anxious. However, we could not keep them apart, and now realize that facing the death of a friend can be worked through. Moreover, the feeling of camaraderie encourages the children to find coping mechanisms.

The parents, too, found support, not only from the staff but from other parents who had faced the same painful problems of coming to terms with an ill, mutilated child. No parents rejected their child, and each found a different way of coping.

It is clear that each individual child reacts in his or her own way to the assault on the body. There seems to be a difference between coping mechanisms and defense mechanisms. On the one hand the child has to cope with a painful and unpleasant reality, on the other he has to defend against the fears and fantasies which this surgery arouses unconsciously. In the clinical management of these cases the role of the child analyst is to intervene only when a defense is becoming ineffective. This intervention is directed toward the support of effective coping mechanisms and to the modification of ineffective defenses.

Splitting is a common defense and appears to be successful in many cases. The child cannot be angry with and hate the person who he feels has saved his life. He therefore displaces his aggression onto the nurses or psychiatrist and in this way is able to begin to work through the trauma of the amputation.

This defense of splitting can, however, put great strain on the staff. Staff from four medical disciplines, plus nurses, social workers, and nonnursing ward staff were involved in the care of these children, in addition to their parents. Rivalries for the children's affection and misunderstandings between these adults could have hindered their ability to care for their patients. One of the ways this was diminished was by the ward staff groups. I met once a week with the nurses and teaching staff of the ward, and we were able to share feelings of distress and to discuss our understanding of what was going on with an individual child and between children on the ward.

Following the amputation most children's pain was relieved, but the cytotoxic drug regime imposed unpleasant effects on the children. It was hard for the doctors and nurses to subject the children to regular injections causing nausea and other disagreeable bodily effects, when doctors and nurses usually aim to make patients feel better. At times decisions had to be made to stop the treatment and accept that the child could not be cured but would require drugs for the relief of pain from secondary spread of the tumor. Some children who were dying were nursed on the ward, and others were discharged home; this was decided with the parents, but for all of us facing the death of a child is very hard.

Denial was also shown at various stages, particularly by Sharon, but it was not a successful defense. The side effects of the cytotoxic drugs produce further body changes but may also serve as a "second chance" to work through loss, both of body parts and of the body image. Sharon showed the defense of grandiosity in relation to her identification with a war hero, but appeared to be able to use this defense constructively in her return to physical activity. For John, the possibility of identifying with a hero held no comfort and made him more anxious about loss of control.

Catherine primarily used displacement; having dealt with her anxiety about dying, she was able to face some of her fears about the loss of her limb. The natural phenomenon of a phantom limb which slowly reduces in size was used by John as a way of his being in control of his amputation. He did not have to accept passively the massive trauma which was imposed on him.

Although it is evident that the child's previous experience, especially in relation to loss of an important object, affects the way in which he reacts to loss of a limb, we cannot predict which defenses will be the most prominent. I have not been able to expand on the reactions of the parents and caretakers to the child's loss, but clearly this profoundly influences the way in which the child copes. If the adults encourage denial or react with horror, the child is likely to identify with these defenses. One father described how ashamed he was to take his son to the swimming pool because the boy had to take off his wig and limb and hopped bald-headed like Kojak into the pool. The boy was of subnormal intelligence, but happily identified with Kojak.

This paper is based on clinical observations made during crisis work with adolescents undergoing amputation of a limb and long-term chemotherapy. It would be interesting to compare their reactions with those of children and adolescents who lose a limb through physical trauma. The hypotheses put forward need to be substantiated with more formal psychological tests. Our team now includes a psychologist who will be able to compare the children's drawings of a person before and after surgery and obtain their responses to the Rorschach test. Because of the distance which many children have to travel and the rigors of the treatment regime, it seems unlikely that any of these children will ever be in intensive psychoanalytic treatment, which would give us the best insight into the mental functioning of amputees.

In any event, it is essential to follow these youngsters into adulthood and see if the adaptations they have made are adequate or break down at a later stage.

BIBLIOGRAPHY

Bailey, A. A. & Moersch, F. P. (1941), Phantom Limb. *Canad. Med. Assn. J.,* 45:37–42.

Becker, R. D. (1972), Therapeutic Approaches to Psychopathological Reactions to Hospitalization. *Int. J. Child Psychother.,* 1:65–97.

Bergmann, T. & Freud, A. (1965), *Children in the Hospital.* New York: Int. Univ. Press.

Ewalt, J. R., Randall, G. C., & Morris, H. (1947), The Phantom Limb. *Psychosom. Med.,* 9:118–123.

Freud, A. (1952), The Role of Bodily Illness in the Mental Life of Children. *This Annual,* 7:69–81.

——— (1956), Comments on Joyce Robertson's "A Mother's Observations on the Tonsillectomy of her Four-Year-Old Daughter." *This Annual,* 11:428–432.

Freud, S. (1917), Mourning and Melancholia. *S.E.,* 14:237–260.

Gardner, R. (1971), *Therapeutic Communication with Children.* New York: Science House.

Gilder, R., Thompson, S. V., Slack, C. W., & Radcliffe, K. B. (1954), Amputation, Body Image and Perceptual Distortion. Naval Medical Research Inst. Project N.M. 004 008 04 03.

HEALY, M. H. & HANSEN, H. (1977), Psychiatric Management of Limb Amputation in a Preschool Child. *J. Amer. Acad. Child Psychiat.,* 16:684–692.

JORRING, K. (1971), Amputation in Children. *Acta. Orthoped. Scand.,* 42:178–186.

KAGEN-GOODHEART, L. (1977), Re-entry: Living with Childhood Cancer. *Amer. J. Orthopsychiat.,* 47:651–658.

KAUFMAN, R. V. (1972), Body-Image Changes in Physically Ill Teenagers. *J. Amer. Acad. Child Psychiat.,* 11:157–170.

KESSLER, H. (1951), Psychological Preparation of the Amputee. *Industrial Med. & Surg.,* 20:107–108.

KOLB, L. C. (1952), The Psychology of the Amputee. *Collected Papers of The Mayo Clinic,* 44:586–591.

——— (1959), Disturbances of the Body-Image. In: *American Handbook of Psychiatry,* ed. S. Arieti. New York: Basic Books, pp. 749–769.

KYLLONEN, R. R. (1964), Body Image and Reactions to Amputations. *Conn. Med.,* 28:19–23.

LUNN, V. (1948), *Om Legemsbevidstheden.* Copenhagen: Munksgaard.

LUSSIER, A. (1960), The Analysis of a Boy with a Congenital Deformity. *This Annual,* 15:430–453.

MAHLER, M. S. (1968), Comments on Dr. Löfgren's Paper. *Int. J. Psycho-Anal.,* 49:410–412.

NOBLE, D., PRICE, D., & GILDER, R. (1954), Psychiatric Disturbances Following Amputation. *Amer. J. Psychiat.,* 110: 609–613.

NORTON, A. H. (1965), Management of Catastrophic Reactions in Children. *J. Amer. Acad. Child Psychiat.,* 4:701–710.

PARKES, C. M. (1973), Factors Determining the Persistence of Phantom Pain in the Amputee. *J. Psychosom. Res.,* 17:97–108.

——— (1975), Psychosocial Transitions. *Brit. J. Psychiat.,* 127:204–210.

PLANK, E. N. & NORWOOD, C. (1961), Leg Amputation in a Four-Year-Old. *This Annual,* 16:405–422.

SANDLER, J. & ROSENBLATT, B. (1963), The Concept of the Representational World. *This Annual,* 17:128–145.

SILBERPFENNIG, I. & MAHLER-SCHOENBERGER, M. (1938), Der Rorschachse Formdeutversuch als Hilfsmittel zum Verständnis der Psychologie Hirnkranker. *Schweiz. Arch. Neurol. Psychiat.,* 40:302–327.

SOLNIT, A. J. & PRIEL, B. (1975), Psychological Reactions to Facial and Hand Burns in Young Men. *This Annual,* 30:549–566.

Children of Chowchilla

A Study of Psychic Trauma

LENORE C. TERR, M.D.

IN THE SUMMER OF 1976, 26 CHILDREN WERE KIDNAPPED IN CHOW-chilla, a rural community, population 5,000, in the San Joaquin Valley of California. Chowchilla is a middle-class town; there is some poverty, but no affluence. In June and July children attend summer school for morning academic courses and afternoon swimming.

At the time of the kidnapping, I considered volunteering my services, but I did not because no one in the community asked for help. In late November 1976, Dr. Romulo Gonzales, a Fresno child psychiatrist, forwarded to me an article "Chowchilla: The Bitterness Lingers" (Miller and Tompkins, 1976), in which several parents complained that no one was helping their children who by now were suffering from nightmares and fears. The newspaper article was an unmistakable plea for help. I phoned one of the parents who had been quoted in the article, and she responded at once to my offer of limited crisis treatment and a research study. I met with a small group of parents on December 16, 1976. The study, which began with 4 families, included by August 1977 each of the 23 child victims who has remained in

Assistant Clinical Professor of Psychiatry, School of Medicine, University of California, San Francisco.

This work was supported by a grant from the Rosenberg Foundation, San Francisco.

The library assistance of Esther Cagen is gratefully acknowledged.

547

Chowchilla as well as one or both parents. I did not interview the bus driver or the kidnappers.

Aims of the Study: The Chowchilla kidnapping offered an unusual research opportunity. Each child had been subjected to virtually the same external experience. The events had taken place away from parents or familiar adults. No one had died or had been seriously injured. The group was selected at random (by the kidnappers) and mixed in age, sex, and ethnic origins. The children were a "normal" day camp population because the summer school is regarded in the community as recreational, not remedial.

I undertook this study with two goals in mind: (1) to provide short-term treatment to the victims and to identify those who would require long-term intensive psychotherapy; (2) to learn more about the effects of a single traumatic event upon children and their families.

Freud's original theoretical constructs regarding psychic trauma are useful and durable. Stimulated by the study of individuals as well as group reactions to catastrophes in World War I, Freud (1920) defined

> 'traumatic' as any excitations from the outside which are powerful enough to break through the protective shield . . . there is no longer any possibility of preventing the mental apparatus from being flooded with large amounts of stimulus which have broken in and of binding them [p. 29f.].

In 1926, he added that the essence of the traumatic situation is the "experience of helplessness" on the part of the ego, which is suddenly and unexpectedly overwhelmed.

The application of Freud's theory to the understanding of group catastrophes has led to innovative approaches and advances in the understanding and treatment of individuals who have been traumatized as well as in the prevention of more long-lasting or serious disorders in those who have experienced disaster or who may face extreme danger in the future (Kris, 1941, 1944; Anna Freud and Burlingham, 1939–45; Lifton, 1967; Krystal, 1968; Kai Erikson, 1976).

Waelder (1960) stated, however, that Freud

looked forward to later investigations, by psychoanalysts, of the traumatic neuroses, and of the probable relationship between shock, anxiety, and narcissism.

But there was little follow-up along this line. The war neuroses disappeared with the war, and the interest of psychoanalysts was concentrated on the psychoneuroses, from there to expand, later, to character neuroses, behavior disorders, and . . . the psychoses, rather than to the traumatic neuroses [p. 166].

In fact, few, if any opportunities like the Chowchilla kidnapping have presented themselves for study of the effect of a psychic trauma upon an entire group. In order to gain a further understanding of the effects of trauma, especially upon children, I observed and interviewed the children of Chowchilla. The suddenness, the intensity, and the duration of the life-threatening conditions that were imposed upon 26 children make this study particularly applicable to the psychoanalytic theory of trauma.

Method of Study: During the first 5 months after the kidnapping, the victims received no psychiatric help. Three of the children moved out of the community. Over an 8-month period, I interviewed each of the remaining 23 children and one or two parents from each family at least once. Most interviews lasted approximately 1 hour. Seven children preferred group interviews with siblings and/or parents. Longer blocks of time were provided for family interviews, which elicited developmental data and recent historical material. Interviews took place in the junior high school science room in the winter, and at a picnic table in the town park in the summer.

Group meetings were offered for those parents who wished to discuss mutual concerns. A consistent group of 5 or 6 families attended these informal meetings for about 3 months, and 3 more formal general meetings for all parents were held subsequently. In view of the traumatic nature of the kidnapping and the press coverage, I chose to write notes during the interviews rather than to use a tape recorder. I discussed my interpretations with the child and with a parent. The interviews were both investigative and therapeutic. I asked the parents not to discuss the study with reporters in order to insure that the evaluations could proceed without interference. The parents and children guarded the study well. Two recent books by reporters about Chowchilla make no mention of direct psychiatric contact with the children (Miller and Tompkins, 1977; Baugh and Morgan, 1978).

General Group Characteristics: The group consists of 17 girls and 6 boys, ranging in age from 5 to 14 years. There were 7 sibling and 2 cousin groups. The 14 families ranged from extreme poverty to middle class. There were 16 Caucasian youngsters, 6 Mexican-American children, and 1 American Indian child (see table 1).[1] In regard to serious preexisting family problems, the

Table 1

Age Groupings, Sibling and Cousin Groupings

Latency (5–8)	Late-Latency, Prepubertal (9-11)	Pubertal (10–14)
Mary (5)[a]	Jackie (9)[e]	Terrie (10)
Susan (5)	Celeste (9)[fx]	Rachel (12)[cy]
Benji (6)[b]	Barbara (9)[g]	Janice (12)[g]
Ellen (6)[cy]	Elizabeth (9)[a]	Bob (14)
Sally (7)[cy]	Debbie (10)[cy]	
Leslie (7)	Alison (10)[x]	
Mandy (7)	Sammy (10)	
Tania (8)[b]	Carl (10)[dy]	
Louis (8)[dy]	Sheila (11)[fx]	
	Johnny (11)[e]	

[a-g] Indicate sibling groups.
[x-z] Indicate cousin groups.

children can be divided into three groups: 5 children whose families had had no serious problems, 8 children whose families had had one; and 10 children whose families had exhibited two or more major difficulties. By "serious problems" I am referring to separation or divorce, alcoholism, major mental illness, vio-

1. The ages cited in the examples of the children are their ages when kidnapped. Only common American fictionalized names are used in order to protect the children's identity. Names of towns, states, and community members are also fictionalized.

The quotes used are direct quotes from my handwritten notes. For brevity's sake, ellipsis points have been eliminated.

lence, death, frequent moves from place to place, or a chronically ill sibling in the family. Families were viewed in one additional way: the strength of family bonding to the community. The families of 10 children had strong communal bonds prior to the kidnapping, mostly due to the presence of large extended families nearby.

Preexisting Problems in the Children: Only 1 child of the 23 had been considered by parents to have an emotional disorder prior to the kidnapping, Benji (6). There was no phase of development he had "sailed" through. Teachers considered him very bright, but hyperactive. He had been spanked at home for stealing, lying, and playing with matches. About 1½ years prior to the kidnapping, he saw a psychiatrist, who told the parents that Benji did not require treatment, but the family had been dubious about this opinion, and asked their family physician to consider medicating the child. Benji had been placed on pemoline (Cylert) and had improved, but he remained impulsive and difficult to manage.

In reviewing the children's histories, it could be reconstructed that 3 other children (Louis, Leslie, and Janice) had had unrecognized emotional disturbances before the kidnapping. Louis (8) had fallen on his head several times. His family migrated between two states, often living without enough heat, water, or food. Louis had "silly" habits, such as repeatedly sticking out his tongue. He had been promoted to third grade, although he could not read at all. ("I need glasses," Louis explained.)

One year prior to the kidnapping, Leslie's mother had decided to cut off all contact between Leslie (7) and her natural father. Mrs. L. suffered from severe asthma, and Leslie feared that she might lose her mother as well. She was a serious child and probably had been depressed for some time.

Janice (12) at age 7 had discovered the body of her younger brother who had been accidentally electrocuted. She stopped learning for 2 years, and experienced repeated nightmares and daydreams of her dead brother's face for 5 years. At the time of the kidnapping, Janice already had a chronic posttraumatic stress disorder!

Two children suffered from serious physical disorders. Sammy (10) was legally blind. He studied Braille, rode a bike (much to his mother's pride and fear), but was unable to participate in sports. His nystagmus worsened whenever he was "nervous." Alison (10) has had rheumatoid arthritis and asthma almost all her life. On many occasions she has required joint aspirations, steroid injections, splints, and emergency treatment for wheezing.

Some parents noted less persistent difficulties in their children's development. Debbie (10) earlier had been willful and demanding. Celeste (9) did not talk at all until 2, was stubborn, and unable to discuss her feelings, but she was a brilliant student at school and popular with peers. Sheila (11), Celeste's sister, had been fussy as an infant and demanding later in childhood, often threatening to run away if she didn't get her own way. Jackie (9) had not been a cuddly baby, but became more affectionate in recent years. Bob (14) has never been able to speak about his feelings. Elizabeth (9) was overconcerned about her parents' problems. Carl's stepfather often beat him for "lying" or for his "bad attitude."

Manifestations of these preexisting problems were observed in the children's initial as well as in their long-term reactions to the traumatic event.

THE KIDNAPPING

On July 15, 1976, 3 men wearing stocking masks kidnapped 26 children, who were riding a school bus home from summer school. They held them for 27 hours, at which point the children and their bus driver escaped. The kidnapping took place in stages: (1) A white van blocked the right-hand lane, and as the bus slowed down to pass, a gun-carrying stocking-masked man forced the driver to open the door. Two masked men jumped onto the bus, one ordering the bus driver and the first three rows of children to the back, and the other driving the bus. The kidnapper who had originally stopped the bus followed in his van. Both vehicles pulled into a slough, or dry creek bed, where an empty green van was already parked. (2) The youngsters were transferred from the bus into two vans; the older children from the front of the bus into the white van, and the younger children and the bus driver into the green van. Siblings were separated in many instances. The van windows were painted or boarded over. (3) The children were driven around in total darkness for 11 hours with no opportunity to eat, drink, or make a bathroom stop. A barrier separated the children from the kidnapper-driver. (4) At about 3:30 A.M. the youngsters were transferred one by one from the vans into a "hole," actually a buried truck-trailer. Under a tentlike canopy, a stocking-masked man asked each child's name and, in most cases, took from the child a personal possession such as a shirt, a pair of glasses, or a toy. The child was then sent down a ladder into "that hole." (5) The children were now reunited in a large space eerily lit with flashlights. There were stale breakfast cereals, potato chips, peanut butter, and water. "Bathrooms" were two wheel-wells, one for boys, the other for girls. A few heard a kidnapper say he'd be back. Sounds of shoveling and dirt falling above the "hole" were then heard for about an hour. (6) The children remained buried in the "hole" for 16 hours. A "crisis" occurred when Louis (8) knocked away a supporting post and the roof began to collapse. This led the bus driver and a few boys to examine the roof where they discovered that a metal plate and two 100 lb. batteries could be moved from an enclosed space at the top. The boys could just squeeze into the space and attempt to pry up the top of a wooden cubicle the kidnappers had constructed over the original entry area. Considerable amounts of dirt had to be scooped down into the trailer as the top was lifted. (7) The labor went on for hours, during which time many children slept or were passive. The active children included 2 boys, Bob (14) and Carl (10), who "dug"; 2 boys, Johnny (11) and Sammy (10), who removed dirt; and a girl, Terrie (10), who held the flashlight. The bus driver helped move the metal plate and batteries, "dug" for a short time, and he lifted children when they escaped. (8) The children egressed one by one into twilight. Bob and Carl, who had dug the others out, hid when they emerged from the "hole," fearing that the kidnappers were waiting nearby. The bus driver located a phone, called the police, and the entire group was taken to a nearby prison for questioning and sporadic sleep. The stay away from home extended into the next morning. Each child was met by his or her own family, as well as by a gathering of townspeople, officials, reporters, and TV cameras.

The children had spent about 36 hours away from the community. During this time the families of the kidnapped youngsters anxiously awaited word of what had happened to the children. For 27 hours no word was received. Then the families had to wait until the children were examined and "debriefed." Thus the total period of separation was approximately 43 hours.[2]

THE CHILDREN'S INITIAL RESPONSES

The events during the kidnapping itself were reconstructed through my interviews with the children 5 to 13 months after the kidnapping. Their descriptions of their own behavior and of their peers' behavior were vivid and detailed and corroborated each other to a remarkable degree.

Reactions to the Masked Men with Guns: At the moment of the bus take-over, 8 boys and girls were immediately aware of the danger. They recognized that the guns were real. Because hunting is a popular pastime in central California, guns are often kept at home. Mary (5) recognized them at once: "I knew guns. I thought they'd shoot." Tania (8) recalled, "I thought it might be a joke, but the guns were real, and I was scared." Johnny (11) looked at the guns and felt "a tingle in my back." Leslie (7) remarked, "I knew it was a kidnapping and I cried." In fact, Leslie was the only child in the group who remembered knowing throughout the 27 hours that they had been kidnapped!

Other children recognized the guns and the danger, but were unable to conceptualize the entire procedure as a kidnapping. For example, Susan (5) in her interview consistently referred to the kidnappers as "crooks." She complained, "The crooks took my lunch pail and my brand-new swimming suit. I thought they were robbing the whole bus." Several children used the word "robbers" instead of "kidnappers" in their interviews. Tania (8) did not say "kidnap" until October 1976. Mrs. C. stated that Celeste (9) used the phrase "when we were gone" instead of the word "kidnap." Celeste told me, "I shut off my mind and try not to think about

2. Because the kidnappers did not testify at their trial, their motivation for kidnapping these youngsters is unknown.

it." Louis (8), who is afraid of drowning, was convinced the men had entered the bus in order to "kill us and throw us in the ocean." Jackie (9) and Johnny (11) thought initially that they were victims of a joke. When the masked men entered the bus, Johnny mocked with his hands raised, "We didn't do it." Quickly, he realized it was not funny. Sammy (10), who is legally blind, was totally confused about what was happening. Terrie (10) at first believed the men were sheriffs, and later felt confused.

Misperception of the kidnappers' appearance was an early stress response. Four children misidentified the men immediately, one misidentified a kidnapper later, and one "saw" an imaginary fourth kidnapper. These misperceptions contributed to the "fourth kidnapper hypothesis" which terrified many of the victims long after the kidnappers had been arrested. When the bus was taken over, Jackie (9) saw "a man with one leg who used his shotgun as a cane." Celeste (9) saw a "lady" from whom she hid. "It looked like her hair was curled. My cousin Alison thinks it was a lady too." Sammy, hampered by his feeble vision, perceived a "bald man" driving the bus after it had been taken over. Benji (6) thought "one guy was black." Debbie (10) "saw a fat chubby man when they took our names." Tania saw "someone sitting in the green van when we got off the bus." No other child saw such a "person."

Janice (12) reacted to the kidnappers' faces with immediate fear. For 5 years Janice had dreamed and daydreamed about her dead brother's face. When the kidnappers entered the bus, Janice was horrified by their mask-covered faces. Since the kidnapping, she often dreams of their faces, and these are entirely separate from the continuing dreams about her brother's face. During the day at school Janice thinks of "the guys—what they looked like. I stop doing my work. My grades have gone down bad. I used to be a C or better, now I'm C's and D's."

Reactions to Transfers: Transfers from bus to vans and from vans to "hole" led to several anxious reactions, especially in the group age 8 or above. Since moving from one place to another involved unanswerable questions about what would happen next, several children imagined horrifying possibilities. Seven children in both vans (Bob, Jackie, Johnny, Debbie, Sheila, Tania, and

Carl) believed they would be shot as they were moved one by one out of the bus or vans. They had seen or heard about movies in which soldiers were told to get out of trucks, only to be shot as they exited. Because of a discussion in the older children's van about being shot, some youngsters vied for position of exit. Debbie (10) recalled, "In the van, I thought they'd shoot the first 2, the middle 2, and the last 2, so I went third to get out." Jackie (9), who imagined being lined up and shot, remembered, "I had seen *Serpico;* there was a charter bus which pulled into a garage and they said they'd shoot them and then drove off. Well, maybe not *Serpico.*" The children's fantasies of being shot have become the basis for repetitious traumatic dreams.

During the second transfer from vans to the "hole" the kidnappers asked each child his or her name and took a personal object. Sammy (10), though legally blind, was forced to give up his glasses. He related, "The man who drove the van tried to touch me. I threw my shoes at him when I was going into the hole—brand-new ones, one day old. I hit him in the arm. I aimed at his face. It bounced off his arm and hit me in the forehead." Mandy (7) was forced to give up a towel she had borrowed from a friend, and worried subsequently about her friend's reaction. Elizabeth (9) was forced at gunpoint to surrender a new tee shirt which ironically read, "I'm a lover not a fighter. Be nice to me." No children objected to or worried about giving the kidnappers their names. Benji (6) warned the men when they asked his name, "Don't hurt Susan or I'll get you!"

Reactions to the Van Ride: The 11-hour ride on the vans was bumpy, dark, hot, smelly, and tiresome. Jackie (9) fainted three times. Terrie (10) suffered a nosebleed. Because no bathroom stops were made, the problem of continence vs. incontinence was a major dilemma for each child. Janice (12) and Celeste (9) did not urinate through the 27-hour ordeal, even when the wheel-wells of the buried moving van were designated by the children as bathrooms. Six additional children were dry throughout the van ride— Mary (5), Susan (5), Benji (6), Louis (8), and Sammy (10). Ellen (6) and Debbie (10) reported waiting a "very long time" prior to wetting themselves. Of the children who attempted continence, Ellen, Susan, and Janice subsequently experienced urgency and daytime accidents; Sammy and Mary suffered cramps. Terrie (10) and Rachel (12), who had allowed themselves to wet their under-pants, continued to experience urinary urgency. After their return, Terrie (10) had a bladder infection which cleared rapidly with treatment. Leslie (7) and Alison (10) were enuretic, but improving prior to July 1976; the kidnapping set both girls far back in their achievement of bladder control. The 7 child victims who experienced newly acquired bladder problems the year after the kidnapping, did so most likely on psychological basis. It has been shown that acutely stretched bladders regain elasticity in a short time following the insult (Campbell, 1970).

Two episodes during the van ride were particularly frightening for the group: when the kidnappers filled the gas tanks with gasoline, and when they backed up the vans. Alison (10), who is asthmatic, believed that she was being asphyxiated during the refueling. "People cried, but I cried the most. I felt I couldn't breathe in there. When they put gasoline in, it made everybody cough and I felt I was suffocating. In the hole I couldn't get air. There was only one fan and everyone was gathered around it. I went back to the fan once in a while." One year after the kidnapping Alison's mother related, "The new car makes her go crazy. She says in the back of the car it doesn't get cool enough. She huffs and puffs and says she can't breathe." Carl (10) and Sheila (11) also reacted with fantasies to the refueling of the van. Carl thought the gas was going to be used to "burn us up." Sheila thought the gas would "smother us." When the van was backed up, Alison, her cousin Sheila, and Bob (14) believed that the men had placed a rock on the gas pedal to back it off a cliff. The 3 of them awaited their free fall to death. (A TV or movie stunt may have inspired this fantasy.)

Group reactions were evident in both vans. One younger child remarked, "If one started to cry, everyone did." Peep holes were sought to figure out where they were, but no one found a good peep hole. Older children tried to gauge curves and bumps to figure out their locations. The younger children sang, "If You're Happy and You Know It, Clap Your Hands, Clap Clap." No one clapped.

Reactions to the "Hole": The 16-hour ordeal in the truck-trailer was the most terrifying part of the episode for the majority of the kidnapped youngsters. They heard the sounds of dirt being shoveled above them, and they realized that they were being buried. They begged and shouted to the diggers to no avail. The near collapse of the roof made them aware for the first time that they might die. Several children began to fear that they would never see their families again.

Louis (8), who moved the wooden stake, knew he was in a truck, but was unaware of the danger in moving the stake. On the other hand, 8 youngsters mentioned the near collapse of the roof as the most frightening aspect of the kidnapping; each of these 8 was fully aware that they might die at any minute. Five additional children pointed out that their major worry in the hole was that they would never see their parents again. Two children were preoccupied with concern about separation from siblings.

In the entire 27-hour ordeal, the only opportunity for activity occurred in the hole after the roof almost collapsed. Sammy (10) had suggested digging several hours earlier, but the bus driver and the older boys rediscovered this idea following Louis's accident. Bob (14) and Carl (10) did the digging. Sammy (10) tried to dig blindly with his fists, but he hit his head on "something" and fainted. After recovering, Sammy removed the dirt. About 8 months after the kidnapping, Sammy reported, "I got a headache and fell on the ground for a few minutes on Wednesday. I haven't told anybody." Bob (14) fainted twice, but the bus driver poured water on him and Bob continued digging. Johnny (11) believed the others thought he was too chubby and too weak to dig. After a brief attempt at digging, he helped clear dirt away. Terrie (10) "asked Jack to help, but he said 'no,' [so] I held the flashlight for all the boys." Sheila (11) and Janice (12) helped by keeping the younger children quiet and out of the way.

There was a mental hazard in being a "hero." Bob (14) hallucinated during the hours of solitary clawing at wood and dirt in a confined cubicle. He related, "There was a wooden box over us; I didn't know where we were. I went up there, kicked and tore apart mattresses for tools—got one corner up and looked through there. It looked like a blue rug, white bedspread, bureau, and a TV. I almost fainted when I saw it. I was positive I was going into their [the kidnappers'] trailer. This happened when I was alone. I didn't tell more than one person. Then I stopped looking there at all. I made a bigger hole and saw rocks and trees and maybe heard a river. This made me want to do a lot more. When I got out, it looked like a very different place. I saw green trees, and the trees actually were brown. I had heard running water, but there was no water when I got out. I saw daylight through the crack, but I came out at dusk or dawn." Bob's hallucinations had been auditory (running water) and visual. They had reflected mental attitudes on Bob's part about his exhausting labor. The terrifying vision of the kidnappers' trailer symbolized Bob's fear of further stress. The encouraging vision of green trees and a peaceful meadow reflected Bob's later optimism about the possibility of successful escape. Bob believed for months after the kidnapping that "I had lost my mind." He told his mother about the hallucinations, but was unable to accept her reassurances. At the end of his psychiatric interview, Bob expressed enormous relief, stating that he had not known before that normal people could hallucinate.

There were two other hallucinatory phenomena during the kidnapping. Susan (5) saw the kidnappers lying across the top of the buried moving van. "I saw the men took their masks off on top of us. They were lying down for a nap. I could see them on top of the hole. They didn't see us getting out." It is highly unlikely that Susan actually could have seen this because the trailer was deeply buried in dirt. Tania's extra kidnapper in the green van also was imagined or hallucinated.

The passive children in the hole were uninvolved in the escape process. Debbie (10), who is bright and strong-willed, deeply resented that she had not been allowed to dig or move dirt. Susan (5) and Tania (8) took naps, but woke up when the roof started to collapse. Benji (6), Elizabeth (9), and Celeste (9) had to be awakened to leave the buried truck once the escape route had been established. Elizabeth recalled one year later, "I fell asleep in the hole, I didn't know they were digging. They woke me up to get out. I thought the guys [kidnappers] were there and *they* made us get out." The uninvolvement of the sleeping youngsters may be denial, but it also must be remembered that by the time of escape any nonsleepers had been awake for about 35 hours.

Reaction to Escape: After the escape, the children continued to be afraid. Carl (10), a digger, refused to put his head out of the hole because it might be shot off. Bob crawled out on his belly, fearing gunfire from the kidnappers. After the others were released from the hole, Bob hid in the bushes because he believed that the kidnappers were lurking somewhere nearby. Debbie recalled, "I thought the men would be out there. I hid behind the mattress." Janice (12) was so frightened escaping from the hole that she described it as the most terrifying event in the entire kidnapping!

All transfers, including the transfer from captivity to freedom, were ventures into the unknown. There was no way to know, except in retrospect, that the nightmare was indeed over.

Reactions to Rescue: The children did not consider their stay in prison at all traumatic. They were pleased to receive clean pajamas, and they were mildly annoyed that their sleep was interrupted for questioning, but no child pointed to the stay in prison as frightening. As a matter of fact, few realized they were actually in a prison. There have been no signs of posttraumatic reactions to the prison stay.

MAJOR FEARS EXPERIENCED BY CHILDREN DURING THE EPISODE

There were three major fears in retrospect expressed by the children: (1) separation from parents or from siblings; (2) death; (3) further trauma. Only one child expressed a fear of injury of body parts (Benji, 6). No child expressed concern about loss of love or about matters of conscience.

Past anxieties which related to the kidnapping created additional stress for those youngsters who made those mental associations. Louis's fear of the water, Alison's fear of her asthmatic attacks, Benji's fear of spanking, and Johnny's concern about his weight are examples of anxieties which were magnified by association to the traumatic event.

Retrospective Significance: For some children, the last contact with their parents, the school day itself, or a physical item they noticed prior to the kidnapping assumed a special significance during the traumatic event. Five children had had angry confrontations with their mothers the morning of the kidnapping. During the 36-hour ordeal, the unpleasant exchange with his or her mother became mentally associated with the stress itself.

Tania (8) had been angry because her parents were about to leave for a family reunion in the mountains. "I was angry they left. I never told them that since I got back." Throughout the kidnapping episode, Tania believed that her parents were enjoying themselves on their camping trip. At the prison following the escape, Tania arranged for another child to take her home. Actually, Tania's parents had heard the news and were anxiously waiting in Chowchilla.

Two sisters, Celeste (9) [3] and Sheila (11), and their cousin, Alison (10), argued with their mothers the morning of the kidnapping. They wanted to "skip school." Sheila left her mother, who had insisted she attend school, with the parting statement, "You're the meanest mother in the world!" Sheila did not consciously think about her "parting shot" during the kidnapping episode, yet it became indelibly associated with her perception of trauma. On the other hand, Alison, who felt she had been "shoved out the door" by her mother, remembered this scene during the kidnapping itself, "I knew it wasn't my mother's fault, but I still felt angry. I wished I could have stayed home."

The School Day and Its Later Significance: Alison (10) recalled an uneasy feeling at school. "There was a new bus driver and he kind of scared me. I was scared just that day. Sometime during school." Alison's "premonition" can be reconstructed as follows: Alison noted the new bus driver with apprehension. Her mother indicated that Alison for years has been quiet and shy around strangers. During the kidnapping, Alison's mind retrospectively linked her anxiety about the new bus driver to the psychic trauma itself, leading Alison to believe she had had foreknowledge of disaster.

Bob (14) had been so slow getting ready for school in the morning that his mother, who usually drove him, insisted that he take the bus home. He tried to arrange a ride with a friend, but at the last minute the plans did not materialize, and he was forced to take the school bus. He had to run for the bus and flag it down

---

3. Celeste's early morning argument with her mother probably led her initially to misperceive a kidnapper as "a lady" (see above).

in order to be a passenger on the subsequently terrifying ride. Bob turned out to be a "hero," and he has ruminated at length about the significance of the preceding chain of events.

For several children, the bus ride up to the kidnapping point took on retrospective significance. Some children had already been let off the bus. Sheila (11) remembered, "It was strange how we asked Jack to take the 'town kids' home first. We were stopped on the way to *our* stop." Other children thought about *why* they had chosen a particular seat. Jackie (9), who usually did not sit with her brother Johnny (11), worried during the kidnapping about *why* they chose to sit apart. In her interview 6 months after the kidnapping, Jackie contemplated, "Most of the kids went with their sisters, but Johnny was up front. I was bothered because I wasn't with Johnny. I think about it mostly at night before going to sleep. That day I decided to sit in back. Usually I sit in front near Johnny. Johnny doesn't like me. He's always mad at me." Elizabeth (9) also worried about her separate seating placement from her sister, Mary (5). (Since the kidnapping, Elizabeth's concern for Mary's safety has been repeated in the older girl's hovering, overprotective behavior to her sister.) Sally (7) recalled that the van blocked the road near her church. Afterward, on Sundays at church when Sally fell asleep during the sermon, she dreamed of the kidnapping. For Sally, seeing the church immediately preceded the trauma, and the perception of "church" became firmly linked to the traumatic anxiety itself.

THE MENTAL FUNCTIONING OF CHILDREN DURING A TRAUMATIC EVENT

In 1967 Anna Freud stated, "What I would consider as evidence for the occurrence of a traumatic event is, as an immediate reaction to it, a state of paralysis of action, of numbness of feeling; in the case of a child, a temper tantrum, physical responses via the vegetative nervous system taking the place of psychic reactions" (p. 238). Furst (1967) hypothesized, "The acute traumatic state takes one of two forms: the traumatized child may appear immobilized, frozen, pale, becoming extremely infantile and submissive in behavior; or else the trauma may be followed by an emotional storm, accompanied by frenzied, undirected, disorganized behavior bordering on panic. Signs of autonomic dysfunction may contribute further emphasis to either picture" (p. 40).

None of the physical responses or emotional reactions anticipated by Furst or A. Freud were noted in the 23 children who sustained purely psychic trauma in Chowchilla. The kidnapped youngsters remembered quite vividly how they themselves and their peers had responded at the moment of stress. At the instant of the bus take-over, they remembered crying, but they reported no "paralysis of action," numbness, flailing about, amnesia, or vegetative responses. Some children experienced brief, fleeting denial ("it's a joke" or "it's the sheriff").

Misperceptions and hallucinations were dramatic evidence of ego malfunction at the instant of trauma. Eight children misperceived or hallucinated during the ordeal. Since only one had been previously considered emotionally disturbed, cognitive dysfunction was a reaction of the normal ego to "a breach in the stimulus barrier."

Further evidence of ego malfunction is the repeated attempt to gain retrospective mastery or control through the discovery of "omens." Some of the kidnapped children could remember that in the midst of the extremely stressful events they had become obsessed about an early morning exchange with their mothers, placement in the bus prior to the kidnapping, or the fact that some children had already been let off the bus. The child's ego, temporarily unable to master the overwhelming traumatic event, retreated to less-threatening episodes just prior to the trauma. In doing so, the ego interprets prior events as omens, and reconstructs the day's happenings in a way that would have avoided or prevented the trauma.

This phenomenon is, in my opinion, a new finding. If confirmed, it may be important in other traumatic conditions such as grief following sudden unexpected death. Cain and Fast (1972) described children's retrospective obsessions about the day before the suicide of a parent, but they ascribed this phenomenon to the child's superego. I believe that the ego's struggle for mastery during a traumatic event may also be an important factor in the obsessive thinking by child survivors of parental suicide.

Finally, during the traumatic event the ego exhibits its malfunctioning by developing an immediate "fear of further trauma." The child victims recalled that during the kidnapping, they feared separation, death, and further shocks or surprises. The discomfort of ego disruption was so intense that the children dreaded further repetitions of this sensation. The fear of further psychic trauma may be similar to Rado's (1942) "traumatophobia" proposed during World War II to account for the prolongation of traumatic war neuroses. "Fear of further trauma" is a term which better describes the findings in Chowchilla because the classical mechanisms of phobia (Freud, 1909) were not apparent.

It is difficult to decide whether some of the misunderstandings during the traumatic episode were due to age-adequate misinterpretations,[4] whether the defenses normally available to the children had been put out of action, or whether they represented a mixture of naïveté and some use of denial. Those children who repeatedly referred to the men as "robbers" and "crooks" exhibited misunderstanding of the purpose of the episode as well as some denial. It is important to note, however, that these were only *partial denials*. Each child interviewed was able to tell a fully detailed story of what had happened. None exhibited the repression, amnesia, memory lapses, emotional numbing, or blurring of consciousness described in adults after extreme stress (Janis, 1958; Horowitz, 1976). Massive denial of segments of the external events was not observed in the Chowchilla victims.[5] It will take further research to determine whether children experience massive denial or altered consciousness states under other traumatic conditions.[6] In this regard E. Sterba (1968) makes an interesting point in her

4. One would expect that the younger children might have been unable to conceptualize "kidnapping," but, in fact, 7-year-old Leslie, one of the youngest, was the only child who fully understood what had happened to the group.

5. Bob's hallucinations were based on denial in fantasy, but this is not the form of denial mentioned in the literature in adults, which stresses the denial of parts of the event.

6. A recent clinical example from my practice again illustrates the difference in the use of denial between traumatized children and adults. Caroline was 8 when she was attacked by a German shepherd dog, who slashed open her throat. Mrs. C. was in her home during the attack, but came outside and rescued her daughter. Caroline very nearly died, and required surgery and

study of adolescents freed from concentration camps: "Unlike adults, who had a symptom-free period, the children survivors . . . developed emotional disorders as soon as they were settled in this country" (p. 57f.).

Psychoanalytic theory considers denial one of the "primitive" defenses seen in the youngest individuals or the most immature egos (Anna Freud, 1936). This view of "denial" is based upon retrospective reconstructions during psychoanalysis. It is very curious that adults have been reported to use the most massive forms of denial during traumas, yet the few children of Chowchilla who did exhibit some form of denial employed only partial denials of a subtle sort (failure to use the word "kidnap" or believing for an instant that the kidnapping was a joke). Why do adults exhibit massive use of a "primitive immature defense," whereas children do not? Is denial truly an immature defense? Only firsthand observation of infants and prospective studies of children similar to the Chowchilla study will answer these questions.

THE CHILDREN'S LONG-TERM REACTIONS

The interviews and observations of the kidnapped children established that each of the 23 children was affected by this traumatic event. The children developed a variety of persistent fears and unsuccessfully attempted to cope with them. Unconscious anxiety manifested itself in play, behavioral reenactments, and repetitive dreams. The children showed changes in their cognitive functioning and some developed lasting personality changes.

FEARS

Every child in the group of 23 exhibited kidnap-related fears at the time of psychiatric examination. Twenty children feared being

---

hospitalization. Four years later the child remembered every detail of the attack and rescue (verified by witnesses, because it was a legal case). She recalled that her mother pulled the dog back from further attack. Mrs. C. cannot remember how she got the dog off or how she held it off. That part of the episode is completely forgotten by the adult, but remembered by the child.

kidnapped again; [7] 12 were afraid of a fourth kidnapper; 6 believed that the arrested kidnappers themselves were coming back; and 10 believed there would be a second unrelated kidnapping.

Twenty-one children experienced common "mundane" fears: 10 were afraid to be left alone; 15 feared sounds; 3 feared confined spaces; and 3 were afraid of open spaces. Eight children experienced attacks of such acute anxiety that they screamed, ran, or called for help.

Fear of Another Kidnapping: Six children originally "misidentified" a kidnapper during the 27-hour kidnapping experience. They "saw" a bald man, a peg-legged man, a "lady," a black man, a fat man, and a fourth man in a green van. This misidentification "spread" through families. Other children rethought the kidnapping on their own, and decided there must be a fourth kidnapper. The "fourth kidnapper hypothesis" eventually affected 12 youngsters.

Family spread of the "fourth kidnapper hypothesis" occurred in Jackie's and Celeste's cases. After Jackie misidentified the "peg-legged man," her brother, Johnny, feared that a "mastermind" would plot again to kidnap them. Johnny recalled wistfully, "At 10 I went through an earthquake. I was thrown out of bed. I never continued scared. I never played or dreamed about it." Alison, Sheila, and Celeste, who are cousins, were affected by Celeste's belief that a "lady" had kidnapped them. Alison stated, "Celeste says she saw a woman with a gun. I worry maybe there's a woman involved in it. I'm afraid about it. Since the kidnapping I don't like to walk too far because I think someone may try to kidnap me." Both Benji (6) and his sister Tania (8), who had misidentified a kidnapper originally, continued to be concerned about a fourth kidnapper. "Did you ever see a guy with a long nose?" Benji inquired. "Sometimes I think spies are watching me." Tania, who fears the original kidnappers as well as "the fourth man," noted, "One night I heard something in my room. I thought it was someone outside. Sometimes I worry one would come back."

Some children independently came to the "fourth kidnapper

7. In clinical practice with latency-age youngsters, fears of being kidnapped are not at all uncommon. No Chowchilla child recalled having had such fears prior to the kidnapping, but it is possible that the traumatic event did reaffirm unconscious fears of this nature in some.

hypothesis." Terrie (10) mused, "I worry there were more because of all the things they did." Bob (14) developed the same theory. Mandy (7) remembered, "I saw two kidnappers. I thought there were more." Sammy (10), unfortunately hampered by his blindness, confessed, "I'm not sure it's them [in jail]."

Six children feared the three kidnappers who were in jail awaiting trial. Bob (14), one of the "heroes," concluded, "Sometimes I think they did it to let us get out, so that they'd get caught and go to jail a couple of years, and then start killing us one by one like in the movies. I think about what they're going to do if they get out when they do get out." Susan, 9 years younger than Bob, independently developed the same fear, "I think the men are coming back." Louis (8) related, "I think about bad stuff everywhere. I think that they're going to kill us with a knife. I want the men here so I can slap them. Will you take me to the jail to hit them? Can we bring a papaya to hit them with?"

Ten children feared a new kidnapping by kidnappers unrelated to the original group. Carl (10), a hero, told me, "In the night I get scared going to bed, hearing sounds—mouses and dogs. I'm worried they might be men walking outside." Janice (12) mentioned, "If strange men come to the school, I stick with friends. I'm afraid they're coming for me." Rachel (12) noted, "I don't like to turn off the lights. I'm afraid someone would come in and shoot and rob us. When I wake up I turn on the light. I've been in Bakersfield helping my brother—at night in Bakersfield it feels like someone broke in. Nothing is there. I hear footsteps again. I keep going to check. I check where the sound is coming from. I'm very frightened of the kitchen because no one's there at all. I completely avoid it. At home I kept feeling someone was looking in and watching me. I kept the light on. I was afraid they'd come in and kill us all or take us away again."

Small children as well as the older ones feared another kidnapping. Mary (5) was interviewed in an empty classroom of her own school on a windy day in early summer. She interrupted her interview several times with "What's that?"

"Just the wind," I reassured her.

Again, "What was that knocking? I thought it was a car, maybe kidnappers."

"Only the wind."

"I had nightmares and dreams about it. When I think they were in jail. And a van kept parking and stopping and the fan was on." In Mary's case, a harmless sound associated with the horrors of the van ride and the hole has now "contaminated" all wind. Again and again, Mary asked, "What's that? What's that?" as the wind gusted outside our school room. No reassurance was accepted.

Ellen (6), her sister Sally (7), and Elizabeth (9) were the only youngsters who did not mention fear of another kidnapping. Yet, Elizabeth avoided the school bus by hiding in the bushes, complaining of knee, head, and stomachaches, or walking home before the bus arrived. Throughout the year Mrs. E. had to drive the child to the bus stop, stand there with her until she entered the bus, and watch as the door closed behind her.

Fear of the "Mundane": Widespread fears of mundane or ordinary experiences (21 cases) were due to the belief in and avoidance of signals or omens of the kidnapping-to-come, to the avoidance of any perception which could evoke the original traumatic anxiety, to cognitive errors, to loss of trust, and to regressions. From the quotes in the preceding section, it is evident that the children's fear of another kidnapping affected their attitudes about their ordinary environment: motor vehicles, the dark, the wind, "mouses and dogs," "hippies," the kitchen, etc. Many of these items were believed to be signals or warnings of an impending kidnapping. Children remained continuously on the alert. Johnny (11), who needed a baby-sitter because he feared being left alone, stayed up watching the baby-sitter when she fell asleep. He explained to his parents that someone should be "on guard." Janice (12) commented, "I still stay away from strangers. I cross the street to get away from them. I might be scared tonight at our graduation dance because of so many strangers there."

From the children's point of view the kidnapping began when an innocent-looking van blocked the road and the school bus stopped. The white van did not alarm any children. Yet in the aftermath of the kidnapping, 15 children exhibited persistent fear of unfamiliar vehicles. The perception of the parked van and the perception of stress were associated in the children's minds so that vans, cars, or buses subsequently symbolized extreme danger in the present [8] as well as for the future. In part, cars, vans, and buses were so widely feared because they might signal another kidnapping. Alison (10), according to her mother, "has fits if we won't take a friend [along] for a ride." Terrie (10) is uneasy whenever she spots from her living room window "cars I don't know." Terrie's father agreed, "I'm glad she's more cautious."

The fear of reexperiencing traumatic anxiety also underlies "fear of the mundane." Certain sensory stimuli associated with the original psychic trauma are avoided by the group because they evoke the original overwhelming anxiety, similar to the "traumatophobia" hypothesized by Rado (1942) in cases of adult war neurosis. Bob (14) stated, "When I go into a basement, I want to get out of there fast. It reminds me of the stale air in the hole." Carl (10), who had dug for hours in the cubicle, hated the confinement of elevators. Many children refused peanut butter, the main staple food in the hole. Sammy's blindness forced him to link smell and auditory perceptions to his perception of overwhelming anxiety. He explained, "I think about it [the kidnapping] when hippies are drinking and going in cars. The kidnappers were drinking in the white van. I smelled pot in the white van and heard them popping their cans." Sammy (10) has exhibited intense anxiety near "hippies."

Panic Attacks: Eight children suffered from attacks of such overwhelming anxiety that they had to flee or call for help. Ordinary "mundane" stimuli precipitated these episodes. Susan (5), whose dreams indicated that she accepted her own death (see below), announced to her mother one morning, "Laverne [her toddler sister] is dead! She's not up yet." Mandy (7) twice screamed that her little brother had been kidnapped when he was actually playing next door or trying on clothes in a store dressing room. She insisted the episodes had occurred *before* the kidnapping, but Mrs. M. reported that they occurred *after* it.

A year after the kidnapping, Terrie (10) awoke to find her parents gone, and a strange white car outside her house. Johnny's and Jackie's mother rushed over in response to Terrie's urgent phone call and sat with her until Terrie's parents returned home.

8. A particularly poignant example of the intensity of this fear of vehicles is described on p. 584.

Sixteen months after the kidnapping, Terrie became so over-whelmed with emotion while testifying in the criminal trial that the judge ordered a recess. Despite Terrie's relative calm during most of the postkidnapping period, she demonstrated extreme anxiety and emotionality twice when an external stress evoked vivid sensory memories of the original trauma.

Exactly one year after the kidnapping, Johnny (11) refused to sleep in his bedroom for many nights because he believed the ceiling was collapsing. Elizabeth (9) "shook and cried" on several occasions when the school bus approached to take her to school. Debbie (10) fled from a white van parked in an alley on the an-niversary of the kidnapping. Sammy (10) experienced two panicky episodes, according to his mother. "Before Christmas during vaca-tion he was biking with a friend riding sandhills. A station wagon, two guys, and a dog were there. He abandoned his bike and ran home. He said he didn't want to be kidnapped again. He cried a lot. I advised him not to panic and run. Just before the Fair in May, there were strangers on the road, and he gave up biking there and refused to go further."

Discussion

Destruction of Trust: The vast majority of child victims be-lieved they could be kidnapped again. Each of them in some way listened and watched for signs of danger in the dark, when alone, near cars, strangers, when confined, or when out in the open. They remained permanently on guard. No matter what anyone told them, they were unable to trust again. Bob (14) summarized, "I'm much more cautious now. I know it can happen to me. Before I thought it only happens to other people." Lifton and Olson (1976) have referred to similar phenomena in adults as "shatter-ing of the illusion of invulnerability." In children this effect is so marked that it appears to be a destruction of basic trust.

Many of the Chowchilla children had been well parented and well loved. Even so, after the kidnapping they never again could fully trust the world. E. H. Erikson (1950) has pointed out how basic trust is established in infancy by consistent gratification of the child's needs. The child develops a general optimism that the future will be pleasant and that the world is a relatively friendly, safe place. When an overwhelming trauma like the Chowchilla kidnapping generates so much anxiety that the ego cannot deal with it, trust is shattered. Ordinary routine is fraught with fears. No parental reassurance can be accepted.

Johnny's mother once reassured him long before the kidnapping, "Those kind of people just don't live around here!" Now she feels powerless to offer him any new reassurances; nor would he accept them. Tania's mother noted, "She had been very easy to get along with. Loving. When she first came back, she wouldn't kiss me. She wouldn't sit on our laps. My mother pointed out that now she's fearful of closeness because she might lose it." After the kidnapping, Tania was an angry little girl with a night light, fear of vehicles, and fear of the sound of her own heater. Her trust was shattered completely.

Fear of the Mundane: One of the particularly interesting findings in this study is the frequent occurrence of fears of ordinary routine stimuli. "Fear of the mundane" is evoked by auditory, visual, olfactory, gustatory, or tactile senses. It is multicausal, relating to the erosion of basic trust, establishment of omens, fear of further trauma, and cognitive malfunction (see below).

Bowlby (1973) delineated certain situations which arouse fears in infants and animals. He defined the earliest fears of childhood as fears of noise, strangers, strange objects, heights, looming objects, animals, and the dark or being alone in the dark. In the Chowchilla kidnapping, fear of noise, strangers, and the dark or being alone in the dark were encountered frequently. This could be interpreted as a regression in the victim whose ego had been compromised, causing a return to the most primitive fears; however, since the kidnapping itself involved dark, being "alone," strangers, strange noises, and strange objects, it is more likely that the fears were derived from the traumatic circumstances themselves. Further studies may determine if regression, allowing return to the most primitive fears, actually occurs in psychic trauma.

COGNITIVE FUNCTIONS

Misperception, a striking immediate response in 8 of the children, affected an even larger group later. Overgeneralization and time confusion also occurred long after the kidnapping. Impaired school performance at a cognitive level was surprisingly uncommon. Finally, flashbacks, which have been described in adults as unbidden intrusions into ordinary cognitive functioning, did not occur in the children.

Distortions of Perception: In the section on initial responses to trauma, it was pointed out that 8 children misperceived or hallucinated during the kidnapping itself. Some children who did not originally misperceive did so much later. For example, Barbara (9) remarked, "If I see three 'hippies' I say, 'Mom, *they* kidnapped us.' One time I was sure I saw him in a Western movie." Mary (5) misperceived the wind to be the kidnappers coming in a car. Carl (10) heard men's footsteps in the sounds of "mouses and dogs," and Alison (10) and Rachel (12) heard footsteps at night. Tania (8), who during the kidnapping had "seen" a fourth kidnapper, later believed she had spotted one of the kidnappers wearing a stocking mask on a TV show and, on another occasion, the same one performing in a cowboy movie.

Overgeneralizations: Concrete traumatic perceptions were later "overgeneralized," so that a large class of objects came to represent the original specific perception. In reenactment and in panic attacks, stress signals based on overgeneralized perceptions worked as portents or omens. Bob "heroically" reenacted when he saw a strange car in trouble outside his home (see section on reenactments). The perception of "white van" had been overgeneralized after the kidnapping to any vehicle encountered unexpectedly.

Overgeneralization often accounted for startle responses to noise. During her interview at home, Barbara (9) jumped when her father's motorcycle pulled into the yard, even though she had been expecting him to arrive. The sound of the vans, Barbara's original traumatic perception, had been generalized to include any vehicular noise.

Six-year-old Ellen overgeneralized from her traumatic perception of the collapse of the roof of the hole to the ceiling of her own house. She had a panic attack when a leak developed in her roof. Alison's family car smelled like the van and stimulated her asthmatic attacks. Any confined space felt like a cubicle to Carl. The dark felt like the hole or the vans to many children.

Distortions in Sense of Time: Eight children made crucial mistakes in time-sequencing, most of which had to do with when in relation to the trauma symptoms had developed. Alison (10) and

Jackie (9) expressed anxiety about "predictive" dreams. Johnny (11) believed he had started collecting guns *before* the kidnapping; Celeste (9) believed her dreamy immobility had begun prior to her captivity. Carl (10) insisted his fear of elevators and closed spaces had begun *before* he "dug" in the tiny cubicle. Sheila (11) thought her dreams of the caged monkey occurred prior to the kidnapping, and Sammy (10) and Mandy (7) confused the timing of their anxiety attacks. Most of the postkidnapping timing of the above episodes was verified through parent's history, but the onset of Carl's fear of elevators or Sheila's and Alison's dreams could not be verified. Since they were so similar to the other children's postkidnapping fears and so well connected to Carl's, Alison's, and Sheila's individual experiences during the kidnapping, I assumed that they occurred after the trauma.

"Time-skew" generated more anxiety than it relieved. The child who experienced time-skew had to worry whether the episodes he or she believed had preceded the kidnapping were warnings or omens that should have been heeded.

School Performance: Changes for the worse in school performance were observed in 8 children, and changes for the better occurred in 2.

Most worsening in school performance occurred because of personality changes which affected the child's conduct (Tania, Sammy, Johnny, Sheila, and Janice) or because of school avoidance (Elizabeth and Susan). The major cognitive factor in poor school performance was failure to concentrate (Ellen, Elizabeth, and Janice).

Mrs. E. recollected, "Ellen's teacher called that she couldn't stay still. She had no attention span, and she was excellent in kindergarten. This was until about January. It took her 5 months to finish the first book and then she read 7 or 8 books in the spring. She got her attention back." Elizabeth (9) who, like Ellen (6), could not concentrate, explained, "Sometimes I daydream at school about getting in the hole and sitting in the dark. I don't like the teacher. He yells a lot. He says the work only once and talks very low. I sit at the end of my table. I've had a terrible year at school. Sometimes I sneak and try not to go. I may flunk the grade. I don't know."

The children who improved in school did so because of factors unrelated to the kidnapping. Mary (5) repeated kindergarten the year after the kidnapping and was much improved the second time. Carl (10) had a better year in school, probably because he was separated most of the year from his stepfather, with whom he did not get along. The remaining 13 kidnap victims showed no change in their school performance the year after the kidnapping.

Flashbacks: The Chowchilla children did not exhibit the type of daytime intrusive "visions" reported in the literature dealing with psychic trauma or grief in adults (Parkes, 1970; Horowitz, 1976). The child victims seemed to have control over whether or not they "saw" the scenes of the kidnapping. Johnny (11) related, "I dwell on it once in awhile. A kid brings it up in some way." Bob (14) reported that before going to sleep he often "browsed" through the whole event, but this was done at will and not as an intrusion. Terrie (10) also described this process. "I get to thinking about it on the way to sleep. Sometimes during school. The whole idea of it." Elizabeth (9) reported picturing herself in the hole during school, and Janice (12) recalled seeing the men's faces at school, but these thoughts occurred at times when they were disinterested in the work. Alison (10) remarked, "I think of it once in awhile without expecting to. I think of the hole and when they first got us into the vans. I think a lot about those [2 predictive] dreams" (see below).

Six older children (ages 9–14) reported daytime visions of the episode. They used "voluntary" verbs such as "browse," "think," or "dwell." There was no evidence of the type of sudden involuntary flashbacks previously reported in adults. Since the group younger than 9 did not complain of "seeing" the kidnapping at all, the "voluntary" vision may be a transitional phase. Perhaps because no child employed massive denial, sudden intrusions could not occur. Furthermore, since there is a sequential development of the ability to daydream or fantasize (A. Freud and Burlingham, 1942), the intrusive "flashback" may not develop until late adolescence.

Discussion

Stress Signals: Certain experiences the children had had years earlier (e.g., the movie *Dirty Harry;* see p. 598), the morning before (arguments), immediately before (the church), during the kidnapping itself (the stuffiness, peanut butter, dark), and even afterward (dreams) were reconstructed by them in retrospect to be "omens" of terror-to-come, and/or they became permanent trigger mechanisms for the sensory evocation of traumatic anxiety. Stimuli that were inaccurately perceived and objects or persons that were overgeneralized became permanently associated with the stress in the predictive sense. Once formed, these stress signals provoked fear of the mundane, panic attacks, repetitive play, reenactments, and psychophysiological symptoms.

Relevance of Traumatic Misperception to the Child Witness in Court: The possibility of misperception during stress must be considered when deciding on the use of courtroom testimony by child witnesses, and perhaps adult witnesses, who have themselves been traumatized. If a child is so severely traumatized by an event that he or she may have visually distorted or hallucinated, it is important that verifying evidence such as fingerprints, ballistics reports, or another witness's account be used to corroborate the traumatized child's identification of the perpetrators.

PLAY

During my first meeting with a small group of mothers and fathers, I asked about play and received no response until I explained that the parents might not see a direct connection to the kidnapping. At that point, the group produced a torrent of Halloween behaviors, hobbies, strange games and interests, all of them very much related to the trauma.

From the first meeting on, it was necessary to ask adults and children very direct specific questions about play and unusual behaviors because their connection to the kidnapping was unconscious. (Personality change, from the beginning, was much easier for families to "see" in relation to the trauma.)

For the purposes of this study, I have defined "play" as an activity the child feels he or she enjoys, alone or in a group. I have included "hobbies" as a type of play. Eleven children repeatedly "played" the kidnapping experience. Even though the games lacked subtlety, only 1 of the 11 realized that the play was related to the kidnapping. Such "traumatic" play was repeated monotonously with no relief of anxiety.

A month or 2 after the kidnapping, Leslie (7) developed a "bus driver" game, which she played with her toddler sister two to three times a week. Leslie placed two chairs on top of the kitchen table: one in front for herself and one behind for 3-year-old Marjorie. Leslie proceeded to "drive" her bus and to stop at each "passenger's" stop. She explained that Marjorie usually was a passenger, but "I pretend there are other kids too." When asked if she thought the game might be related to the kidnapping, Leslie quickly retorted, "Oh, no. I drive a *safe* bus. No one on my bus ever gets kidnapped!"

Sheila's mother remarked that she could not trust 11-year-old Sheila with her younger sister "for a minute." Sheila repeatedly frightened the little girl by jumping out of hiding places, saying, "You'll never see Mommy again." Whenever her mother left the room, Sheila contrived a way to make the 5-year-old believe that she was all alone in the house. Sheila recalled that her own worst fear during the kidnapping was: "We'd never see our parents again." Sheila's traumatic fear and her "game" were strongly linked, yet she was unaware of any connection.

Johnny (11) felt fat, weak, and ineffective during the kidnapping. He had been relegated to removing dirt. In his postkidnapping "hobbies" Johnny's concern about weakness and helplessness was evident. He began an extensive collection of toy guns. Even though he insisted that the collection existed prior to the kidnapping, neither his mother nor his sister confirmed this. In the spring following the kidnapping, Johnny sent away for a Charles Atlas body-building course, using money he had saved for himself. When the booklets arrived, Johnny was furious to read that it was not recommended to begin the program until age 14. In a fit of dismay and frustration, he burned the entire packet in the fireplace.

After the kidnapping, Susan (5) began playing with guns, and Mary (5) and Elizabeth (9) played almost daily "tag" against imaginary "bad guys." These 2 girls reported having seen Sammy (10) frequently playing the same game, but Sammy did not remember it.

Janice (12) engaged in a complicated chase-and-tag game during recess periods at her junior high school. This game was the only instance in which the connection of play to kidnapping was conscious. Janice consistently played the part of kidnap victim, while up to 20 fellow students interchanged roles of kidnappers, policemen, and bus driver. Janice had been one of the originators of the game, which was played daily for several months. A teacher finally intervened and officially terminated the game. Janice's group play had been a direct repetition of the kidnapping.

Carl (10), a "hero" to the other youngsters, could not remember any postkidnapping play, but his mother did remember. "Two times he's put stockings on his face and he's said, 'Look Mamma!' He's frightened the sister [his aunt] and her children. One time he jumped out of the closet, maybe more times. He looked terrible! His little brother [3] was afraid. One time he played bus driver." In the hole, Carl had been a "hero" capable of taking action to secure the release of the others, yet he was unprotected from the need to defend against his own anxiety and helplessness.

Mary (5) and Elizabeth (9) each indulged in highly individualistic play. Mary, early in her interview, stated, "I thought the hole was just down in the ground. I heard them put on dirt and I started crying. I wouldn't go to sleep or nothing. I thought they [the kidnappers] would come in there too. The hole was the scariest part!" Later, Mary confided, "There is a cement place at my grandma's which is like a hole. I put clothes in it and my Barbie dolls. I pretend they're stuck in the hole." Mary was unable to see a relationship between her play and her fear of the hole. The longer I discussed it with her, the less she admitted to this kind of play.

Following the kidnapping, Elizabeth (9) became a "prank" telephoner. Quite by accident, because she phoned the parent of another kidnap victim who recognized her voice, Elizabeth was caught. She told me that she breathed hard on the phone, whispering, "Help me, help me," and then hung up. Elizabeth had repeated her calls again and again in a vain attempt to diminish her anxiety about helplessness and isolation.

Louis (8) doodled. Even though he was engaged in an unsuccessful struggle to learn to read, his schoolwork was covered with quickly drawn sketches of campers, trailer trucks, and moving vans. During his psychiatric interview, Louis doodled as he spoke. "I thought the hole was a trailer or one of those trucks. It had two wheels. I draw it a lot. I draw another one almost every day. After the kidnapping was coming, I drew and drew one of those pictures. Sometimes I draw people in the trucks. Sometimes I make drivers and I scratch through his face," Louis grimaced. Louis drew a picture of himself with no arms. He said, "They're shooting me right in the heart." He drew another truck, this one "with a papaya to hit the men over the head." He drew a second truck with the driver scratched out, a large hunk of dirt on top, a huge supporting stake in the process of falling down, and two tiny armless children, one black and one white, inside the trailer. Louis's doodles were undisguised pictures of his helplessness, his fear, his burial. He feebly turned passive into active by scratching through the drivers' faces and including a papaya as a weapon, but Louis remained the armless victim, the helpless one in his doodles. Each picture produced more anxiety and no consolation.

Bob (14), the children's "hero," indulged in repetitious play in July 1977, exactly one year after the kidnapping. Bob's mother observed that every night "he takes the cushions off the couch and punches them until he's worn out. We have barbells, but he wasn't using them. It was superaggressive and he looked very intense. He pounded the cushions so hard that he tripped the circuit breakers on the other side. I asked him to stop, but instead he moved the cushions to the other side. I feel better with him gone for the summer." This activity lasted about 2 hours a night for 2 weeks. It ended when Mrs. B. sent Bob away to spend the summer with relatives. Bob's physical-fitness spree, an anniversary reaction, was a repetition of his digging, which had led the group to safety, but which had been originally traumatic for Bob, as evidenced by the hallucinations he had experienced as he dug.

Retelling, a Variant of Traumatic Play: Retelling is repeated storytelling of the kidnapping events, with the same enjoyment which characterizes childhood play. Before I consider retelling, however, it is important to note that there were more children who hated and avoided talking about the experience than those who enjoyed repeating the story.

Five children used talk as a type of repetitive play. Carl (10) was transferred to a different school district shortly after the kidnapping. He quickly let the students at the new school know that he was a kidnap victim. He told his story to his church choir, and frightened his cousins with his tales. Carl related, "Someone said, 'Were you kidnapped?' The kids said, 'I saw you on TV.' Lots of kids asked me questions. I told the story five, six times. Sometimes people ask about it. I told different classes about it. I told the fifth graders and they asked lots of questions. They liked the stories." When I interviewed Carl, he was unable to tolerate an interruption of his stories, which he delivered rapidly in a monotone. He impatiently dispensed with my interjections and went on with his story from exactly the place where he had been stopped.

Jackie (9) and Johnny (11) enjoyed speaking on TV. They were often present fortuitously when reporters were around. Both relished the opportunity to talk to the microphones and recorders. It had become a kind of game for them, but their symptoms continued unrelieved despite their repeated opportunities to talk to "the world."

Benji (6), at home or in interviews, elaborated detail upon detail in a steady stream of fact and fantasy. In about 5 minutes of interviewing, Benji blurted, "They were so ugly. I thought they were pigs! They asked me my name and age. I was about to tell them a lie. They told us when we got out, 'Don't be mad or we'll hurt you!' I thought they'd hurt us. I'm glad I watched the cartoons. It got my mind off those dumbos. I was going to call them fatties. If that guy had laid a hand on me, I would have flipped him over my head." There was seemingly no end to Benji's repetitious elaborations and no relief from the anxiety he expressed.

To summarize, 14 of 23 kidnap victims played or retold kidnapping-related material in a repetitious manner. These children did not stop playing spontaneously. They had to be told to stop, to be moved to another place, or to accept a psychiatric interpretation before they were able to give up their monotonous, quasi-enjoyable pursuits. The major defenses in traumatic play were turning passive into active, displacement, identification with the aggressor, denial, and isolation of affect. Much play, however,

was simply repetition of a traumatic episode with little elaboration or defense at all. Instead of relieving anxiety, traumatic play
stirred up more anxiety.

Halloween "Play": Halloween is a traditional time for children
to frighten others with the very fears they harbor themselves. Two
of the Chowchilla victims dressed as kidnappers for Halloween.
Carl (10), one of the diggers who had rescued the group, was reported by his brother to have worn a stocking mask. Johnny (11)
dressed in a stocking mask and jumped out of a closet, pointing a
toy gun at his terrified sister, Jackie (9), and another frightened
kidnap victim, Susan (5).

Two other kidnap victims were sought out and terrorized by a
nonkidnapped Chowchilla youngster on Halloween. An older
boy, dressed as a kidnapper, jumped out at Benji (6) and Tania
(8), who were "trick or treating." Benji reverted to "baby talk"
for several months. Tania had repressed the entire incident by the
time she was interviewed 3 months later.

Discussion

Ordinary play is a child's laboratory; in play he or she experiments with future coping, masters previously unresolved conflicts,
tries out various defensive possibilities, and obtains relief. Waelder
(1932), A. Freud (1945), Levy (1945), and Klein (1955) pioneered
in the understanding of the play of normal children, neurotic
youngsters, and those children who had undergone such stress as
hospitalization, birth of a sibling, and death in the family. In
fact, Freud (1926) said: "It is certain that children behave in this
fashion towards every distressing impression they receive, by reproducing it in their play" (p. 167).

During World War II, A. Freud and Burlingham (1942) described the play of a traumatized 4-year-old, Bertie. The only
distinctions they drew between his play and that of the others
was his denial of his father's death and the compulsive repetition
of his play activity. Bertie's denial, they stated, "was never completely successful, the play had to be repeated incessantly—it became compulsive. The games of the other children remained
transitory. Bertie stopped playing in this way when, half a year
later, he at last gave up his denial and was able to tell his story"
(p. 197).

Before I consider the traumatic play of Chowchilla, let us consider the play of a normal child who meets an ordinary life stress such as hospitalization. He plays "doctor" a few times, identifies with the doctor's feelings, understands that the doctor meant him no harm, and is able to achieve lessening of anxiety about the hospitalization. The identification with the doctor, or the displacement of the "victim" role to a doll or younger sibling, enables the child to see that the playmate victim is taking it calmly, that the doctor is not attacking the patient for revenge; thus the play achieves a corrective denouement to the originally stressful occurrence. Anxiety is relieved and the child has no further reason to "play" the occurrence.

In contrast to this, consider the normal child who encounters a true emotional trauma, a stress that cannot be fully handled by the ego, a stress which would not have been expected in the course of an ordinary lifetime. This "normal child" uses the same play to practice coping with the trauma; the same displacements, identifications with the aggressor, turning passive into active, and denials. But the play no longer works; it is ineffective in warding off anxiety, and instead it creates more anxiety. Even though the play is ineffective, it is tried again and again partly because ordinary play has always "worked" before for the child. But traumatic play does not allow corrective reworking or working through. The "playing" child cannot find a retrospectively corrective ending to a true psychic trauma, nor can he experiment with other methods which could have helped him meet the stress with poise.

Can a child gain relief in play by identifying with aggressors that an entire community believes to be evil monsters? Pretend to be a bus driver who himself was a weeping, praying victim? Call for help, when in reality no one could have heard? Pretend to drive a "safe" bus, when dreams remind the child that the bus was highly "unsafe"? Learn to achieve comfort with the idea of being kidnapped?

Ordinary childhood play offers no way to re-prepare for extraordinary stress, no way to rework the loss of trust, no way to reassure the self that such things will not happen again. The child who has found previous solace in ordinary play cannot achieve comfort in the traumatic play into which ordinary play is converted once it is repeated frequently and monotonously. The more the traumatic game is played, the more the child perceives that there could have been no way, even in a hundred practice sessions, that such an uncommonly stressful event could have been met with poise or, for that matter, in a different fashion. Traumatic play must be stopped by an outsider—through an interpretation or, if none is available, by a command.

REENACTMENTS

Many of the child victims exhibited unusual behaviors which were found to include segments of motor activity or fantasies which had originally taken place during the kidnapping itself. These unusual postkidnapping behaviors were direct reenactments of attitudes, fears, or actions which had originally taken place just before or during the kidnapping. These reenactments are a specific form of the repetition compulsion (Freud, 1920). There was little or no defensive elaboration. The original traumatic thought, behavior, physical response, or fantasy simply was repeated. It is amazing that the vast majority of parents and children who mentioned unusual behaviors were unaware of the repetition. Reenactments occurred singly, sporadically, or frequently. Frequent reenactments were often considered by parents to be personality changes. A review of the postkidnapping behavior of the Chowchilla youngsters revealed that 14 of the 23 children reenacted.

Psychophysiological Reenactments: Sammy's fainting on the playground and Alison's wheezing in her family car are physical reenactments of physiological occurrences which originally took place during the kidnapping. Furthermore, the 7 children who complained of daytime wetting, cramping, urgency, or urinary withholding were undergoing, at least in part, reenactments of the bladder discomforts they had endured during the traumatic van ride.

Reenactment of Prekidnapping Behavior: Three girls who had argued with their mothers the morning before the kidnapping developed argumentative personalities after the kidnapping.

Tania (8) had been angry at her parents for going on a trip. Throughout the kidnapping she maintained her anger, picturing them as having a good time. After the kidnapping Tania changed her name to Tony: "It's close to a boy's name. I'm not Tania anymore. I was a little mean in the second grade. Now I'm meaner than before. I got into a fight over a jumprope. I kicked Judy Jones who I don't like and the teacher got mad." Tania's personality changed from a slightly stubborn, but generally pleasant child, into an angry, bickering, and physically aggressive girl. She preferred boys to girls. "I don't know why." Her angry rejection of her mother during the kidnapping may have been displaced to girls her own age. She has organized her personality change around the change of her name from Tania to Tony. "I feel really ugly and mean. I wasn't ugly last year."

When on the day of the kidnapping, Sheila's mother refused to let her "skip school," Sheila (11) left her mother with the parting statement, "You're the meanest mother in the world!" After the kidnapping episode, her mother said, "She slams into my bedroom pouting, saying, 'Mom makes me do everything. Mom doesn't care about me.'" Mrs. S. has overheard Sheila telling her 5-year-old non-kidnapped sister, "Mom is going to tear my ears off!" Sheila was unaware of a link between her accusations of her mother after the kidnapping and her remark to her mother the morning of the kidnapping.

Alison (10), Sheila's cousin, believed she had been "shoved out the door" by her mother. Mrs. A. was puzzled about Alison's argumentative attitude toward her, "Is this a stage, or is this related to the kidnapping? She treats us like we're really mean. We never saw that behavior before the kidnapping."

Finally, one small girl who had pleaded not to go to school the day of the trauma, refused school the entire year after the kidnapping. School refusal had not been a previous problem for Susan (5).

While Tania's, Sheila's, and Alison's reactions are reenactments of prekidnapping behaviors, they also represent personality changes. A minor incident prior to the tramautic event became magnified by the kidnapping, the girls unconsciously holding their mothers responsible for their terrifying experience.

Reenactment of Kidnapping Behavior and Fantasy: The "hero,"
Bob (14), reenacted his heroism dramatically and dangerously 18
months after the kidnapping. One afternoon, Bob's parents
noticed a strange car stopped near their house and asked Bob to
investigate. A few moments later, loud shouts in an Oriental
language emanated from outside. When the family rushed into
the yard, they found a Japanese tourist whose car had broken
down just outside their property. The man gesticulated that he
had been shot. The parents turned to Bob and discovered that he
had shot the traveler with a BB gun. Bob explained that the man's
car was close to their home, and that he believed the man was
about to do the family harm, so he had shot him. Luckily the
tourist was not seriously injured.

This dramatic episode of reenactment was set into motion
through Bob's response to a stress signal or omen. After originally
seeing kidnappers emerging from a benign-looking "van in
trouble," Bob overgeneralized any "vehicle in trouble" to be a
sign of impending disaster. *This* time Bob did not wait for further
developments; he "rescued" his family by shooting the tourist.

Other behavioral reenactments were less dramatic, but equally
interesting. Ellen (6) described the near-collapse of the ceiling of
the buried moving van as her most frightening moment during
the kidnapping. The winter following the kidnapping, it rained
so hard one day that a leak developed in the roof of Ellen's house.
Her mother recalled, "She held on to me so much she wouldn't
let me get a pail."

Sammy (10) reenacted at the schoolyard when without any provocation, he pushed a much smaller girl and slapped her in the
face. He bragged, "I gave them all a rough time. I don't care. It
doesn't bother me." Sammy, a previously unaggressive child, had
been so frustrated when a kidnapper took his glasses, that he tried
to hit him with his shoes.

Elizabeth (9) and Benji (6) reenacted fantasies that they had
originally experienced during the kidnapping. When Elizabeth
was in the hole, she thought, "I wanted to be alone with Mom.
I felt Mom needed me. She wanted me to help her. I am needed
to protect her about the fights. I think I can stop fights by calling
the cops." After the kidnapping Elizabeth developed the habit of

phoning her mother to check "if she's okay." Mrs. E. complained, "Elizabeth gets nervous and phones whenever I go out anywhere. She gets scared and follows me around. She calls other people a lot trying to chase me down. She knows almost everyone in town."

Benji's reenactment of a fantasy occurred in April 1977 when he set fire to a neighbor's yard. Benji had remarked, "I think about it every day, that he [the kidnapper] was threatening the kids. Even at school. I wish I could do what I thought they were going to do; harmful things!" Benji, who had had an impulsive and immature personality prior to the kidnapping, fantasied retaliation and identified with the kidnappers during the 27-hour ordeal, leading to the firesetting episode 9 months later. (In the natural history of hyperactive, immature children, firesetting often occurs. Benji had lit matches, but set no fires, prior to the trauma. Therefore, this example is only a "probable" reenactment.)

Celeste (9), who had argued the morning of the kidnapping with her mother, believed that a "lady" kidnapper was driving the bus (perhaps her mental representation of "the avenging mother"). When the bus stopped, Celeste recollected, "I didn't want the lady to see me. I had my head down. I was on the back of the bus. Then I thought they'd shoot me if they found me, so I came out." Months after the kidnapping, Celeste occasionally behaved in a way which was inexplicable to herself and to her parents. Whenever she encountered a girlfriend or a woman teacher, at the market or on the street, she took cover. Hiding, a reenactment of the original episode which had occurred when Celeste "didn't want the lady to see me," was repeated whenever a female acquaintance was unexpectedly encountered.

Celeste had been forced into immobility, first in the van and then in the hole, where she eventually fell asleep. Celeste recalled, "In the hole I knew I was buried. I was worried I'd never see my parents again. I cried in the hole. The roof was caving in. I thought I'd be killed then. I did nothing. That was the very worst moment in the hole." A year after the kidnapping, Celeste explained, "I sit kind of paralyzed. I get a funny feeling that I have dreamed, but I can't remember. I think I get that feeling every day." Celeste's teacher has pointed out that Celeste is much quieter than last year.

Rachel (12) also had been too passive to become a self-appointed flashlight holder or baby-sitter in the hole. She watched, immobile and helpless. One year after the kidnapping, Rachel explained, "I stare at something and my mind drifts. It's definitely since the kidnapping. I go into trances. I don't know what I've been thinking. I used to talk more. Now I think a lot to myself."

Both Celeste and Rachel reenacted their original helpless paralysis with enough dreamy immobility to account for personality change.

Discussion

Reenactment was a striking finding in many of the Chowchilla children. Single reenactments were grim and dramatic, never consciously connected to the traumatic anxiety which precipitated them. Multiple reenactments in the same child accounted for personality change. Although quite similar to play, there was no associated sense of enjoyment in the reenactments. In contrast to "acting out," there was very little disguise or defensive elaboration.

Some Notes on the "Hero": Bob and Carl, the "child heroes" of Chowchilla, both suffered severe posttraumatic pathology. Publications on trauma have implied that the hero, by taking effective action, might be spared the effects of psychic trauma (Horowitz, 1976; Weiss and Payson, 1967), but this was not the case in Chowchilla. The heroes of Chowchilla suffered posttraumatic effects that were similar to those of the more passive kidnap victims. Their traumatic repetitions (play and reenactment) dealt more with heroics and omnipotence than did most other children's, although nonheroes such as Benji, Louis, Johnny, Sammy, and Terrie also experienced heroic or omnipotent postkidnapping fantasies (see below). Both the "heroes" and the more passive children, however, played, reenacted, feared, and relived in dreams the horrors of being a helpless victim. The "heroes" of Chowchilla were victims first, heroes second.

DREAMS

At the initial parent-group meetings in Chowchilla, a surprising variety of dreams were described by the kidnapped children's parents. Some mentioned that their children spoke or called out in their sleep, but had no later memory of a dream. Others pointed out that their youngsters dreamed exact repetitions of the kidnapping. Other parents remembered that their children had been frightened by a dream that the family or a friend had been kidnapped. Finally, some parents related that their children dreamed, but the dreams had "nothing to do with the kidnapping."

In interviews, each child was asked for dreams about the kidnapping, dreams similar to the kidnapping, dreams which had "nothing to do with the kidnapping," and their associations to such dreams. Furthermore, the child was asked about sleep habits, and the parents were asked about sleep-talking, sleepwalking, and night terrors.

Several different types of dreams could be distinguished by the degree to which the kidnapping experience was disguised in the manifest content of the dream: there were exact repeat playback, modified playback, and more fully disguised dreams. Some children had terror dreams, which they did not remember; others dreamed of their own deaths, and 2 children believed they had predictive dreams.

All the 23 children had dreams relating to the kidnapping after the event. Some children dreamed just one type of dream throughout the postkidnapping period; others began dreaming variant-repetitive dreams almost at once. There were some differences in the timing of the types of dreams. Terror dreams and exactly repeated dreams occurred more frequently in the early postkidnapping period, whereas many months later the disguised dreams were more common, as were the repetitive dreams in which there are variants in people, place, or conclusion.

Four Dreams of One Child: Jackie (9) described four dreams which exemplify each of the types noted above. They were dreamed in several successive nights one year after the kidnapping. Jackie's mother wrote me the following note, "It began with Jackie on July 5th. She came into our room in the middle of the night sobbing. She was not awake although her eyes were open. She began telling me that she was going to die, 'I'm going to die. I know I am going to die.' She said it several times, and it was quite awhile before we could get her completely awake. The next morning she said she did not remember coming into our room." The dream Jackie's mother described is a nonremembered terror dream.

In her interview on July 15, Jackie described the other dreams she had had "two weeks ago." In one dream, "Me and Johnny got kidnapped. Two guys who looked like two of the guys, the two oldest ones, who kidnapped us—they shot and killed both of us. I went in and told Mom I had a dream. I got up and crawled into bed with her." Jackie had fantasized during the kidnapping that she would be lined up and shot. The dream she described was an exact repetition of this fantasy.

Jackie went on. "I had another one. A store in town was getting robbed. Me and Mom were going to call the police. The same guys [two older kidnappers] saw us call the police and they shot us." This is a modified repeat dream. Mother is now a victim. She and Jackie ary trying to obtain effective help, a solution not possible in the actual kidnapping. They are caught and shot, again the dreaded fantasy of being shot, which had so frightened Jackie in the transfer from van to the hole.

When asked for a dream from the same period which had "nothing to do with the kidnapping," Jackie replied, "I had a dream in a castle. I was a princess with a big giant catching me, grabbing me. He grabbed my shirt and ripped it off."

"Which shirt?" I asked.

A look of utter amazement came across Jackie's face. "The shirt I wore and they [the kidnappers] took in the kidnapping!"

Unremembered Terror Dreams: Fourteen children's parents reported the occurrence of dreams in which the child called out, moaned, or got out of bed with no conscious verbalization or later memory of the experience. Their sleep-talk is indicative of thought which had occurred during the kidnapping itself. Sheila (11) cried out "no" in her sleep on several occasions. Susan (5) said, "Give it to me" (probably her new lunch pail the "crooks" had taken), and Jackie (9) said she was going to die. Elizabeth (9), who regretted that she had not sat with her younger sister on the bus, called out, "No, you can't have Mary!" Bob cried out, "Let us out" or "Leave us alone."

Eight children who experienced terror dreams have had other

types of dreams as well. Six had only terror dreams. Mandy (7) had only one episode of crying in her sleep about 2 months after the kidnapping. Celeste (9) reported daily dreams of which she had no memory. Ellen (6) slept with her mother because of unremembered nightmares. Carl (10) walked in his sleep several nights, but could not recall any dream content. Tania's mother reported, "Tania is dreaming. She's afraid to go to sleep—all along since it happened. I hope moving to a new house will straighten it out," but moving did not solve this problem. Bob (14) cried out and often moaned in his sleep, but he could remember nothing beyond the feeling that he had dreamed.

Exact Repeat Playback Dreams: These occurred in 12 children. Sally (7) reported that she experienced repeated dreams of the kidnapping only when she slept through church services. "I dream when the man gets on—when we get on the vans. I thought we were near the church when I was kidnapped." The church was the first mental association between "mundane" observation and the trauma itself that Sally had made during the kidnapping.

Janice (12) told me one year after the kidnapping that she had dreams of the men's faces, "being on the bus," her transfer from the van, and her escape from the hole. She had such dreams two or three times a month. She continued to dream of her electrocuted brother's face several times a month. The two sets of dreams were completely separate. Faces were prominent in Janice's dreams, most likely because of her horror upon seeing her electrocuted brother's face 5 years previously; thus when she was kidnapped, she feared and later dreamed about the men's faces.

Five children dreamed of the taking of the school bus by masked men; 3 dreamed of the vans, 2 dreamed of getting into the hole, and 1 dreamed about the escape from the hole. Such dreams portray the part of the kidnapping that was most frightening to the child. Benji (6) and Sheila (11) told of many exact repeat dreams, but did not identify the specific aspects that were repeated.

Four children experienced exact playback dreams of fantasies originally conceived during the kidnapping. Jackie's dreams of being lined up and shot have already been described. Louis (8), who originally had thought the men would throw him into the ocean, recalled, "I have bad dreams. Somebody will get me and take me far away in the ocean. I'm afraid you'd go down, down with the fish. The shark would eat me. I been learning how to swim, but I can't swim. I dream every night."

Elizabeth (9) initially believed she was needed to protect her sister, Mary. "After I got back [from the kidnapping] I had bad dreams every day for a few weeks. Then none at all. The bad dreams were in the hole. When they put us there, they took my shirt. I dreamed about going down the ladder. Mary wasn't going to come down. They would have taken her with them, I thought. I called Mary and she came down. I dreamed about that part." Elizabeth's mother believed that Elizabeth dreamed every night 12 months postkidnapping.

Mary (5), Elizabeth's sister, stated, "I had dreams about the hole. I thought they were down in there with us and I slept with my Mom that night and I got scared and I hid under the covers." In another dream, Mary "thought they [the kidnappers] were sleeping and I got scared." During her confinement in the hole, Mary had imagined that the kidnappers were in there too, a fantasy which subsequently became the theme of her dreams.

Modified Playback Dreams: Dreams with changes in characters, settings, or outcomes were reported by 14 children. Unlike the exact playback dreams, the modified dream was usually a single, unrepeated dream.

Dreams in which changes of protagonists occurred almost always included members of the family or friends. Johnny (11) was particularly upset about a dream in which his father was taken away and hung in a sack by the kidnappers. He had had an argument with his father the night before the dream. Terrie (10) dreamed twice that the kidnappers took her and her brother (an older boy, who had not been kidnapped) into the slough and killed her brother. Terrie recalled that during her captivity in the hole, she had worried whether her older brother could show at a local fair the swine that they had raised together. (In reality, of course, he never did exhibit the swine.) Alison (10) dreamed she was on a bus and that the kidnappers were "after" her father and little brother. Janice (12) dreamed her mother and father were kidnapped.

In some dreams, the place where the child was sleeping that night replaced the original kidnapping setting. Sheila (11) dreamed that men came into her aunt's house (where Sheila actually was sleeping that night) and were going to take her away. Debbie (10) dreamed the kidnappers were breaking into neighbors' houses. Sammy (10) the first night he slept home after the kidnapping thought, "The guys lived there [the quarry]. I thought they could have followed us. I dreamed someone covered my mouth and took me." After that, Sammy dreamed about ten dreams that the kidnappers were breaking into his bedroom to get him.

Changes in dream outcome also occurred: retribution or wishful-thinking outcomes, terror-filled suspenseful terminations, new conclusions to frightening fantasies which had occurred during the kidnapping, and death to the kidnap victim.

Benji (6) and Mary (5) experienced wishful-thinking retributive outcomes. Benji dreamed several "good dreams" in which he hit the kidnappers in the back or in the nose. Mary dreamed the kidnappers were in jail.

Terror dreams with uncertain, extremely frightening outcomes occurred in several instances. Rachel's (12) dreams of paralysis are particularly poignant. "I had one a few months later. We were at our house, outside. A guy was in our parking lot. Our door was shut. My sister-in-law was there. Someone else. The man had a gun. He told us to get in. They got in. I ran out, but *I couldn't move*. He shot me. I woke up." Rachel went on, "I had another dream. A man had come and was robbing an old next-door neighbor, who died about 3 years ago. He was taking everything from her house. I saw him and I couldn't identify him. I tried to get in and call the police, but *I couldn't move*. He was coming to our house. He had already killed everyone else. I woke up." Rachel is the girl who experienced dreamy paralysis as a reenactment of her inability to take any action during the kidnapping. Her modified playback dreams reveal the same terrifying paralysis.

Fantasies which actually concerned the child during the kidnapping itself turned up in dreams, sometimes with a new conclusion. Sheila (11), whose worst fears during the experience had been of smothering and of not seeing her parents again, dreamed that she, 7 friends, and the bus driver were taken off the school bus and buried by the kidnappers in little individual tents. One child was killed.

Disguised Dreams: In response to my request, "Tell me a dream

you had recently which has nothing to do with the kidnapping,"
Leslie (7) laughed and said, "I know a dream which has nothing
to do with it. I dreamed I ate ice cream!" She immediately associated, "We didn't get to eat ice cream at Disneyland." [9] Leslie had
experienced depression following her loss of contact with a man
who had hosted her at Disneyland. The dream is a wish-fulfillment
dream in which ice cream symbolizes Leslie's friend.

Disguised dreams dealt with the same types of content as the
repeated exact replay dreams and the modified playback dreams.
For instance, Sheila (11) dreamed a monkey had been caged by a
trainer, who "bossed it around." The monkey stood for the kidnapped child. The sequence ended retributively with release of
the "monkey" and retaliation upon the trainer (kidnapper). Sheila
could not remember if the dream appeared before or after the
kidnapping because her traumatic symptoms involved a distortion
of her sense of time. Several children could not remember whether
play, dreams, or fears, obviously connected to the trauma, had begun before or after the kidnapping, but parents were usually able
to corroborate that play and fears had developed afterward.
Dreams, on the other hand, could not be corroborated by parents.

Holes and underground places appeared in disguised dreams.
Elizabeth (9) dreamed that a friend's mother "would come and cut
everyone up and put us in a glass-deal. She sliced me with a knife.
She had already killed [her daughter] and she was still alive. We
went in a little hideout underground and her mother couldn't
find us." Leslie (7) dreamed, "I was in an alligator hole and an
alligator bit me. I woke up and was glad." She also "had a bad
dream about someone being in a big hole—one of those round
ones—a friend fell in."

Sammy's disguised dreams included corrective endings. He
stated, "Last night I dreamed I was king and told them to stop
ruling the world. And I got them on my side and I got the world
clean without anything bad going on. No drinking, smoking dope,
or anything." Sammy (10) went on to say he had "had a whole
bunch about making the world good or being happy."

Dreams in Which the Child Dies: Five Chowchilla children had

9. The kidnapped children were taken to Disneyland shortly after the
event.

dreams which are highly unusual in clinical practice: terrifying dreams of the child's own death. These death dreams occurred either in modified playback or in disguised form. Barbara (9) dreamed, "Three men stopped the kidnapped kids on the road and they killed us and then they put us in a hole." During the kidnapping Barbara realized she had been "buried" underground. To Barbara, burial is a mental representation of death. In another of Barbara's dreams, "We [her family] were riding in a car. Men in a van got us, kidnapped us, killed us, and put us in a grave." She went on to associate, "We were at the cemetery where my grandma is buried. We don't go there much. I don't remember my brother."

Jackie (9) repeatedly dreamed of being lined up, shot, and killed. She related, "I was the last one off the van. I was really scared. I thought they'd shoot the first and last person. I didn't expect to live when I got off the van." Jackie had imagined and accepted her own impending death; hence her ability to dream it.

Louis (8) remembered two recent dreams in which he had died. "A dinosaur stabbed me, and a wolfman got me and ate me." During his interview Louis had drawn a picture, "They're shooting me in the heart." Susan (5) dreamed, "A little big black dog bit me while I was asleep and I was dead." Susan also died in two other dreams in which a bat and a dracula killed her. During the stay in the hole, Susan had "tried to take a nap, but Louis got a little block [the stake holding up the roof] and he wouldn't put it back. Everybody woke up." Susan's experience of taking a little nap in the hole and waking up with the ceiling collapsing was, in her mind, being bitten while asleep and dying.

Predictive Dreams: Two girls experienced what they felt to be predictive dreams, which extremely frightened them. Alison (11) remembered, "Just before the kidnapping I had two dreams, both of them the same. I had them about two days before—one, one week before and one two days before. Me and Sheila were walking home. We went into the cafeteria. Two or three guys came in and locked it and said we'd never get out. I heard a ghost-dream after each dream [another repeated dream]. I don't know what those guys looked like. Sheila is my cousin. She was also kidnapped. Me, Sheila, and Celeste didn't want to go to school. Our mothers said 'no' and they pushed us out the door." Alison had said nothing about a "dream" when she argued with her mother about going to school the day of the kidnapping, but she mentioned her "predictive dreams" to her mother some time after the kidnapping. Alison's dreams were probably postkidnapping, modified playback dreams, which in retrospect seemed to Alison to have occurred prior to the kidnapping. As already noted, several children exhibited a distorted time sense related to the trauma (Johnny's gun collection and Sheila's caged-monkey dream were both thought to have occurred prior to the kidnapping).

Nineteen months after the kidnapping, Jackie (9) phoned about what she felt to be a "predictive" dream. Her class had gone on a ski trip and on the way back, Jackie had fallen asleep just as the school bus entered a mountain tunnel. "We [the ski-bus group] were in a hole, and men came in and shot us all. We were all dead. Is that going to happen? Did I dream the future?" Jackie was greatly relieved to hear my opinion that she had dreamed what had already happened, rather than what would occur later. The intensity of the dream was remarkable. The child felt so close to the trauma 19 months later that she could not be sure whether it was about to happen now or in the future.

Discussion

The repetitive dream is a hallmark of "traumatic neurosis," or "posttraumatic stress-response syndrome" (American Psychiatric Association, 1978) in adults. In sleep or dream laboratories, there have been attempts to produce such dreams experimentally, thus far, without success (De Koninck and Koulack, 1975).

In studies of adults from concentration camps, the battlefield, or peacetime stress, all the types of dreams found in the Chowchilla children have been described. For example, "Jane," one of the Horowitz's (1976) stressed patients, described her own nonremembered terror dreams. Exact repetitions and modified repetitions are noted by Mercier and Despert (1943), Rappaport (1968), and Krystal and Niederland (1968). An example of a disguised traumatic dream is described by Horowitz (1976) in the case of "Daniel."

Like other traumatic dreams, the dreams of the Chowchilla victims are an expression of the compulsion to repeat (Freud, 1920) and brought no relief. It was only the interpreted dream that offered the child an opportunity for abreaction and understanding. In this way, traumatic dreams were like traumatic play; interpretation was the primary mechanism of relief.

Dreams of Death: In clinical work with children, dreams of their own death are highly unusual. Fraiberg, in a personal communication,[10] has suggested that death dreams may be the repetition of the child's past experience with what he or she believes to be death itself. For many children, burial underground means death. They cannot conceptualize death beyond being put in a box and placed under the earth. A child who has been placed in a hole and has heard dirt shoveled on top dreams death as a past experience for which the mental representation is accepted into dream life. On the basis of the idea that one dreams one's own death if one has already experienced "one's own death," it can be postulated that children who have fainted, who have experienced seizures, who have been in comas, or who have been emotionally unprepared for anesthetic induction might also dream their own deaths.

A second mechanism enabling a child to dream about his or her death may be based on the child's belief during a psychic trauma that death is close at hand and the child's acceptance of impending death. Once death is accepted as a reality, not to be fought, but to be allowed in, the image of death is incorporated into the mind and is available for dreaming.

One might view death dreams as similar to examination dreams and interpret them along the lines indicated by Freud (1900): in the past what was dreaded most did not come to pass, a reassuring thought with regard to the future. On the other hand,[11] the profound dread and terror with which the children reacted to their death dreams lessens this possibility. Rather than a sense of relief upon waking up alive, at least one child, Jackie (9), believed the

10. I wish to thank and acknowledge the help of Selma Fraiberg, Ann Arbor, Michigan, for her review of my original draft, and for her thoughts on death dreams.

11. A letter from Freud (1930) to Elizabeth Lancaster (published in 1970, see Lancaster) indicates that he believed traumatic dreams as a class to be quite different from examination dreams.

death dream to be "predictive." Since the kidnapped children as a group were so resistant to reassurance, this explanation of their death dreams does not coincide well with their other observable characteristics.

Finally, dreams of death and dreams of paralysis may occur in part because the traumatized child is readily able to perceive while dreaming the motor paralytic effects of REM sleep. If this perception (Hobson and McCarley, 1977) occurs in the psychically traumatized child, there may be some posttraumatic change in the nature of dreaming which enables the psychically stressed child to perceive REM paralytic effects more readily than the nonstressed child.

Dreams and Verbalization: While evaluating the Chowchilla children, I rated their ability to verbalize their feelings, based upon behavior in interviews and material from parents' histories. Seven children were particularly nonverbal about emotion. Six of these children experienced only unremembered terror dreams; Terrie (10), the exception, remembered only two dreams, both modified playback dreams about her brother being killed in a kidnapping.

In contrast to this, the 9 particularly verbal children experienced at least two types of dreams. They had multiple and repeated dreams. They remembered what had occurred in most dreams, and they used their dream associations to gain relief in their psychiatric interviews.

Infants exhibit large amounts of REM sleep (Anders, 1978), but nothing is known about the content of their dreams. Since dreams do not depend upon verbalizations, we cannot expect the nonverbal youngsters actually to have dreamed less. On the other hand, the type of dreams the kidnapped children related depended upon their ability to verbalize. Some ability to verbalize emotion is required for a disguised or a playback dream to be dreamed and to be remembered. Without the ability to speak about emotional material, the major dream type available to the child is the terror dream. The night terror is a well-described phenomenon of the toddler-age child (Niederland, 1957). One explanation for the commonness of this type of dream in 2- and 3-year-olds may be their inability freely to verbalize emotion. As the child acquires this ability (Katan, 1961), night terrors tend to disappear. Six of the 7 Chowchilla youngsters who never fully acquired the ability to verbalize emotions, like toddlers, dreamed dreams for which no words could later be found. Without words, it was difficult to remember. Without words, there was only nameless terror.

Predictive Dreams and Time-Skew: The notion that dreams actually predict future events will not be dealt with here. I feel that the explanation for "predictive dreams" lies in the ego's belated attempt at mastery following a traumatic event. The psychically traumatized child searches for ways the stress could have been avoided by obsessing about prior events, episodes during the trauma itself, and even posttraumatic occurrences such as dreams. These episodes are connected because the ego's attempts at mastery and control require answers to "Why did it happen to me? How could I have been warned?" In the child's search for ways he or she would have been prepared, the child pays little attention to visual perceptions or to time sequences. If a dream happened after the trauma, it may be snatched up and used associatively as an omen, or a portent, "I should have known. I had a dream first."

COMPENSATORY FANTASIES

Revenge fantasies were observed in 6 youngsters. Bob (14) emphatically stated, "I get revenge thoughts. I would put them back down there where we were. They'd have as much food and water. I'd put hinges and a padlock on that [metal] plate. If they'd done that, we couldn't have gotten out. I'd like to turn them loose in Chowchilla for a day. Everybody'd take care of them. My dad said, 'They've lived toooooo long!' " Benji (6), far less sophisticated than Bob, put it this way, "I still hate them. I double hate, I mean 'twiple' hate 'em. I think about 'em once a week. Like I'm going to kick 'em. After Sunday, it'll be a few days until I get this cast [broken leg] off, then I'm going to kick them in the mouth."

In January 1977, as Leslie (7) walked home from school, a man stopped her and showed her his genitals. Leslie's comparative thoughts about the kidnappers and the exhibitionist are interesting. "I think all the guys are on Death Row and they'll get executed. I think he [one of the kidnappers] should get executed [she sighed], he probably won't [sighed again]. Maybe a firing squad or a gas chamber. I wish they'd use a firing squad. It's faster. It'll be over and they won't do it again. I think they wanted money and they wanted to shoot us. I think a little about the man I saw [the exhibitionist]. I have no dreams about the man. I think he should be put in jail for 2 years."

Susan's mother reported that Susan (5) wanted the prison officials to "starve them to death. They didn't feed us." Louis's revenge fantasies were less specific, "I'm driving and crashing with cars and everything." Jackie (9) suggested to her mother that the kidnappers "ought to be kept in the hole until the trial."

Fantasies of heroism or omnipotence were observed in 5 youngsters. Terrie (10) retrospectively fantasied that she had been unafraid during the kidnapping. Actually, she had been very confused and anxious about separation from her brother. Terrie recalled, "I believed we'd be able to get out. If they set their mind to it, anybody can do anything." Bob (14) told his mother he'd like to "show" the kidnappers by winning the world rodeo championship. Louis (8) asked me, "How do you grab guns?"

Johnny (11) felt he had failed by not being a "hero." A long time before the kidnapping, Johnny and his father had seen the movie *Dirty Harry,* in which a school bus and its passengers are held hostage by an escaping criminal. As they watched the movie, "Dad kept saying, 'What would you do if you got kidnapped like that?' " Johnny never answered. During the kidnapping Johnny felt he did nothing special. Later he retrospectively reconstructed his father's question to be a warning. He believed he should have prepared himself. In response to the disappointment of failing himself and failing his father, Johnny indulged in heroic fantasies as well as actual preparations for heroism.

Sammy (10) similarly indulged in large-scale heroic and religious daydreams. He insisted upon taking part in Barbara's and Janice's scheduled interview, but then asserted, "I don't need to talk to you. I have faith." He observed, "I've had a whole bunch [of daydreams] about making the world good or being happy. [During the kidnapping] I worried about the *other* kids. I hoped nothing would happen to them. I didn't care about myself."

In this context, it is interesting to note a posttraumatic fantasy of Bob (14), who in reality had been the "hero" of the incident. It will be recalled that the kidnapping inadvertently was Bob's "punishment" for dawdling that morning. Mrs. B. had punished him by refusing to drive him home from school. Later Bob felt he was placed on the bus "by chance" in order to help the children escape. He mentally reversed the "punishment" into the "privilege" of heroism (a "heroism" which he dangerously and inappropriately reenacted 18 months after the kidnapping).

Mandy's postkidnapping wish never to have to separate from her mother again was somewhat analogous to the omnipotent wish-fulfillment fantasies noted above. Mrs. M. related, "Once she told me she'd never get married and she'd live with me for the rest of her life. Another time she said she'd marry a rich guy, build me a house to live in, and get me to baby-sit. She told me she'd give me a penny for it!"

Two children experienced fantasies of parental hostility, most likely displacements of the kidnappers' motives to parents. Mandy (7) accused her mother during an argument of wishing she were back in the hole. Benji (6) had moved into a new house a few months after the kidnapping. He very seriously stated, "They'll fix my room when I die." This is a highly unusual statement for a young child. Benji had accepted his own death, as had the child victims who dreamed their own deaths.

Discussion

Altogether, 10 children's fantasies have been reported in this section. It is surprising that there were not more. However, considering the brevity of my contact with these children and the much more pressing realities, fears, dreams, and behaviors they wished to discuss, the paucity of fantasy material is understandable. Further research studies of a more prolonged and intensive type may shed more light upon the formation of unconscious fantasies that link the external trauma to phase-specific internal conflicts.

PSYCHOPHYSIOLOGICAL SYMPTOMS

Some of the physical symptoms experienced by the children after the kidnapping, such as urinary urgency and/or incontinence, often associated with cramps, as well as Alison's asthmatic attacks and Sammy's fainting spells, can be considered reenactments of physical responses which originally had occurred during the psychic trauma itself (see above). Dillon and Leopold (1961) observed 13 cases of enuresis which they attributed to posttraumatic psychological regressions in children who had sustained concussions. Although regression may contribute to the urinary problems of the Chowchilla victims, specific reenactment is a more likely cause.

Other physical symptoms appeared to be associated with the chronic anxiety. Sammy's nystagmus, a sign related to his blindness, worsened appreciably the year following the kidnapping, according to his mother. "His eyes were very dilated and his eyes moved a lot more. They took his glasses from him on the kidnapping. He's had headaches, but I figure it's the eye problem. The headaches have only come up since the kidnapping." Elizabeth (9) also experienced worsening of a preexisting physical symptom. Her knee, chronically painful from a torn cartilage, was far more bothersome the year following the trauma.

Seven children's eating habits and weight changed markedly. Janice (12), Susan (5), and Mandy (7) gained more than 10 pounds, and Tania (8) and Jackie (9) gained weight so quickly they outgrew their clothes. The latter 2 girls tapered off to more ordinary size, but the first 3 remained overweight. Carl (10) stopped eating and lost weight, although he is now fairly well proportioned. Johnny (11), who had been accused of being too chubby to be a "digger," recalled, "My eating cycle was off when I got home. I couldn't eat dinner." Johnny valiantly tried to lose weight and gain strength after the kidnapping. When I last saw him in late summer 1977, he looked leaner and his voice had changed. He had spent the entire summer doing hard physical labor outdoors.

PERSONALITY CHANGES

In other sections of this report, I have referred to behaviors and attitudes that led to lasting personality changes in the children. Here I shall summarize those findings and present some additional observations.

Four types of personality changes were noted by parents: hostile or irritable personalities (6 children): dreamy or immobile personalities (3 girls); clinging or regressive personalities (6 girls); and show-off or clownish personalities (4 boys). Some of the personality changes consisted of frequently repeated reenactments; in others, the child's behavior was not a repetition of behavior or fantasy which had occurred during the trauma, but rather was the repetition of an attitude developed during the kidnapping. A third group of personality changes could not be considered repetitions at all, but instead were the end product of severe chronic anxiety or depression.

"Mean" behavior or persistent irritability were observed in Barbara (9), Tania (9), Sammy (10), Alison (10), and Sheila (11). Janice (12) was expelled from school three times the year following the kidnapping for misbehavior and failure to obey the rules. Shortly after the kidnapping she gained over 15 pounds. She explained most of her difficulties the year after the kidnapping as "nervousness." Janice, who suffered from a traumatic reaction prior to the kidnapping, could not handle two simultaneous post-traumatic conditions with enough remaining energy to cope with ordinary frustrations. Barbara (9), Janice's sister, originally had been easygoing, but after the kidnapping she, too, was irritable and prone to bickering. Barbara experienced terrifying dreams of her own death and was fearful of ordinary stimuli. As in Janice's case, Barbara's irritability was probably related to extreme anxiety. Four children demonstrated mean or angry character changes as reenactments (Tania, Sheila, Alison, and Sammy).

Withdrawal and immobility occurred as reenactments in 2 cases (Rachel and Celeste), but a similar personality change affected Leslie (7), because of the worsening of preexisting depression. Leslie was deeply hurt when a man, who had been her host at Disneyland, did not phone or write her afterward. This served to reawaken Leslie's prolonged mourning for her natural father, with whom contact had been broken one year prior to the kidnapping.

Six youngsters regressed. Ellen (6), Sally (7), Elizabeth (9), and Mary (5) continued to sleep in the same beds with their mothers one year after the kidnapping. Susan (5), who the morning of the kidnapping had requested not to go to school, developed a school phobia and clinging and gained 10 pounds in a short time after the kidnapping. Mandy (7) also regressed and gained weight. Her mother explained, "She's always been quiet and bashful. [Now] she gets all nervous when I'm shopping and walk around the corner. She clung in Disneyland. She absolutely clung and pulled on me. Terrie's mother couldn't get over how she would not have anything to do with the group. She still sticks with me." In Mandy's case, an exaggeration of preexisting personality traits occurred after the trauma.

The fourth type of personality change observed was "show-off" or "clownish" behavior. Four boys exhibited this pattern; in each case, there was both exaggeration of preexisting traits and some reenactment. Carl's stepfather complained, "Before the kidnapping he was a little bit show-off. Much more now!" Louis (8), Carl's brother, grimaced or stuck his tongue out whenever he felt anxious. His mother stated, "He is funny and should be in the circus. He does things to look like a crazy guy." Louis had "covered" for his academic difficulties for years by playing the "fool" or the "clown." This "foolish" behavior worsened when he also had to "cover" for his disruption of the stake which had almost resulted in death for the entire group.

Johnny (11), who called himself "Joker Boy," had taken part in a class play the day of the kidnapping. He played the part of Samuel Adams in a production ironically entitled "We Must Be Free." After mentioning the play in an interview, Johnny followed with a joke, "A guy has a 'lucky ring,' looks at it, and falls into a manhole." Johnny's retrospective association of the ironic play title to the trauma itself was one factor in the inappropriate clownishness he exhibited for at least 8 months after the kidnapping. Furthermore, he had wisecracked during the bus take-over itself. When the kidnappers took his shoes, Johnny commented to his fellow victims, "Poor guys [the kidnappers]. Maybe they'll smell them." When the kidnappers told him, "Get down in the hole," he mimicked, "a 'hole'?" Since the kidnapping, Johnny's behavior is replete with wisecracks. At midyear, his teacher complained of this to Johnny's parents.

Benji (6), like Johnny, had attempted to "talk back" to the kidnappers. He told his parents 2 weeks after the kidnapping that "it was a bravery test and he passed." There is now a show-off quality in Benji's attitude. He calls his parents "Dummy" and "Stupid." He brags about the damage he could do to the kidnappers.

Nineteen children exhibited personality changes. Only 4 youngsters were spared (Bob, Terrie, Jackie, and Debbie). Girls and boys tended to establish different personality problems. Although there were only 6 boys in the study group, 4 took on "wise-guy" or "clownish" attitudes, 1 acted "mean," and 1 was spared personality difficulties. On the other hand, of 17 girls, 6 regressed, 3 were immobilized, and 5 became "mean" and/or irritable. Three girls were spared personality change. The sex difference observed may in part be due to the different roles the children were assigned during the kidnapping: activity to the boys and passive waiting for the girls. Girls, who were allowed to do nothing in the hole, later were immobile or regressed. Boys, on the other hand, who had dared a wisecrack or who had helped remove dirt, were overly sarcastic or mean afterward. Girls, who were hostile or irritable after the kidnapping, were reenacting morning fights with their mothers or exhibiting debilitating anxiety.

SUMMARY OF LONG-TERM EFFECTS

Every one of the 23 children was affected by the psychic trauma of the kidnapping. For clarity, I have tabulated major findings. Table 2 presents the important posttraumatic symptoms and signs and the number of children affected by each. In table 3 I have clinically rated the severity of the children's symptoms. The correlations between severity of stress-related symptoms and characteristics of the group appear in table 4.

Age, presence of siblings or cousins during the kidnapping, and family pathology has no apparent effect upon the severity of posttraumatic symptoms. Although there were fewer boys, 5 of the 6 had severe symptoms and the 6th was clinically very close to the severe group, whereas the 17 girls divided evenly in severity. The reason for the severe symptoms in boys is uncertain, but it may be related to the weaker community ties in the boys' families. There seems to be some protective function in family bonding to the

Table 2

Symptoms and Number of Children Affected

Symptom	Number of Children Affected
Personality change	19
School decline	8
Reenactment	14
Play	11
Retelling	5
Dreams (total)	23
Death or predictive	6
Only unremembered terror dreams	6
Time-skew	8
Initial misidentification	5
Hallucination	3
Fears	23
Compensatory fantasies	10

Table 3

Severity of Posttraumatic Symptomatology

Severity	Number	Children
Asymptomatic	0	
Mild	0	
Moderate	6	Ellen (6), Leslie (7), Sally (7), Jackie (9), Debbie (10), Terrie (10)
Moderately severe	7	Mary (5), Mandy (7), Louis (8), Celeste (9), Barbara (9), Sheila (11), Rachel (12)
Severe	10	Susan (5), Benji (6), Tania (8), Elizabeth (9), Sammy (10), Alison (10), Carl (10), Johnny (11), Janice (12), Bob (14)

community; 8 children in the severe group come from families with weak community ties.

There also appears to be a correlation between prior major physical or emotional vulnerability of the child and posttraumatic

Table 4

Symptom Severity and Group Characteristics

Number in Group	6 Moderate	7 Moderately Severe	10 Severe
Age Range	5–10	5–12	5–14
Sex	6 girls	6 girls 1 boy	5 girls 5 boys
Siblings or Cousins present	4	6	8
Family pathology			
No problems	0	3	2
One problem	4	1	3
Two problems	2	3	5
Relationship to Community			
Strong	4	4	2
Weak	2	3	8
Prior Vulnerability of Child (Physical or Emotional)			
Major	1	1	4
Minor	3	2	2
None	2	4	4

symptoms. Only 2 children with major vulnerability were not in the most severely affected group. Leslie (7) suffered from a depression prior to the kidnapping. Although her stress-related symptom severity was only moderate, she exhibited worsening of her depression after the kidnapping experience. Louis was on the borderline of the most severely affected classification. It is important to note that *every* child was moderately to severely affected.

THE FAMILIES' AND COMMUNITY'S RESPONSE

Because my major research interest in the Chowchilla study was to observe the reactions of individual children to a single psychic trauma, information about community responses to the trauma was obtained informally and at times parenthetically. By the time the study ended, a surprisingly large amount of data about community response had accumulated. The most productive source of information was the parents' group meetings, but data were also obtained in the children's and parents' interviews as well as in talks with the school superintendent, district attorney, and sheriff. Parents and children were candid about their feelings about one another, about the community, and about their understanding of the community's response to them.

RESPONSE OF FAMILIES

Traumatic Responses of Individuals: During the kidnapping family members suffered definite stress-related symptoms. Families were initially confused when their children did not return, and in general they denied to themselves that any foul play could have occurred. Many families attributed the bus delay to a flat tire or a minor accident. No family immediately believed a "disaster" had taken place. The second state, severe apprehension, occurred for each family when they made contact with the school superintendent, the sheriff's office, or another informed individual, and learned that the bus and children were missing.

The apprehensive period was emotionally traumatic. Some parents with many relatives in the Chowchilla area were able to group together with their extended families, which served some protective function. The situation was worse for families without many friends or relatives. Mrs. L., Louis's and Carl's mother recalled, "I was waiting for the kids. Someone had said the bus broke down. At first I was not scared. Then at 10 o'clock someone from the school came. They told me that they [the boys] had been kidnapped. No one came to stay with us. I couldn't sleep at night. I cried."

During the traumatic wait, some parents reacted just as the kidnap victims were reacting themselves in the vans and hole. They thought back to the morning before. These parents experienced guilt about interactions with their youngsters. How could they have insisted that their children go to school against their wills, or as a punishment? Susan's mother sounded almost as though she had written this article herself when she puzzled, "On the day of the kidnapping she said, 'I don't want to go swimming.' I think Susan may have had a presentiment. I was going to pick her up at noon. Now I kick myself that I got too busy and didn't get her at noon." Mrs. J. said, "Jackie had kissed me good-bye and then called me and kissed me again. That stuck in my mind." Mrs. J. believed throughout the absence of the youngsters that Jackie may have sensed an omen or a presentiment. She stated, "Every day I see them off now [to school], 'you guys have a nice day' even when I'm angry. Every day." Bob's mother, who had punished him by insisting that he take the bus, volunteered, "When they were missing I considered it *my* fault and I felt terribly guilty."

Long-term individual responses of nonkidnap victims within families bear strong similarities to the victims' later reactions. Stress-response symptoms were experienced by parents, some siblings, and grandparents as well. A few nonkidnapped siblings became willing, or at least passive, participants to kidnap play. Some parents experienced kidnap-related dreams. Leslie's mother told of a repeated dream that her "father was going away and never coming back again. I was in a foster home from 4 to 8. The dream was that he was leaving me there. The place was a dump." In this situation, Leslie's mother's identification with her own child's helplessness reawakened in her the long-dormant traumatic anxiety about her own "abandonment" at age 4. Susan's and Tania's mother talked in her sleep after the kidnapping, "I don't care what you say. It's too dark to see what they're doing." These dreams are the result of the mothers' intense identifications with their children. A grandparent also identified with the victims. In February, Benji's and Tania's mother stated, "My father is obsessed with it. He can't sleep, still. He says, 'Try to put yourself in their [the victims'] place.' He's almost 72. He just retired; he had been retired 2 months when it happened. He wants to write a book to get it out of his system." Leslie's little sister, Marjorie, is an interesting example of dreams by identification. In 1978, long after the data-gathering was complete, Leslie's mother phoned to tell me that Marjorie, then age 4, had recently begun experiencing repeated frightening dreams, "I'm in a hole." These were the first dreams that the little girl had ever told her mother.

Family members reacted to the episode with overprotectiveness often mixed with hostility toward "outsiders." Alison's mother reported, "I hold back on things she could do, like going to a friend's house, or if she's 5–10 minutes late." Sammy's mother stated, "I feel fearful of who they [Sammy and his sister] talk to. I back off from strangers." Terrie's 17-year-old brother, according to Mr. T., "was hostile to anyone who offended Terrie. Reporters were all over her sticking microphones in her mouth. He hit one of them."

Many family members felt they needed to express their overwhelming feelings in writing or by speaking a great deal. This is evident in the parents' "books" and interviews to the press about the kidnapping. Jackie and Johnny's mother "wrote a minute-by-minute account" of the occurrences of the first several days. Benji's and Tania's father told me, "I thought of a song all about the kidnapping and I have written it down." (Unfortunately I never heard it.)

The "fourth kidnapper hypothesis" spread into the parents' realm of fears and, of course, this did not help to stop the theory, which had originated with their own children. Sammy's mother spoke for both herself and her husband, "We are still fearful that someone else could have been involved. Maybe women. They [the kidnappers] were staying in a house in the country. I felt there were more people involved than just those three. At a parents' meeting, several parents pointed out that one adult witness had noted four vans and that another citizen of Chowchilla had seen three vans the afternoon of the kidnapping. Even as they mentioned their concern about extra vans, the parents' consensus was that "the kids came up with the story [of the fourth kidnapper], rather than the adults." At another parents' meeting, Johnny and Jackie's mother noted several murders and fatal accidents which had occurred in Chowchilla in the past few months. Her statement,

"So much is happening in Chowchilla," carried with it the terrifying idea of a "master plan." Finally, Janice's and Barbara's mother required hospitalization in May 1977. "Last month I was in the hospital for 3 or 4 days for 'nerves.' I still think someone in town is letting people know everything that's going on. I feel someone is telling private secret things. The guys who kidnapped the kids, they took off, they had planned to go back. How did they know all this mess? They didn't have radios or anything. My thoughts stopped hanging together. I thought all along that there is another person."

Just as the children had convinced themselves that the jailed kidnappers might come back, Louis's and Carl's mother worried, "When I saw the one with glasses [a kidnapper shown on TV after the arrest], I looked in the windows and thought I saw one of them; sometimes still!" Mandy's mother, a person from a close-knit family, was in no way spared the fears or vicarious "flashbacks" of the kidnapping. "I get awfully scared, and scenes from the kidnapping flash through my mind every time I miss one of them" (her two children, one a kidnap victim).

In summary, those parents who were willing to disclose their response to the kidnapping exhibited with less intensity many of the same traumatic reactions the children had exhibited. They searched retrospectively for omens, and they experienced guilt about everyday ordinary interactions with their children. Some of them exhibited traumatic dreams. Many feared a fourth kidnapper or a return of the original kidnappers. They wrote and talked repeatedly about the event to try to expel its repetitious influence.

Traumatic Responses of Families: Three kidnap victims were moved by their families out of the Chowchilla community within weeks to a month or two. Carl and Louis, who often migrate to another state for a few months each year, stayed away from Chowchilla longer the year after the kidnapping. As a matter of fact, Carl was left in another state for the entire school year, even though his family returned to California in early spring, 1977.

Since the study finished, two additional families (3 victims) have left the Chowchilla area. The parents of 2 other kidnapped youngsters are contemplating a move to a far distant state. Almost a year before they moved, the father of one victim told me, "I'd like to leave and tell no one where we are. Our words have been twisted. Parents are resenting things that were supposed to have been said which we haven't said. Reporters have misquoted me. They blew everything up and exaggerated."

Moves occurred for realistic reasons, such as better jobs or loss of privacy in Chowchilla, but also for emotional reasons. These were: (1) fear of another kidnapping in Chowchilla; (2) fragmentation of the parents' community and their relationship to the community at large (see below); (3) realization by some families that they would prefer being near extended families at times of great stress.

Three temporary separations between parents occurred within months of the kidnapping, and I did brief marriage counseling for each of these couples. Two of the marriages reconstituted and have remained stable since then. In the third case, other separations had previously taken place between the parents and their relationship remains tenuous. Although there were a great many preexisting problems in each of the 3 couples, there is no doubt that the acute stress of the kidnapping precipitated the separations. None of the 3 couples had strong ties to the Chowchilla community, nor did they have extended families nearby.

THE FAMILIES AND THE COMMUNITY

Victims and Nonkidnapped Peers: Many kidnap victims retained their good relationships with nonkidnapped Chowchilla children. However, there were trends which caused problems between the victims and their nonkidnapped peers: jealousy, scapegoating, and attempts to create more fear in the victims. Sammy's blindness, which until then he had been able to hide, was exposed in the newspapers. "It was in the paper about my blindness. They went around saying, 'You're blind.' Kids felt they didn't want to go around with a blind kid." Sally (7) worried that at show-and-tell in summer school, 1977, "a boy told about a very big gun that could kill 8 people and Miss Percy told about it too. They did that because I was kidnapped." Johnny complained that children who "mentioned" the kidnapping set off immediate daydreams. Janice related, "Kids say I'll go to summer school and get kidnapped."

Leslie complained, "A little girl named Nancy said there'd be a kidnapping in the cafeteria after that. She said she'd known that first. It makes me worried it'll happen. Someone else'll do it maybe at summer school. I might not even want to go. Darlene thinks it will happen again. Everytime she says it, she makes me cry. She won't leave me alone. And just I thought it would happen again."

Many nonkidnapped youngsters were jealous of the victims' attention, notoriety, and Disneyland trip. Sammy mentioned, "Some on the bus say, 'Man, I wish I was in it!' I don't think it's so lucky." Tania complained, "Everybody asks me things. I don't know what. I don't like to talk about it."

The Families and Their Relationship to Each Other: The parents of the victims, many of whom had not really known each other prior to the kidnapping, were thrown into an immediate relationship in which they shared in common their horrible experience. A massive fragmentation of the parents' unity had, however, already taken place by the time I arrived in Chowchilla in December 1976. The process of the development of the parent-group splintering began with their relationships with reporters. Hundreds of reporters had descended on the town within hours of the news. Some parents were willing to talk to reporters; some of them were misquoted. Furthermore, reporters inserted their own opinions in the articles, such as the opinion that Chowchilla is a poor, hot, dusty town. Parents, nonkidnapped townsfolk, and town authorities resented "bad mouthing" of the town, and afterward blamed the parents who had been willing to talk to reporters. Social workers, teachers, psychiatrists, or general physicians were not mobilized. News reporters were thus the recipients of the parents' and children's verbalizations, much of it subjective and highly emotional. The end product of the "talk" was mutual suspicion. Terrie (10) said, "I feel the kids talk too much. I think some people are trying to get something off of this."

The second external factor in the splintering of the parental community was the parents' attempts at general meetings after the kidnapping. After a relatively smooth first meeting, a second meeting took place at which they tried to elect a slate of officers; discussed how to distribute money which had come into the community as voluntary contributions; and mentioned a possible civil lawsuit. A few parents dominated the meeting. As a result of these very innocent mistakes, some parents believed that a kidnap "social club" was being formed, certainly not the intention of the parents who had organized the meeting in order to express their feelings and "compare notes" on the progress of the children. Furthermore, some parents deeply resented any talk of money, although the distribution of voluntary contributions was indeed a realistic problem. One father complained, "About 15 people were there and we couldn't get in a word. I got up and told them when my daughter was gone, I would have given anything to get her back, and I got her back for nothing. I didn't want anything from anyone because I got what I wanted." He resented the others "trying to get money out of it." Money issues, which later were discussed with more calm, could not be handled at all a few months after the kidnapping.

The Reactions to Local Officials: After discussing the stories of the kidnapping with their children, many parents disagreed with the media's and the town's designation of the bus driver as the sole hero of the affair. In addition, they questioned the handling of money and the news media by town officials and school administrators. They experienced unhappiness about their churches and ministers as well. Terrie's father explained, "I used to go to church before this happened. After it happened, our minister wanted to have a special program for Terrie. He had 5 or 6 reporters there with cameras set up in the church. I was embarrassed. We felt tricked. Terrie was embarrassed. We didn't want publicity. I didn't appreciate them in church when we were there to give thanks."

The disintegration of parent-community unity occurred because the parents of the victims experienced so much unchanneled internal hostility that they were ready to turn on each other and on all the community authorities at the smallest "insult" or "embarrassment." The hostility had been stirred up by the senseless attack upon their children for which no motivation had then or has yet been discovered. With the kidnappers safely in custody, revenge fantasies could not successfully channel all the anger.

Relation to Law Enforcement Officials: The major force in the community which eventually began to unify the parents and also provided them some outlet for their anger was the law enforcement team of sheriff and district attorney. These men were willing to listen and to record the injuries done to the children. They had the singleminded purpose of presenting the state's, and therefore the parents', case in criminal court. Some parents, who had originally shied away from any psychiatric intervention, arranged appointments after the district attorney pointed out that the psychiatric reports would help him to establish that "bodily harm" had been done.

Relation to Mental Health Workers: The town of Chowchilla was unprepared to handle a psychiatric emergency. The day after the children returned, the director of Family Service of Fresno phoned the Madera County Sheriff's office offering large-scale help, and was told everything was under control. Family Service of Fresno was never contacted after that.[12] The director of the Madera County Mental Health Clinic consulted immediately with the Superintendent of Schools. However, the only direct contact between some parents and children and professionals of the community mental health service occurred at a meeting a few months after the kidnapping. Some parents might eventually have sought out the mental health facility, but the workers did not approach the individual parents directly. Furthermore, one set of parents who felt disappointed about a prior contact with the clinic expressed their opinion to other parents. "We had several visits with a psychiatrist in Madera. They sat on the floor playing cars. They never told me much. They were trying to teach us how to live with him." Another mother told others that she had phoned the clinic, "talked to the lower-downs, and it's baloney!" Finally, parents may have hesitated to ask for help because at their meeting with the mental health center staff, "they said maybe 1 in 26 would experience problems. They assured us nothing would be wrong." Which parent could admit that his child was the 1 in 26?

THE TREATMENT OF CHILDREN AND FAMILIES

During the course of this study, brief treatment produced noticeable improvements in some of the children. These were brought about primarily by abreaction and understanding attained through

12. Personal communication, Mary Amacher, Director, Family Service of Santa Cruz and formerly Director, Family Service, Fresno.

interpretation or clarification. Most traumatic play was curtailed by the end of the study period. Reenactments continued, as did personality changes. Terrifying dreams were less frequent, although still present. Fears of other kidnappings continued unabated. At the end of the study period, Benji's mother had arranged for him to enter long-term psychotherapy. Elizabeth's mother had planned to enroll her as a patient in the local community mental health center, but there is no indication that she did so. No other parents were interested in obtaining psychiatric help on a long-term basis for their youngsters.

It would be interesting to interview these children again 2 to 3 years from now to determine which, if any, traumatic effects still remain.

Discussion

In Chowchilla, in response to a strictly psychic trauma without death, mutilation, or loss of property, family members exhibited reactions that were similar to, but less intense than, those of the victims themselves. There are two mechanisms which account for this. (1) Families were psychically traumatized from the beginning by the realization that their children were missing and helpless. They experienced the guilt described by Lindemann (1944), and the "search for meaning" defined by Chodoff et al. (1964). Furthermore, they struggled for ego mastery through the retrospective search for omens and portents. (2) Because of strong identification between parents and children and because of the regressive tendency in normal parents which allows them to reexperience their own developmental stage as their child experiences it (Benedek, 1959), the parents put themselves in their children's places and experienced the trauma just as the youngsters did. Examples of the traumatization by identification are 3 mothers' dreams of being victims, the parents' fears of strangers, and the spread to parents of the "fourth kidnapper hypothesis." Leslie's little sister's dreams of holes is an example of symptom spread by a younger sibling's identification.

Washburn and Hamburg (1965) reported the spreading effect of fear among African baboons following the shooting of 2 animals by a local scientist. Even though the entire band of baboons had not witnessed the shooting, the fearful behavior of some dominant animals led the others to follow suit for 8 months. The spreading effect of psychic trauma was reported in the Buffalo Creek disaster. It was possible in the civil lawsuit to collect damages for psychiatric disturbances in relatives of the victims or members of the community who had been far distant from Buffalo Creek at the time of the flood (Stern, 1976). In Chowchilla, the spread of fear was unique, in that it was the children's fears which spread to the parents, rather than the reverse, which has been previously reported many times.

The second important point in considering the families is the fragmentation which occurs in a psychically traumatized community. Chowchilla illustrates that fragmentation occurs because of psychic trauma; and that death, mutilation, or property loss are not required for the disintegration of community unity to take place. Kai Erikson (1976) first observed and recorded the fragmentation which occurred under the very different traumatic conditions (death and loss of whole towns) in Buffalo Creek. When Chowchilla also exhibited fragmentation of community, it could more definitely be concluded that *psychic* trauma is central to the loss of community unity. Undirected hostility accounts for the fragmentation in Chowchilla. Several authors point out that a manmade catastrophe arouses more aggression than a natural disaster (Lifton and Olson, 1976; Luchterhand, 1971; Rangell, 1976). Because there was no way for the Chowchilla parents, children, or town officials adequately to express hostility to the kidnappers, nor was there any way to understand why the event had happened, parents and children began to express hostility in situations they could understand. The church, the school, the town administration, and the other parents became the recipients of displaced hostility.

DISCUSSION

The Chowchilla kidnapping provided a unique research opportunity: (1) 26 "normal" youngsters had experienced *the same trauma;* (2) the trauma was *purely psychological* with no concomitant serious physical injury to any child; (3) *none of the children had*

died, thus eliminating the factors of mourning (Barnes, 1964;
Lacey, 1972) or "survivor's guilt" (Lifton, 1967); (4) the study was
prospective in that it began 5 months after the traumatic stress and
continued as symptoms developed; and (5) *parents were not present* during the traumatic event. In descriptions of children during
World War II the point had been made that their reactions to
bombings or air raids depended strongly upon the reactions of
their parents or guardians (A. Freud and Burlingham, 1942;
Solomon, 1942). In this case, only one adult, the bus driver, was
present during the traumatic experience. Most of the children had
not known him well, and by their accounts, he was quiet, passive,
and relatively neutral during most of the kidnapping. Toward the
end, he exerted leadership in discovering, along with some of the
older boys, a route for escape from the hole. According to the
children, the older boys actually dug the escape route. During
the 11-hour van ride, half of the children had no contact with any
adult at all. Thus, the trauma was experienced by children virtually alone.

The important findings in this study and their significance have
been previously discussed. In this final discussion I will comment
only upon three aspects of the study which have not been emphasized up to now: the effect of the child's age and a comparison of
children's and adults' reactions to traumatic events; the significance of omens in psychic trauma; and some proposals for the
handling of disasters affecting children.

AGE OF THE TRAUMATIZED CHILD

In 1920 Freud defined psychic trauma as "an extensive breach
being made in the protective shield against stimuli" [p. 31]. This
definition was reaffirmed by Anna Freud (1968). Implicit in this
definition is the idea that response to trauma depends upon ego
maturity. All of the Chowchilla children were old enough to understand that they were in life-endangering peril. Since the age
range was 5 to 14, one might expect to find important differences
in their responses to trauma based on their stages of development.
Such, surprisingly, was not the case. There was an amazing similarity of response across the entire age range.

For instance, traumatic play was a feature not only of latency but of adolescent posttraumatic response (Bob and Janice). As a matter of fact, it was surprising to observe adolescents using play at all as a mechanism of handling anxiety. Hallucinations were observed in a 5-year-old, an 8-year-old, and a 14-year-old. Misidentification and time-skew, striking cognitive malfunctions of the ego, occurred in children over a 6-year spread.

Not only did the children's responses to trauma remain relatively uniform across a wide range of ages, but there were several similarities to traumatic responses experienced independently of the children by their parents. Omens, repetitive dreams, fears of another kidnapping, "fears of the mundane," failure to develop group cohesiveness, and anniversary reactions were experienced both by the children and by their parents.

While much of this has been discussed previously, the children's failure to achieve a feeling of communality requires some elaboration. Very few of the kidnap victims sought out further relationships with one another. Despite a group trip to Disneyland and a winter skating party arranged by parents, the bus driver, and the school superintendent about 8 months after the kidnapping, the children did not interrelate. The only exceptions were Sammy and Janice and Barbara (siblings) and Debbie and Jackie, who remained friends. This finding differs from the typical annual reunions of army units, probably because the group training in the armed forces builds morale and group closeness *prior* to (and preventing some) psychic trauma experienced on the battlefields. In Chowchilla, the children's failure to relate communally was very similar to that of their parents and to that described by Kai Erikson (1976) in adults at Buffalo Creek.

Finally, anniversary reaction is a type of behavior noted in the children that has been previously described in adults. Four children showed this reaction:

Jackie (9):   Extensive series of dreams—2 weeks
Debbie (10):   Panicky "escape" from white van—one episode
Johnny (11):   Fear of ceiling collapse—about 2 weeks
                     Fear of being left alone—1 month
Bob (14):   Play; punching couch for 2 weeks

This tabulation, however, is incomplete because not all families were seen after one year; unless they requested an interview at that time, there was no way to learn of anniversary behaviors in their youngsters.

On the other hand, this study also disclosed several differences between adult and child reactions to trauma. Since I have discussed them in the preceding sections, I shall only summarize them here: (1) no amnesia or haziness about the experience takes place in children; (2) no denial of the actual event alternating with intrusive repetitive phenomena occurs in children; (3) no true flashbacks are observed in children; (4) children "play" their trauma in a manner similar to the repetitive dreams of both children and adults; (5) major signs of ego dysfunction in traumatized children are cognitive malfunction: misperception, overgeneralization, and time distortions; (6) reenactment is an important finding in children. Although there is some mention of adult traumatic reenactments in the literature (Wangh, 1968), the literal repetition of actual event-related behaviors and thoughts has not been emphasized in descriptions of traumatized adults and may be a finding characteristic of children.

OMENS OR STRESS SIGNALS

When a sudden unexpected danger occurred in Chowchilla, no child or adult could understand its motivation or its meaning. Because the healthy mind struggles to control its environment, the "trapped" youngsters and waiting parents struggled to master or control what had happened to them. Many children in their struggle to understand believed consciously or unconsciously that arguments and/or punishments from mother, the school day itself, or seating arrangements on the bus had some relationship to the trauma. The intense need to know WHY? or HOW COULD I HAVE BEEN WARNED? could only be answered subjectively from their own experiences. Their subjective "clues" or partial answers were to become lastingly and firmly associated with the mental representation of the trauma itself. Many children and several mothers retrospectively attributed to commonplace, ordinary occurrences the power of portents or signals of terror to come.

In ancient or primitive societies, omens and portents were commonly held to be warnings of disaster. The mechanism for this may be the same as that observed in the Chowchilla victims. Homer in *The Iliad* and Coleridge in *The Rime of the Ancient Mariner* described the behavior of birds as warnings of disaster to come. Perhaps when societies were unexpectedly traumatized, they too, like the Chowchilla victims, tried to achieve mental control by searching for small incidents prior to the disaster which should have been warnings or motivations. When the flight of the bird was retrospectively linked to the trauma, the association of the "signal" and the stress remained indelibly fixed. A warning, omen, or portent was thus assigned by looking backward.

The psychiatric literature on trauma includes descriptions of episodes in which victims panic or behave as if undergoing the trauma again, usually in response to a perception which is similar to the conditions of the original trauma (Grinker and Spiegel, 1945; Archibald and Tuddenham, 1965). This occurs, I believe, because of the retrospective establishment of omens or stress signals. This concept is not found in the psychiatric literature, but literary works from Shakespeare to Hawthorne and Mosel (1961) are replete with portents, clues, or signals of terror to come. These are not only literary devices to prepare for climactic occurrences, but they represent sound psychological mechanisms as well. The audience or reader, just as the Chowchilla victim did, comes across the central disaster and remembers back to the ordinary occurrences, which now are firmly associated with the major catastrophic event itself.

PROPOSALS FOR RESPONSE TO DISASTERS

Based upon my findings concerning the reactions of the Chowchilla children and their families, I offer some suggestions for the handling of disasters. Additional community approaches are presented by Barton (1969), Grosser et al. (1964), and Parad et al. (1976).

1. The waiting period is very important. Before the news is in (in cases of hostages, kidnappings, or a distant disaster), community mental health workers should contact families. They can introduce themselves, sit with families who have no one to help them, and

form a relationship prior to the relief or the despair which will take place once the results of the disaster are known.

2. Mental health workers should immediately evaluate the victims, once they are released. This is as important as the physical examination. The general physicians who examined the Chowchilla victims at Santa Rita Prison testified at the trial that the children had not been seriously affected. Since general physicians do not yet have expertise in judging the effects of psychic trauma, psychological evaluations should be in the hands of behavioral scientists or a "team" of physicians and mental health workers. In any event, psychological assessments should be performed as *routinely* as physical examinations.

3. *Continued individual* contact with children and parents is to be encouraged. Initially, the interviews may be entirely devoted to the expression of feelings. Parents may have to be interviewed first, before they allow their children to be extensively evaluated (Block et al., 1956). Early group meetings are to be avoided because they may speed community fragmentation. Rather than immediate group meetings, professional contact with the individual families allows verbalization and an opportunity to discharge anxiety and hostility to qualified experts rather than to reporters or the community-at-large.

4. Long-term traumatic effects in the children may not be observed by parents for 6 months to a year. Once parents become aware of the stress-related symptomatology, group meetings as well as individual interpretive therapeutic interviews are in order.

5. The general reputation and availability of a community's mental health facilities will have an important role in whether families are willing to accept its therapeutic intervention during and after a disaster.

BIBLIOGRAPHY

American Psychiatric Association (1978), *Draft, Diagnostic and Statistical Manual of Mental Disorders, 3rd ed.* Washington, D.C.

Anders, T. F. (1978), Home-Recorded Sleep in 2- and 9-Month-Old Infants. *J. Amer. Acad. Child Psychiat.,* 17:421–432.

Archibald, H. & Tuddenham, R. (1965), Persistent Stress Reaction After Combat. *Arch. Gen. Psychiat.*, 12:475–481.

Barnes, M. (1964), Reactions to the Death of a Mother. *This Annual*, 19:339–357.

Barton, A. (1969), *Communities in Disaster.* Garden City, N.Y.: Doubleday.

Baugh, J. & Morgan, J. (1978), *Why Have They Taken Our Children?* New York: Delacorte Press.

Benedek, T. (1959), Parenthood As a Developmental Stage. *J. Amer. Psychoanal. Assn.*, 7:389–417.

Block, D., Silber, E., & Perry, S. (1956), Some Factors in the Emotional Reaction of Children to Disaster. *Amer. J. Psychiat.*, 113:416–422.

Bowlby, J. (1973), *Attachment and Loss,* vol. 2. New York: Basic Books.

Cain, A. & Fast, I. (1972), Children's Disturbed Reactions to Parent Suicide. In: *Survivors of Suicide,* ed. A. Cain & I. Fast. Springfield, Ill.: Charles C Thomas, pp. 93–111.

Campbell, M. (1970), Urinary Obstruction. In: *Urology,* ed. M. Campbell & J. Harrison. Philadelphia: Saunders, 2:1772–1793.

Chodoff, P., Friedman, S., & Hamburg, D. (1964), Stress, Defenses, and Coping Behavior. *Amer. J. Psychiat.*, 120:743–749.

Coleridge, S. T. (1798), *The Rime of the Ancient Mariner.* New York: Dove Publications, 1970.

De Koninck, J. & Koulack, D. (1975), Dream Content and Adaptation to a Stressful Situation. *J. Abnorm. Psychol.*, 84:250–260.

Dillon, H. & Leopold, R. (1961), Children and Post-Concussion Syndrome. *J. Amer. Med. Assn.*, 175:86–92.

Erikson, E. H. (1950), *Childhood and Society.* New York: Norton.

Erikson, K. (1976), *Everything in Its Path.* New York: Simon & Schuster.

Freud, A. (1936), The Ego and the Mechanisms of Defense. *W.*, 2.

—— (1945), Indications for Child Analysis. *This Annual*, 1:127–149.

—— (1967), Comments on Trauma. *W.*, 5:221–241.

—— (1968), Acting Out. *Int. J. Psycho-Anal.*, 49:165–170.

—— & Burlingham, D. (1942), Report 12. *W.*, 3:142–211.

—— —— (1939–45), Infants Without Families. *W.*, 3.

Freud, S. (1900), The Interpretation of Dreams. *S.E.*, 4 & 5.

—— (1909), The Analysis of a Phobia in a Five-Year-Old Boy. *S.E.*, 10:3–149.

—— (1914), Remembering, Repeating, and Working-Through. *S.E.*, 12:147–156.

—— (1920), Beyond the Pleasure Principle. *S.E.*, 18:7–64.

—— (1926), Inhibitions, Symptoms, and Anxiety. *S.E.*, 20:77–175.

Furst, S. S. (1967), Psychic Trauma. In: *Psychic Trauma,* ed. S. S. Furst. New York: Basic Books, pp. 3–50.

Grinker, R. & Spiegel, J. (1945), *Men Under Stress.* Philadelphia: Blakiston.

Grosser, G., Wechsler, H., & Greenblatt, M., eds. (1964), *The Threat of Impending Disaster.* Cambridge, Mass.: M.I.T. Press.

HAWTHORNE, N. (1846–49), *The Scarlet Letter*. In: *Four Great American Novels*, ed. R. Short. New York: Henry Holt, 1946.

HOBSON, J. & McCARLEY, R. (1977), The Brain As a Dream State Generator. *Amer. J. Psychiat.*, 134:1334–1348.

HOMER, *The Iliad*, tr. A. Pope. New York: Hermitage Press, 1943.

HOROWITZ, M. (1976), *Stress Response Syndromes*. New York: J. Aronson.

JANIS, I. (1958), *Psychological Stress*. New York: John Wiley.

KATAN, A. (1961), Some Thoughts about the Role of Verbalization in Early Childhood. *This Annual*, 16:184–188.

KLEIN, M. (1955), The Psycho-Analytic Play Technique. In: *New Directions in Psycho-Analysis*, ed. M. Klein, P. Heimann, & R. Money-Kyrle. New York: Basic Books, pp. 3–22.

KRIS, E. (1941), The "Danger" of Propaganda. In: *The Selected Papers of Ernst Kris*. New Haven & London: Yale Univ. Press, 1975, pp. 409–432.

———— (1944), Danger and Morale. *Ibid.*, pp. 451–464.

KRYSTAL, H., ed. (1968), *Massive Psychic Trauma*. New York: Int. Univ. Press.

———— (1978), Trauma and Affects. *This Annual*, 22:81–116.

———— & NIEDERLAND, W. G. (1968), Clinical Observations on the Survivor Syndrome. In: *Massive Psychic Trauma*, ed. H. Krystal. New York: Int. Univ. Press, pp. 327–348.

LACEY, G. (1972), Observations on Aberfan. *J. Psychosom. Res.*, 16:257–260.

LANCASTER, E. (1970), The Dreams of Traumatic Neurosis. *Amer. J. Psychoanal.*, 30:13–18.

LEVY, D. (1945), Psychic Trauma of Operations in Children. *Amer. J. Dis. Child.*, 69:7–25.

LIFTON, R. J. (1967), *Death in Life*. New York: Random House.

———— & OLSON, E. (1976), The Human Meaning of Total Disaster. *Psychiatry*, 39:1–18.

LINDEMANN, E. (1944), Symptomatology and Management of Acute Grief. *Amer. J. Psychiat.*, 101:141–148.

LUCHTERHAND, E. (1971), Sociological Approaches to Massive Stress in Natural and Man-Made Disasters. *Int. Psychiat. Clin.*, 8:29–53.

MERCIER, M. & DESPERT, L. (1943), Effects of War on French Children. *Psychosom. Med.*, 5:266–272.

MILLER, G. & TOMPKINS, S. (1976), Chowchilla: The Bitterness Lingers. *Fresno Bee*, November 14.

———— & ———— (1977), *Kidnapped at Chowchilla*. Plainfield: Logos International.

MOSEL, T. (1961), *All the Way Home*. Based on J. Agee: *A Death in the Family*. New York: Obolensky.

NIEDERLAND, W. G. (1957), The Earliest Dreams of a Young Child. *This Annual*, 12:190–208.

PARAD, H., RESNIK, H., & PARAD, L., eds. (1976), *Emergency and Disaster Management*. Bowie, Md.: Charles Press Publishers.

Parkes, C. (1970), The First Year of Bereavement. *Psychiatry,* 33:444–467.

Rado, S. (1942), Pathodynamics and Treatment of Traumatic War Neurosis. *Psychosom. Med.,* 4:362–368.

Rappaport, E. (1968), Beyond Traumatic Neurosis. *Int. J. Psycho-Anal.,* 49: 719–731.

Rangell, L. (1976), Discussion of the Buffalo Creek Disaster. *Amer. J. Psychiat.,* 133:313–316.

Shakespeare, W., *Julius Caesar.* In: *The Complete Signet Classic Shakespeare.* New York: Harcourt, Brace, Jovanovich, 1972.

Solomon, J. (1942), Reactions of Children to Black-Outs. *Amer. J. Orthopsychiat.,* 12:361–362.

Sterba, E. (1968), The Effects of Persecutions on Adolescents. In: *Massive Psychic Trauma,* ed. H. Krystal. New York: Int. Univ. Press, pp. 51–60.

Stern, G. (1976), *The Buffalo Creek Disaster.* New York: Random House.

Waelder, R. (1932), The Psychoanalytic Theory of Play. *Psychoanal. Quart.,* 2:208–224.

——— (1960), *Basic Theory of Psychoanalysis.* New York: Int. Univ. Press.

Wangh, M. (1968), A Psychogenic Factor in the Recurrence of War. *Amer. J. Psychoanal.,* 49:319–323.

Washburn, S. & Hamburg, D. (1965), The Study of Primate Behavior. In: *Primate Behavior,* ed. I. DeVore. New York: Holt, Rinehart & Winston.

Weiss, R. & Payson, H. (1967), Gross Stress Reactions. In: *Comprehensive Textbook of Psychiatry,* ed. A. Freedman & H. Kaplan. Baltimore: Williams & Wilkins.

Bibliographical Note

S.E.   *The Standard Edition of the Complete Psychological Works of Sigmund Freud,* 24 Volumes, translated and edited by James Strachey. London: Hogarth Press and the Institute of Psycho-Analysis, 1953–1974.

W.   *The Writings of Anna Freud,* 7 Volumes. New York: International Universities Press, 1968–1974.

Index